Reconstruction Options in Otolaryngology

Editors

JAYNE R. STEVENS
KIRAN KAKARALA

OTOLARYNGOLOGIC CLINICS OF NORTH AMERICA

www.oto.theclinics.com

Consulting Editor
SUJANA S. CHANDRASEKHAR

August 2023 • Volume 56 • Number 4

ELSEVIER

1600 John F. Kennedy Boulevard • Suite 1800 • Philadelphia, Pennsylvania, 19103-2899

http://www.oto.theclinics.com

OTOLARYNGOLOGIC CLINICS OF NORTH AMERICA Volume 56, Number 4
August 2023 ISSN 0030-6665, ISBN-13: 978-0-443-18382-9

Editor: Stacy Eastman
Developmental Editor: Malvika Shah

Otolaryngologic Clinics of North America (ISSN 0030-6665) is published bimonthly by Elsevier, Inc., 360 Park Avenue South, New York, NY 10010-1710. Months of issue are February, April, June, August, October, and December. Business and Editorial Offices: 1600 John F. Kennedy Blvd., Suite 1800, Philadelphia, PA 19103-2899. Customer Service Office: 6277 Sea Harbor Drive, Orlando, FL 32887-4800. Periodicals postage paid at New York, NY and additional mailing offices. Subscription prices are $468.00 per year (US individuals), $1117.00 per year (US institutions), $100.00 per year (US & Canadian student/resident), $599.00 per year (Canadian individuals), $1416.00 per year (Canadian institutions), $653.00 per year (international individuals), $1416.00 per year (international institutions), $270.00 per year (international student/resident). Foreign air speed delivery is included in all *Clinics'* subscription prices. All prices are subject to change without notice. **POSTMASTER:** Send address changes to *Otolaryngologic Clinics of North America*, Elsevier Health Sciences Division, Subscription Customer Service, 3251 Riverport Lane, Maryland Heights, MO 63043. **Telephone: 1-800-654-2452 (U.S. and Canada); 314-447-8871 (outside U.S. and Canada). Fax: 314-447-8029. E-mail: journalscustomerservice-usa@elsevier.com (for print support); journalsonlinesupport-usa@elsevier.com (for online support).**

Reprints. For copies of 100 or more of articles in this publication, please contact the Commercial Reprints Department, Elsevier Inc., 360 Park Avenue South, New York, NY 10010-1710. Tel.: 212-633-3874; Fax: 212-633-3820; E-mail: reprints@elsevier.com.

Otolaryngologic Clinics of North America is also published in Spanish by McGraw-Hill Interamericana Editores S.A., P.O. Box 5-237, 06500 Mexico D.F., Mexico.

Otolaryngologic Clinics of North America is covered in *MEDLINE/PubMed (Index Medicus), Current Contents/Clinical Medicine, Excerpta Medica, BIOSIS, Science Citation Index,* and *ISI/BIOMED.*

Contributors

CONSULTING EDITOR

SUJANA S. CHANDRASEKHAR, MD, FACS, FAAOHNS
Consulting Editor, *Otolaryngologic Clinics of North America*, President, American
Otological Society, Past President, American Academy of Otolaryngology–Head and Neck
Surgery, Partner, ENT & Allergy Associates, LLP, Clinical Professor, Department of
Otolaryngology–Head and Neck Surgery, Zucker School of Medicine at Hofstra/Northwell,
Clinical Associate Professor, Department of Otolaryngology–Head and Neck Surgery,
Icahn School of Medicine at Mount Sinai, New York, New York

EDITORS

JAYNE R. STEVENS, MD
Assistant Professor, Department of Otolaryngology–Head and Neck Surgery, San Antonio
Uniformed Services Health Education Consortium, JBSA-Fort Sam Houston, Texas

KIRAN KAKARALA, MD, FACS
Professor, Department of Otolaryngology–Head and Neck Surgery, University of Kansas
School of Medicine, Kansas City, Kansas

AUTHORS

AARTI AGARWAL, MD
Department of Otolaryngology, Thomas Jefferson University, Philadelphia, Pennsylvania

CARLY E.A. BARBON, PhD
Assistant Professor, Department of Head and Neck Surgery, The University of Texas MD
Anderson Cancer Center, Houston, Texas

DONALD DAVID BEAHM, MD
Department of Otolaryngology, University of Kansas Medical Center, Kansas City, Kansas

SCOTT BEVANS, MD
Associate Professor, Department of Otolaryngology, Tripler Army Medical Center, Hawaii;
Uniformed Services University, Bethesda, Maryland

STEVEN CHINN, MD, MPH
Department of Otolaryngology–Head and Neck Surgery, Rogel Cancer Center, University
of Michigan, Ann Arbor, Michigan

JOSEPH CURRY, MD
Department of Otolaryngology, Thomas Jefferson University, Philadelphia, Pennsylvania

DANIEL G. DESCHLER, MD
Department of Otolaryngology–Head and Neck Surgery, Massachusetts Eye and Ear,
Harvard Medical School, Boston, Massachusetts

PETER DZIEGIELEWSKI, MD, FRCSC
Department of Otolaryngology–Head and Neck Surgery, University of Florida School of Medicine, Gainesville, Florida

CANDACE A. FLAGG, MD
Department of Otolaryngology–Head and Neck Surgery, San Antonio Uniformed Services Health Education Consortium, JBSA-Fort Sam Houston, Texas

JOHN FLYNN, MD
University of Kansas Medical Center, Kansas City, Kansas

NEERAV GOYAL, MD, MPH
Department of Otolaryngology–Head and Neck Surgery, The Pennsylvania State University, College of Medicine, Hershey, Pennsylvania

EVAN M. GRABOYES, MD, MPH
Associate Professor, Department of Otolaryngology–Head and Neck Surgery, Department of Public Health Sciences, Medical University of South Carolina, Charleston, South Carolina

DANIEL HAMMER, DDS, FACS
Associate Professor, Department of Oral Maxillofacial Surgery, Naval Medical Center San Diego, San Diego, California; Uniformed Services University, Bethesda, Maryland

MATTHEW M. HANASONO, MD
Professor and Deputy Chair, The University of Texas MD Anderson Cancer Center, Houston, Texas

CURTIS HANBA, MD
Department of Head and Neck Surgery, The University of Texas MD Anderson Cancer Center, Department of Otolaryngology–Head and Neck Surgery, Houston, Texas

ANDREW J. HOLCOMB, MD
Department of Head and Neck Surgical Oncology, Estabrook Cancer Center, Nebraska Methodist Hospital, Omaha, Nebraska

ANDREW T. HUANG, MD, FACS
Associate Professor, Department of Otolaryngology–Head and Neck Surgery, Baylor College of Medicine, Houston, Texas

EVAN A. JONES, MD
Resident Physician, Department of Otolaryngology–Head and Neck Surgery, Baylor College of Medicine, Houston, Texas

KIRAN KAKARALA, MD, FACS
Professor, Department of Otolaryngology–Head and Neck Surgery, University of Kansas School of Medicine, Kansas City, Kansas

HANNAH L. KAVOOKJIAN, MD
Department of Otolaryngology–Head and Neck Surgery, University of Kansas, The University of Kansas Medical Center, Kansas City, Kansas

ALEXANDRA E. KEJNER, MD, FACS
Associate Professor, Head and Neck Oncology/Microvascular Reconstruction, Medical University of South Carolina, Charleston, South Carolina

GREGORY I. KELTS, MD
Assistant Professor, Department of Otolaryngology–Head and Neck Surgery, San Antonio Uniformed Services Health Education Consortium, JBSA-Fort Sam Houston, Texas

SHANNON M. KRAFT, MD
Department of Otolaryngology–Head and Neck Surgery, University of Kansas, The University of Kansas Medical Center, Kansas City, Kansas

JAMIE A. KU, MD
Head and Neck Institute, Cleveland Clinic, Cleveland, Ohio

CIARAN LANE, MD, MSc
Department of Otolaryngology–Head and Neck Surgery, The Pennsylvania State University, College of Medicine, Hershey, Pennsylvania

BYUNG JOO LEE, DMD
Medical Director, Maxillofacial Prosthodontics and Oral Oncology, Medical University of South Carolina, Charleston, South Carolina

Z-HYE LEE, MD
Assistant Professor, The University of Texas MD Anderson Cancer Center, Houston, Texas

CAROL LEWIS, MD, MPH
Department of Otolaryngology-Head and Neck Surgery, The University of Texas MD Anderson Cancer Center, Houston, Texas

ALICE LIN, MD
Department of Clinical Sciences, Kaiser Permanente School of Medicine, Los Angeles, California

GUANNING NINA LU, MD
University of Washington, Seattle, Washington

HILARY C. McCRARY, MD, MPH
Department of Otolaryngology–Head and Neck Surgery, The Ohio State University Wexner Medical Center, Columbus, Ohio

CAITLIN McMULLEN, MD
Department of Head and Neck-Endocrine Oncology, Moffitt Cancer Center, Tampa, Florida

MATTHEW MIFSUD, MD, FACS
Department of Otolaryngology–Head and Neck Surgery, University of South Florida School of Medicine

TRAVIS R. NEWBERRY, MD
Assistant Professor, Department of Otolaryngology–Head and Neck Surgery, San Antonio Uniformed Services Health Education Consortium, JBSA-Fort Sam Houston, Texas

MATTHEW O. OLD, MD
Department of Otolaryngology–Head and Neck Surgery, The Ohio State University Wexner Medical Center, Columbus, Ohio

MOLLIE C. PERRYMAN, MD
Department of Otolaryngology–Head and Neck Surgery, University of Kansas, The University of Kansas Medical Center, Kansas City, Kansas

PATRIK PIPKORN, MD
Assistant Professor, Otolaryngology–Head and Neck Surgery, Division of Head and Neck Surgery, Washington University, St Louis, Missouri

PABLO QUADRI, MD
Department of Head and Neck-Endocrine Oncology, Moffitt Cancer Center, Tampa, Florida

SAMUEL RACETTE, MD
Department of Otolaryngology, University of Kansas Medical Center, Kansas City, Kansas

NOLAN B. SEIM, MD
Department of Otolaryngology–Head and Neck Surgery, The Ohio State University Wexner Medical Center, Columbus, Ohio

JAYNE R. STEVENS, MD
Assistant Professor, Department of Otolaryngology–Head and Neck Surgery, San Antonio Uniformed Services Health Education Consortium, JBSA-Fort Sam Houston, Texas

AKINA TAMAKI, MD
Department of Otolaryngology–Head and Neck Surgery, University Hospitals Cleveland Medical Center, Case Western Reserve University School of Medicine, Cleveland, Ohio

SRUTI TEKUMALLA, BA
Department of Otolaryngology, Thomas Jefferson University, Philadelphia, Pennsylvania

AARON M. WIELAND, MD
Division of Otolaryngology–Head and Neck Surgery, Section of Head and Neck Surgical Oncology, University of Wisconsin, Madison, Wisconsin

CHAD A. ZENDER, MD
Department of Otolaryngology–Head and Neck Surgery, University of Cincinnati College of Medicine, Cincinnati, Ohio

DAVID I. ZIMMER, MD, DVM
Head and Neck Institute, Cleveland Clinic, Cleveland, Ohio

Contents

Free Flap Donor Sites in Head and Neck Reconstruction   623

Akina Tamaki and Chad A. Zender

> Microvascular free tissue transfer, also referred to as free flaps surgery, is a reconstructive technique that has become a foundational component of complex head and neck reconstruction. There have been considerable advancements in the field over the last 30 years including the number and variety of free flaps. Each of these free flaps has unique characteristics that must be considered for the defect when selecting a donor site. Here, the authors focus on the most common free flaps used in head and neck reconstruction.

Regional Flap Donor Sites in Head and Neck Reconstruction   639

Andrew J. Holcomb and Daniel G. Deschler

> Regional flaps are vital to head and neck reconstruction, allowing surgeons to harvest numerous reliable flaps without the need for microvascular anastomosis. These flaps are very useful in cases of vascular depletion and may prove superior to free flaps as a primary option in certain circumstances. Numerous harvest options are available, and the described harvest techniques are safe and straightforward for an experienced reconstructive surgeon to learn. Donor site morbidity is variable depending on flap selection but minimal in many cases. Regional flaps are an excellent option in resource-limited settings or when minimizing reoperation is a high priority.

Tenants of Mandibular Reconstruction in Segmental Defects   653

Scott Bevans and Daniel Hammer

> The premises of mandibular reconstruction are the restoration of occlusion and mandibular contour for the purpose of preserving the facial identity, oral airway, and effective speech and mastication. Establishing functional occlusion is the primary tenant in all mandibular reconstruction. In cases of segmental defects, particularly in dentate regions of the mandible, there has been a paradigm shift over the past two decades in how surgeons are approaching the restoration of load-bearing mandibular continuity with capacity for dental implantation. Here we discuss considerations for deciding the most effective method of reconstruction in segmental defects.

This summary provides a concise overview of oral cavity reconstruction to optimize functional outcomes in the modern era. Soft tissue and osseous reconstruction options for a wide range of oral cavity sites including lip, oral tongue, floor of mouth, buccal, hard palate, and composite oromandibular resections are reviewed. The appropriate applications of primary closure, secondary intention, skin grafts, and dermal substitute grafts are included. Anatomic considerations, indications, contraindications, and complications of local, regional, and free flaps in oral cavity reconstruction are discussed. Specific defects and the appropriate options for reconstruction of those defects are delineated.

Pharyngoesophageal reconstruction is one of the most challenging reconstructive dilemmas that demands extensive planning, meticulous surgical execution, and timely management of postoperative complications. The main goals of reconstruction are to protect critical blood vessels of the neck, to provide alimentary continuity, and to restore functions such as speech and swallowing. With the evolution of techniques, fasciocutaneous flaps have become the gold standard for most defects in this region. Major complications include anastomotic strictures and fistulae, but most patients can tolerate an oral diet and achieve fluent speech after rehabilitation with a tracheoesophageal puncture.

Midface reconstruction in head and neck cancer or individuals with extensive trauma to the face has evolved significantly over the past few decades with the introduction of free flap reconstruction and virtual surgical planning enabling surgeons to obtain optimal cosmetic and functional outcomes. Traditional methods such as the use of obturators or local flaps still have a role in select situations, but complex defects have been replaced by the advent of microvascular free tissue transfer and virtual planning, which can commonly provide a single-stage reconstruction of the midface with excellent aesthetic and functional results. This article provides an overview of the history and evolution of midface reconstruction, a discussion of how to integrate virtual surgical planning into a surgical practice, an example of a complex midface reconstruction case, and pearls and pitfalls that have been experienced by an experienced reconstructive team.

Reconstruction of the lateral temporal bone with adequate functional and cosmetic outcomes depends on a multidisciplinary approach including the head and neck surgeon, reconstructive surgeon, neurotologist, and anaplastologist. Approaching the defect includes consideration of the location, tissue type, function, and patient/tumor characteristics. Anatomic limitations due to prior therapy also play an important role in reconstructive choices. Here, we review contemporary literature regarding the reconstruction of this complex region.

This article provides an overview of reconstructive options following skin cancer resection broken down by different aesthetic regions and subunits. Although not meant to serve as an all-encompassing source, it provides common indications for using different sections of the reconstructive ladder based on location of defects, tissues involved, and patient factors.

The practicing otolaryngologist frequently encounters consultation for injuries in the head and neck. Restoration of form and function is essential to normal activities of daily living and quality of life. This discussion intends to provide the reader with an up-to-date discussion of various evidence-based practice trends related to head and neck trauma. The discussion focuses on the acute management of trauma with minor emphasis on secondary management of injuries. Specific injuries related to the craniomaxillofacial skeleton, laryngotracheal complex, vascularity, and soft tissues are explored.

It has been demonstrated since the 1990's that surgical outcomes can be improved through protocolized perioperative interventions. Since then, multiple surgical societies have engaged in adopting Enhanced Recovery After Surgery (ERAS) Societal recommendations to improve patient satisfaction, decrease the cost of interventions, and improve outcomes. In 2017, ERAS released consensus recommendations detailing the perioperative optimization of patients undergoing head and neck free flap reconstruction. This population was identified as a high resource demand, oftentimes burdened with challenging comorbidity, and poorly described cohort for which a perioperative management protocol could help to optimize outcomes. The following pages aim to further detail perioperative strategies to streamline patient recovery after head and neck reconstructive surgery.

Virtual surgical planning is a revolutionary tool for the head and neck reconstructive surgeon. As with any tool, there are strengths and weaknesses. The strengths include shorter operative time, shorter ischemic time, streamlined dental rehabilitation, facilitation of complex reconstruction, non-inferior and possibly superior accuracy, and increased durability. The weaknesses are increased up-front costs, potential delays to operative management, limited flexibility on the day of surgery, and loss of familiarity with conventionally planned surgery.

Microvascular and free flap reconstruction are important to the otolaryngology—head and neck surgery practice. Herein, the reader will find an up-to-date discussion of various evidence-based practice trends related to microvascular surgery, including surgical techniques, anesthetic and airway considerations, free flap monitoring and troubleshooting, surgical efficiency, and both patient-related and surgeon-related risk factors that may affect outcomes.

Approximately 50% of head and neck cancer (HNC) survivors are left with dysphagia as a result of treatment sequele, and 25% of survivors experience clinically significant body image distress (BID). Both dysphagia and BID adversely affect quality of life and should be tracked using validated clinician- and patient-reported outcome measures such as the Performance Status Scale for Head and Neck Cancer, MD Anderson Dysphagia Inventory, and Inventory to Measure and Assess imaGe disturbancE-Head & Neck (IMAGE-HN). Subjective and objective evaluation measures are critical to dysphagia workup and management. Building a renewed image after head and neck cancer treatment, a brief telemedicine-based cognitive behavioral therapy, has become the first evidence-based treatment for BID among HNC survivors.

Multiple advances in surgical techniques, technology, and perioperative patient care have revolutionized head and neck reconstruction over the last 40 years. Concurrent with these advances, health systems, patients, and payers have become increasingly focused on value and quality, owing in part to rapidly increasing health care costs. However, there is no consensus on how to define value and quality in the realm of head and neck reconstruction. This review focuses on the past, present, and future of quality improvement efforts in head and neck reconstruction.

OTOLARYNGOLOGIC CLINICS
OF NORTH AMERICA

SERIES OF RELATED INTEREST

Facial Plastic Surgery Clinics
Available at: https://www.facialplastic.theclinics.com/

THE CLINICS ARE AVAILABLE ONLINE!
Access your subscription at:
www.theclinics.com

Foreword

The Necessity of Art and Science in Head and Neck Reconstruction

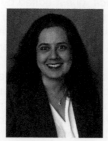

Sujana S. Chandrasekhar, MD, FACS, FAAOHNS
Consulting Editor

Otolaryngologists are acutely aware of our important role in helping patients literally put their best face forward. As skilled as we are with tumor extirpation and managing head and neck trauma, the job is not done until the patient's appearance reaches as close to their expectations as possible.

The father of modern plastic surgery was the New Zealand otolaryngologist, Sir Harold Gillies, born in 1882 and active in practice from 1910 until his death in 1960. His career spanned both World War I and II. It was his experience with the horrors that war inflicts on soldiers that led him to create this multidisciplinary specialty, merging the knowledge and experiences of Otolaryngology, Oral and Maxillofacial Surgery, Dentistry, and General Surgery.[1] Over 21 million soldiers were injured in WWI; 280,000 were left with ghastly facial injuries. All injuries were more severe than in previous wars due to advanced military weaponry; there were also more facial injuries due to trench warfare, which exposed the head to gunfire. On a single day in July 1916, Gilles and his associates saw 2000 war-casualty patients. In Britain, soldiers with facial injuries were called the "loneliest Tommies." When they left the hospital grounds, they were forced to sit on brightly painted blue benches so that the public knew not to look at them. Gillies took on this challenge and said, "Unlike the student of today, who is weaned on small scar excisions and graduates to harelips, we were suddenly asked to produce half a face."

Gillies' younger cousin, Sir Archibald McIndoe, joined him in practice and utilized his charisma, his surgical skills, and his uncanny instinctive knowledge of psychology to care for huge numbers of patients injured in WWII, in particular, veterans who had been burned.[2] Like Gillies, much of this work was by trial and error. The patients with burn injury treated by McIndoe called themselves the Guinea Pig Club and dubbed him "Maestro" or "The Boss." McIndoe recognized early on that the rehabilitation of a

Otolaryngol Clin N Am 56 (2023) xiii–xiv
https://doi.org/10.1016/j.otc.2023.05.001
0030-6665/23/© 2023 Published by Elsevier Inc.

oto.theclinics.com

burned patient was as important as the reconstruction of his physical body. His therapeutic approach to patients with burn injury was mental and physical.

We owe enormous debts of gratitude to the soldiers of the World Wars, not only for the geopolitical outcomes, but also because many of the reconstructive techniques in daily use today can be traced back to the dedicated and innovative surgeons caring for them.[3] Their "guinea pigs," the brave men who were injured in the wars, contributed greatly to the knowledge of head and neck plastic and reconstructive surgery.

This issue of *Otolaryngologic Clinics of North America*, guest edited by Drs Jayne Stevens and Kiran Kakarla, covers the gamut of current reconstruction options in Otolaryngology. The articles in this issue provide a single outstanding resource for the otolaryngologist–head and neck reconstruction surgeon. They cover local and regional flaps, skin grafts, microvascular free flaps, composite grafts, and nerve reconstruction. In keeping with the philosophy of McIndoe and other forefathers, articles focus on tumor and trauma, on optimizing function and appearance, and in providing value. We can now use virtual surgical planning techniques to minimize intraoperative time and maximize outcomes. The reader will be awash in practical tips and innovative ideas to help their patient look and feel the best possible.

Sujana S. Chandrasekhar, MD, FACS, FAAOHNS
Consulting Editor
Otolaryngologic Clinics of North America
President, American Otological Society
Past President
American Academy of Otolaryngology–
Head and Neck Surgery
Partner, ENT & Allergy Associates, LLP
Department of Otolaryngology–
Head and Neck Surgery
Zucker School of Medicine at Hofstra–Northwell
Department of Otolaryngology–
Head and Neck Surgery
Icahn School of Medicine at Mount Sinai
18 East 48th Street, 2nd Floor
New York, NY 10017, USA

E-mail address:
ssc@nyotology.com

REFERENCES

1. Fitzharris L. The facemaker: a visionary surgeon's battle to mend the disfigured soldiers of World War I. New York: Farrar, Straus and Giroux; 2022.
2. Geomelas M, Ghods M, Ring A, et al. The Maestro": a pioneering plastic surgeon—Sir Archibald McIndoe and his innovating work on patients with burn injury during World War II. J Burn Care Res 2011;32(3):363–8.
3. Macrae J. Like your plastic surgeon? Thank a Veteran! Delaware Online. November 6, 2016. Available at: https://www.delawareonline.com/story/life/2016/11/06/like-plastic-surgeon-thank-veteran/93394166/. Accessed April 30, 2023.

Preface

The Innovative Art of Reconstruction in Otolaryngology

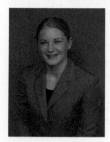 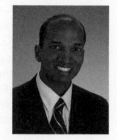

Jayne R. Stevens, MD   Kiran Kakarala, MD, FACS
Editors

Reconstruction in otolaryngology is an incredibly diverse and complex topic. From tumors, both benign and malignant, to trauma from mechanisms as varied as from motor vehicle crashes to self-inflicted gunshot wounds, the surgical defects necessitating reconstruction are vast. Reconstruction of these defects requires both intimate knowledge of anatomy and thorough understanding of normal physiologic function in order to best achieve rehabilitation of form and function. The techniques used in reconstructive surgery of the head and neck require technical knowledge as well as an ability to adapt, as each reconstruction is unique. While some surgical techniques are millennia-old, the last 50 years have seen rapid advances in both reconstructive surgical techniques and associated technologies. Microvascular free-flap reconstruction has allowed surgeons to successfully address defects that were previously out of reach. Technologies such as implantable flap monitoring, virtual surgical planning, and patient-specific implants have been welcome advances to surgeons looking to improve the success, accuracy, and functional outcomes of complex reconstructive efforts.

This issue of *Otolaryngologic Clinics of North America* strives to provide a one-stop reference for surgeons involved in head and neck reconstruction and provides up-to-date information on multiple important topics. We cover major salient topics regarding reconstruction in otolaryngology, from management of trauma and facial nerve reconstruction to free-flap options and optimizing functional outcomes in oncologic resections. Several articles focus on defect-based reconstruction, discussing the full reconstructive ladder for each of these anatomic locations. Other articles focus on advances in our understanding of physiologic recovery, optimization of outcomes, rehabilitation of form and function, and advances in technology that can aid in the planning of complex surgeries and care of often complicated patients with multiple comorbidities. Finally, a brief review of quality and value in head and neck reconstruction

Otolaryngol Clin N Am 56 (2023) xv–xvi
https://doi.org/10.1016/j.otc.2023.04.007
0030-6665/23/© 2023 Published by Elsevier Inc.

provides a possible framework to evaluate and improve our reconstructive efforts. We hope this issue provides the reconstructive surgeon a valuable reference with practical tips on well-known techniques as well as highlighting new and exciting developments in the field.

Jayne R. Stevens, MD
Department of Otolaryngology–
Head and Neck Surgery
San Antonio Uniformed Services
Health Education Consortium
JBSA–Fort Sam Houston, TX 78234, USA

Kiran Kakarala, MD, FACS
Department of Otolaryngology–
Head and Neck Surgery
University of Kansas School of Medicine
Kansas City, KS 66160, USA

E-mail addresses:
jayne.r.stevens@gmail.com (J.R. Stevens)
kkakarala@kumc.edu (K. Kakarala)

Free Flap Donor Sites in Head and Neck Reconstruction

Akina Tamaki, MD[a],*, Chad A. Zender, MD[b]

KEYWORDS

- Free flap • Microvascular reconstruction • Microvascular free tissue transfer
- Head and neck • Head and neck reconstruction

KEY POINTS

- Microvascular free tissue transfer is critical in reconstruction of certain head and neck defects and allow for superior functional and cosmetic outcomes.
- There have been significant advances in the number as well as variations that can be done in these free flaps.
- There are various donor site options with unique qualities, advantages, and disadvantages that must be considered for selection of the appropriate free flap.

INTRODUCTION

Developments and advancements in microvascular free tissue transfer have been critical in the ability to reconstruct complex defects in the head and neck. Before the introduction of free flaps, head and neck reconstructive options included primary closure, local tissue flaps, and nonvascularized bone grafts, often leaving patients with significant cosmetic and functional deficits.[1] The first reported use of microvascular free tissue transfer (MFTT) in humans was in 1959 when revascularized jejunum was used to reconstruct a cervical esophageal defect.[2] Free flap reconstruction has advanced considerably since the 1950s and is now ubiquitous in head and neck reconstruction. In this article, the authors provide an overview of the most common free flaps used in head and neck reconstruction (**Table 1**).

[a] Department of Otolaryngology- Head and Neck Surgery, University Hospitals Cleveland Medical Center, Case Western Reserve University School of Medicine, 11100 Euclid Avenue, LKS 5045, Cleveland, OH 44106, USA; [b] Department of Otolaryngology – Head and Neck Surgery, University of Cincinnati Medical Center, 231 Albert Sabin Way, MSB 6408, Cincinnati, OH 45229, USA
* Corresponding author.
E-mail address: akina.tamaki@UHhospitals.org

Otolaryngol Clin N Am 56 (2023) 623–638
https://doi.org/10.1016/j.otc.2023.04.001
0030-6665/23/© 2023 Elsevier Inc. All rights reserved.

Abbreviations	
MFTT	Microvascular free tissue transfer
OCRFFF	Osteocutaneous radial forearm free flap

DISCUSSION
Anterolateral Thigh

The anterolateral thigh flap (ALT) was first described in 1984 by Song and colleagues.[3] Although originally described as a fasciocutaneous flap supplied by the lateral circumflex femoral artery, further studies revealed that tissue was more frequently supplied by musculocutaneous perforators through the vastus lateralis muscle.[4] Perforators to the flap arise from the descending branch of the lateral circumflex femoral artery or, less frequently, the transverse branch. The ALT flap gained increasing popularity in the 1990s, especially in Asia, and is now one of the most common flaps used for soft tissue reconstruction in the head and neck[5–9] (**Fig. 1**).

Large amounts of muscle and skin can be harvested for the ALT with low donor site morbidity. Maximum width with possibility for primary closure of the donor site ranges from 8 to 12 cm.[10] The thickness of the flap is variable based on patient characteristics including age, gender, body habitus, ethnicity, and flap design and harvesting technique. The proximal thigh is thicker as compared with the distal thigh and generally thicker in women compared to men.[11] Variable amounts of vastus lateralis muscle, in which the descending branch of the lateral circumflex femoral artery supplies and courses through, can be harvested. Other variations include muscle-sparing flaps with dissection of the perforator, thinning the subcutaneous fat of the ALT, and harvest of adipofascial and myofascial ALTs.[12–14]

ALT flaps are one of the most versatile flaps used in the reconstruction of soft tissue defects in the head and neck. Its use for the reconstruction of oral cavity, oropharynx, laryngopharynx, maxilla, skull base, and the external skin is well-documented. In total pharyngectomy defects, ALTs can be tubed for neopharyngeal reconstruction with outcomes comparable to other soft tissue free flaps.[15–17] In addition, vascularized fascia lata can be harvested and used in various static suspensions and reconstruction of structures including the skull base.[18,19] Nerve grafts can also be harvested with sensory branches of the lateral femoral cutaneous nerve or nerve to the vastus.

Weaknesses of the flap include poor skin match with the head and neck and development of leg weakness and seromas from the donor site. The thickness of the flap can also be variable and too thick for certain head and neck defects. Perforator variability can also be challenging as significant variations of perforator location, size, and even absence have been described.[20]

Radial Forearm

The fasciocutaneous radial forearm free flap (RFFF) was first described in 1981 by Yang and colleagues.[21] Arterial supply of the flap is from the radial artery and drained by the cephalic vein and venae comitantes. The vascular anatomy is one of the most consistent and reliable, and there is the benefit of a long pedicle (approximately 18 cm in adults) with large caliber vessels.[22] Venous drainage can be based on either, or both, the deep (vena comitantes), and superficial (cephalic vein) systems[23] (**Fig. 2**).

Several forearm tissues from the antecubital fossa to flexor crease can be harvested. There is individual variability, but the tissue is usually thinner in men and in the distal forearm.[24] An Allen's test should always be done preoperatively to assess collateral blood flow to the hands from the radial or ulnar artery. Flaps can be designed

Table 1
Free flaps frequently used in the head and neck reconstruction

Flap Type	Tissue Type	First Described in Head and Neck Reconstruction	Artery/Vein	Nerve
Anterolateral thigh	Adipofascial, fasciocutaneous myofascial, myocutaneous	Koshima et al,[5] 1993	Descending or transverse branch of lateral circumflex femoral artery/vein	Lateral femoral cutaneous nerve
Fibular	Osseous, osteocutaneous	Hidalgo et al,[45] 1989	Peroneal artery/vein	Lateral sural cutaneous nerve
Gracilis	Myocutaneous, myofascial	Harii et al,[64] 1976	Adductor artery/vein	Obturator nerve
Iliac crest	Osteocutaneous, osteomusculocutaneous	Urken et al,[79] 1989	Deep circumflex iliac artery/vein	
Jejunum	Visceral	Seidenberg et al, 1959	Superior mesenteric artery/vein	
Lateral arm	Adipofascial, fasciocutaneous	Katsaros et al,[52] 1984	Posterior radial collateral artery/venae comitantes	Posterior cutaneous nerve of the arm and forearm
Omentum	Visceral	McLean et al,[83] 1972	Gastroepiploic artery/vein (often right)	
Osteocutaneous radial forearm	Osteocutaneous	Yang et al,[21] 1981 Soutar et al,[32] 1983	Radial artery/cephalic vein and venae comitantes	Antebrachial cutaneous nerve
Posterior tibial artery	Adipofascial, fasciocutaneous	Chen et al,[76] 1991	Posterior tibial artery/vena comitantes	Saphenous nerve
Radial forearm	Adipofascial, fasciocutaneous	Yang et al,[21] 1981	Radial artery/cephalic vein and venae comitantes	Antebrachial cutaneous nerve

(continued on next page)

Table 1
(continued)

Flap Type	Tissue Type	First Described in Head and Neck Reconstruction	Artery/Vein	Nerve
Rectus abdominis	Myocutaneous, myofascial	Hasegawa et al,[67] 1994	Deep inferior epigastric or deep superior epigastric artery/vein	Segmental nerve
Ulnar forearm	Adipofascial, fasciocutaneous	Lovie et al,[42] 1984	Ulnar artery/ basilic vein and venae comitantes	
Subscapular system				
Latissimus	Myocutaneous, myofascial	Fujino et al,[58] 1981	Thoracodorsal artery/vein	Thoracodorsal nerve
Scapula bone	Osseous	Swartz et al,[59] 1986	Angular artery/vein and periosteal artery/vein	
Scapular/parascapular	Adipofascial, fasciocutaneous	Swartz et al,[59] 1986	Circumflex scapular artery/vein	
Serratus	Myocutaneous, myofascial	Harii et al,[60] 1982	Serratus artery/vein	Long thoracic nerve
Thoracodorsal artery perforator	Fasciocutaneous	Guerra et al,[61] 2004	Perforators of thoracodorsal artery/vein	

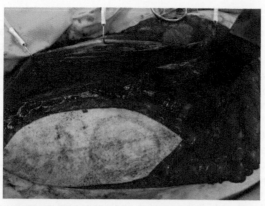

Fig. 1. Anterolateral thigh myocutaneous flap. The descending branch of the lateral circumflex femoral artery supplies the flap and can be harvested with a portion of the vastus lateralis muscle or as muscle-sparing based on perforators.

with separate tissue paddles or a beavertail modification adipofascial extension at the proximal portion.[25] In addition, subcutaneous tissue can be harvested without the overlying skin creating an adipofascial flap; this allows the harvest site to be closed primarily and provides thin tissue that can be used in reconstruction of defects such as the skull base.[26]

The RFFF is one of the pillars of head and neck soft tissue reconstruction given its thinness, reliable vascularization, and pliable tissue. RFFF is frequently used in reconstruction of oral mucosal defects but can be used in many soft tissue defects. It is particularly valuable in total laryngopharyngectomy defects especially when tubbing is necessary and the patient is of larger habitus.[27,28] Variations in design include harvest with vascularized tendon (palmaris longus tendon), muscle (brachioradialis muscle), or nerve (antebrachial cutaneous nerve). The palmaris longus tendon has been particularly valuable in total lip reconstruction and allows for suspension.[29]

Weaknesses of the RFFF include need for skin grafting the donor site, which may have poor take and tendon exposure. There can be sensory loss due to injury to the superficial branch of the radial nerve and transection of the antebrachial cutaneous nerve.[30] In very rare scenarios, harvest of the RFFF may lead to ischemic hand.[31]

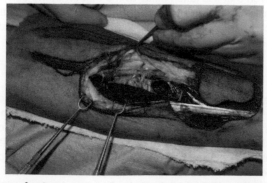

Fig. 2. Radial forearm fasciocutaneous flap. The course of the radial artery, venae comitantes, and cephalic vein are depicted.

Osteocutaneous Radial Forearm

Soon after the description of the RFFF by Yang and colleagues, it was recognized that it was possible to harvest bone from the radius as an osteocutaneous flap (OCRFFF).[21,32] The vascular supply is the same as the RFFF. Perforating vessels to the bone are preserved by maintaining the lateral intermuscular septum. The maximum length of bone that can be harvested is 10 to 12 cm and limited by the pronator teres and brachioradialis muscle. The pronator teres muscle can be detached from the insertion to the radius, but this may increase morbidity and resuspension of the muscle is suggested.[24] It is recommended that no more than 40% to 50% of the cross-sectional area of the radius be harvested.[33] This generally results in less bone than other common bony free flaps including the fibula, scapula, and iliac crest; however, it may be associated with fewer complications when compared with other osteocutaneous free flaps.[34]

OCRFFF can be valuable in head and neck reconstruction by providing bone in addition to all the earlier stated benefits of an RFFF. It is an excellent reconstructive option for limited mandibulectomy and maxillectomy defects. The thickness is usually insufficient to support dental implants, although stacking the bone may open options.[35] It can also be used in nasal, frontal sinus, and airway reconstruction.[36]

Pitfalls include the possibility for radius fractures, although prophylactic plating of the radius has minimized this risk.[37–40] Boat shaped osteotomies were previously advocated to reduce fractures, but right angles osteotomies are now widely done with plating becoming standardized.[41] Radius plate exposure is another disadvantage; this can be minimized with designing the skin paddle with an ulnar bias, preservation of the distal forearm skin at the level of the styloid process of the radius, and closing the muscle (pronator quadratus muscle) over the remaining radius bone and plate.

Ulnar Forearm

The ulnar forearm free flap was first reported in 1984 by Lovie and colleagues.[42] Arterial supply of the flap is from the ulnar artery and drained by the basilic vein and venae comitantes. The ulnar flap is similar in design and use to the RFFF. As much as 10 by 22 cm of skin can be harvested. It is useful in patients who have a failed Allen's test and inability to sacrifice the radial artery. It has unique advantages to the RFFF given different distribution of thickness, less hair-bearing skin, and possible improved cosmesis[43] (**Fig. 3**).

Weaknesses of the flap include a pedicle length that is about 4 to 5 cm sorter than that of the RFFF given that it is taken distal to the takeoff of the common interosseous artery.[24] There is also the chance of injury to the ulnar nerve given the close relationship with the pedicle. Like RFFF, there are similar risks of ischemic hand and poor skin graft take and wound healing.

Fibula

Vascularized fibular bone flaps was introduced in 1975 but was first described in head and neck reconstruction by Hidalgo and colleagues in 1989.[44,45] The blood supply is based on the peroneal artery and vein. The flap provides strong and long bone that can be 22 to 25 cm in length. The 6 to 7 cm of distal and proximal fibula is preserved for ankle and knee joint stability as well as to avoid the common peroneal nerve injury at the head of the fibula. Osseous or osteocutaneous flaps may be harvested. A skin paddle can be harvested, which is perfused by perforators arising from the posterior crural septum (**Fig. 4**).

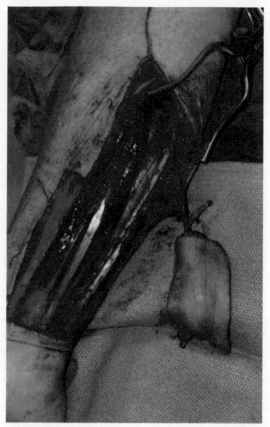

Fig. 3. Ulnar forearm fasciocutaneous flap. The ulnar artery and venae comitantes are depicted. The palmaris longus can be harvested with the forearm flaps, as shown here.

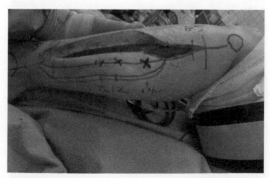

Fig. 4. Fibular osteocutaneous flap. Incisions are marked from the head of the fibula to the lateral malleolus. Multiple perforators to the skin as well as the anticipated skin paddle are marked. Tourniquet can be used during harvest.

Preoperative imaging is necessary to confirm adequate three-vessel (peroneal, anterior tibial, posterior tibial artery) perfusion to the foot. Multiple osteotomies can be done to contour the bone if the periosteum is preserved. Each bone segment should be at least 2.5 cm in length. Variations include double barrel fibulas to augment heights or reconstruct complex bony defects.[46] The lateral sural cutaneous nerve can be harvested and used for sensory supply. The geometry of the flap must be carefully considered especially when a skin paddle is needed to reconstruct an intraoral or external skin defect.[24]

Fibulas are ideal for reconstruction of segmental mandibulectomy and maxillectomy defects. This bone often has adequate thickness for dental implantation.[47] Further advancements include preoperative surgical planning and "jaw in a day" procedures, which allows for immediate dental rehabilitation at the time of the ablative surgery.[48–50]

Limitations include the lack of adequate collateral circulation to the lower extremity and the foot. Functional deficits to the foot including weakness with dorsiflexion may result from peroneal nerve injury and muscle scaring.[51] Common peroneal nerve injury may lead to ankle deformity and anesthesia of the anterior and lateral leg and foot. Pain and weakness with ambulation are possible and may benefit from physical therapy. Skin grafts are often necessary for closure and have the same weaknesses associated with RFFF skin grafts. Forced closure can also lead to compartment syndrome.

Lateral Arm

The lateral arm free flap was introduced in 1982 and described in head and neck reconstruction by Katsaros and colleagues in 1984.[52,53] The flap is supplied by septocutaneous perforators from the posterior radial collateral artery. This is a fasciocutaneous flap with a maximum width from 6 to 8 cm or one-third of the circumference of the arm with possibility for primary closure.[24] The skin flap can be extended distal to the lateral epicondyle and proximal to the deltoid insertion[54] (**Fig. 5**).

The thickness of the flap depends on patient habitus, but it is usually thicker than an RFFF but thinner than an ALT. Variations including harvesting the lateral arm as an adipofascial flap. In this scenario, a greater amount of fascial tissue can be harvested as skin closure is not of concern. In addition, a larger portion of lateral arm skin can be harvested if skin grafting is considered. The lateral arm free flap can be harvested with a segment of the humerus, triceps tendon, and nerve (posterior cutaneous nerve of the arm and forearm).

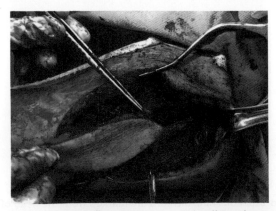

Fig. 5. Lateral arm fasciocutaneous flap. Posterior radial collateral artery and venae comitantes are dissected along the humerus bone.

Lateral arm free flaps are valuable in head and neck reconstruction, particularly of the oral cavity, laryngopharynx, and the external skin. It is particularly ideal for resurfacing head and neck skin defects given its excellent color match and tissue consistency.[55]

One of the major weaknesses of the flap is the small vessel size and short pedicle. The mean diameter of the artery is about 1.55 and 2.5 mm for the vein.[54,56] Other complications include radial nerve palsy, compartment syndrome, lateral epicondylar pain, and lateral forearm numbness.[57]

Subscapular System

There are numerous free flaps derived from the subscapular system, which are based on the subscapular artery or branches from this artery and was first described in the 1980s.[58–61] This includes myofascial, myocutaneous, fasciocutaneous, adipofascial, and osseous free flaps. There is tremendous versatility within this system, and a combination of tissue types is frequently used. The most common free flaps from the subscapular system include latissimus, scapular bone, scapular/parascapular, serratus, and thoracodorsal artery perforator flaps. The various flaps are supplied by the subscapular artery, which branches into the circumflex scapular artery (branches to transverse cutaneous, descending cutaneous, and periosteal artery) and thoracodorsal artery (branches to serratus, latissimus dorsi, and angular artery). Scapula bone can be harvested from the lateral boarder and the scapular tip with a maximum length ranging from 10 to 14 cm.[24] Blood supply to the scapula bone is from both the periosteal artery (circumflex scapular branches) for the lateral boarder and angular artery (thoracodorsal branches) for the scapular tip (**Fig. 6**).

Flaps derived from the subscapular system are extremely versatile and ideal for large defects requiring various tissue types for reconstruction.[62] Soft tissue can vary in thickness based on the type and location, the pedicle is long and large caliber especially when traced proximally, and the soft tissue and bone component have increased separation in comparison to other osteocutaneous flaps, thereby allowing for more freedom in three-dimensional positioning. Chimeric flaps with various components, including mega flaps, can be used for complex reconstruction. Fascio- and myocutaneous flaps can be used in various head and neck soft tissue defects. The latissimus free flap is particularly unique as it provides the largest amount of muscle and is valuable in scalp reconstruction. Bony flaps from the subscapular system can be used in

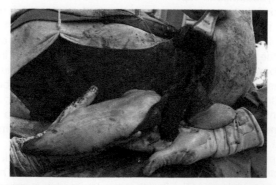

Fig. 6. Subscapular system chimeric flap, also called a mega flap. A myocutaneous latissimus, scapula bone from the lateral boarder and scapular tip, and fasciocutaneous scapular flap are shown. These are all based on the subscapular artery and vein.

various head and neck reconstructions including the mandible and maxilla (including hard palate and orbital floor).

Weaknesses of subscapular system flaps include concern for restriction in two-team approach given the need for positioning. However, with thoughtful positioning, it is very feasible to incorporate a dual two-team approach. Vessel mismatch based on the large caliber of the subscapular vessels when used can be problematic and requires thoughtful recipient site vessel selection. In addition, there is some concern for shoulder dysfunction; however, the extent and clinical significance is debatable.[63]

Gracilis

The gracilis free flap was first described in facial rehabilitation by Harii and colleagues in 1976.[64] The gracilis flap is frequently used for this purpose given the long thin muscle (4 to 6 cm in width) and the availability of a large motor nerve (obturator artery). The vascular supply from the terminal branch of the adductor artery arises from the profunda femoris vessels or, less frequently, the medial circumflex femoral artery.[24]

The flap can be harvested as a myofascial or a myocutaneous flap. These skin perforators usually exit the muscle in the upper third of its length. There is variability in the presence and reliability of perforators to the skin.[65] This flap is much more frequently used as a muscle only flap. By far, the most frequent use of gracilis flaps is for facial rehabilitation. However, it can also be used for external skin and mucosal defects including the lip and oral tongue.[66]

Weaknesses of the flap include small vessel size and short pedicle. Pedicle length is about 6 cm but may be shorter if the vascular pedicle enters the overlying adductor longus muscle and the pedicle is ligated before its entrance to the profunda femoris system.[24]

Rectus Abdominis

The first free rectus abdominis free flap was described in breast reconstruction in 1979 but was not described in head and neck reconstruction until 1994 by Hasegawa and colleagues.[67,68] The flap is based on the deep inferior epigastric or deep superior epigastric vessels. The deep superior epigastric is a continuation of the internal mammary artery, whereas the deep inferior epigastric arises from the deep circumflex iliac vessels. The two vascular systems connect above the umbilicus. However, the inferior system is often preferred due to larger caliber of vessels, and the musculocutaneous perforators are mostly supplied by the inferior system.[69] The flap can be harvested as a myofascial or myocutaneous flap.

The degree of skin and muscle harvested can vary from the entire rectus abdominis muscle to only a small area of the periumbilical region. The term transverse rectus abdominis musculocutaneous flap describes flaps where only the central portion of the muscle with the cutaneous perforator is harvested. The deep inferior epigastric perforator flap is based on a musculocutaneous perforator where muscle is spared.[70] The subcutaneous thickness widely varies based on the patient habitus and location on the abdomen (thinner above the costal margin and thicker in the lower abdomen).[24] Skin can be oriented vertically, horizontally, or obliquely. This flap can incorporate cartilage and bone through harvest of the 6thto10th rib. The segmental nerve can also be used as a vascularized nerve graft.[71]

Long vascular pedicle, large amount of skin, and available muscle make it a good reconstructive option for skull base, oral cavity, and scalp defects. The anterior rectus sheath is a thin but tough layer of the flap that can be used to augment reconstruction including providing a more durable closure of skull base defects and can also be secured to the mandible to maintain bulk of total glossectomy defects.[71,72]

Weaknesses of the flap include consequences of ventral herniation.[73] It is important to understand the fascial envelopes of the rectus abdominis to effectively close the fascial layers. This flap may also not be an option for patients who have undergone major abdominal surgery. Of note, the popularity of the rectus abdominis flap has decreased with increased used of the ALT flap.[74]

Posterior Tibial Artery

The posterior tibial artery flap was first described in 1985.[75] The reported use in the head and neck has mostly been through case reports with the earliest published use in 1991 by Chen and colleagues for esophageal reconstruction.[75,76] Septocutaneous perforators are often found on the medial surface of the distal half of the leg off the posterior tibial artery. It can be harvested as an adipofascial flap or a fasciocutaneous flap.

Large skin paddles off the medial aspect of the lower leg over the transverse intramuscular septum can be harvested. The maximum size of 19 by 13 cm can be safely harvested.[76] Tissue thickness varies with tissue anterior over the tibia being thinner and becomes thicker posteriorly. Other variations include the use of the saphenous nerve harvested with the flap, which can be used for sensation.

The tissue can be large, thin, and flexible with reasonable pedicle length and caliber. Application in head and neck reconstruction is often for shallow mucosal and cutaneous defects.[77] The use is similar to that of the RFFF.

Skin graft is often necessary and has the disadvantage of being over the tibia and risk of poor healing. In addition, like the fibula free flap, one of the three main blood supplies to the foot need to be sacrificed.[24] Preoperative vascularity should be assessed, similar to that for a fibular free flap.

Iliac Crest

The iliac crest flap was first described in 1979 and used in mandibular reconstruction by Urken and colleagues in 1989.[78,79] There are multiple possible arterial supplies to the iliac crest flap, but it is most frequently based on the deep circumflex iliac artery. Skin of the groin, the internal oblique muscle, and iliac bone are harvested.

Uses in head and neck reconstruction include for composite defects involving the mandible or maxilla. Up to 16 cm of bone length can be harvested.[24] The natural curvature of the bone can be considered for reconstruction. The contour is ideal for reconstruction of ipsilateral mandibular angle and body defects. Iliac crest flaps are also harvested with more soft tissue and can be valuable when there is a need to fill large amounts of dead space.[80] It has also been found to have adequate bone for placement of dental implants.[47]

Disadvantages of the flap include donor site complications such as chronic pain, risk of hernia formation, gait problems, and fractures of the anterior superior iliac spine. In addition, it has a short vascular pedicle and increased bulkiness, which need to be considered. There is also concern for the size and reliability of the skin paddle.[81]

Jejunum

The jejunal free flap is a visceral flap and was the first free tissue transfer done in humans. This was first reported in 1959 by Seidenberg and colleagues for reconstruction after a pharyngoesophagectomy.[2] Blood supply arises from the superior mesenteric artery and vein. The jejunum can be used in its tubed form or as a patch.

The use in head and neck reconstruction includes use in pharyngoesophageal defects, especially when circumferential. It can also be used to reconstruct the oral mucosa where there may be advantages of replacing mucosa with mucosa rather than with skin.[82]

Weaknesses include contraindications to use including ascites, significant abdominal surgeries, and patients with chronic intestinal diseases. Also, in comparison to other free flaps, monitoring viability of the flap can be difficult.[24]

Omentum

The omentum free flap was first described by McLean and Buncke in 1972 when it was used to reconstruct a scalp defect.[83] The omentum is folded peritoneum that lays from the greater curvature of the stomach to the transverse colon. It is rich in vasculature and lymphatics. The blood supply is from the gastroepiploic artery, often the right, which is the more dominant.[24] Variations to the flap include harvest of the greater curvature of the stomach, thereby creating the gastroepiploic free flap.[84] This can be used in pharyngoesophageal reconstruction.

Uses in head and neck include closing scalp defects, providing soft tissue bulk, and placement to augment wounds including osteoradionecrosis or osteomyelitis by providing improved vascularity to surrounding tissues.[85]

The biggest disadvantage to the omental flap is the need to perform a laparotomy. This comes with risks including gastric perforations and peritonitis, especially when a segment of stomach is harvested.

SUMMARY

Free flap reconstruction is a foundation of head and neck reconstruction. There are numerous free flaps that are frequently used in the head and neck. This diverse group of donor sites has unique characteristics that must be carefully considered to maximize form and function after ablative head and neck surgery.

CLINICS CARE POINTS

- Microvascular free tissue transfer is a critical component of head and neck reconstruction.
- There are various free flap donor site options with characteristics that should be considered for selection of the appropriate free flap for a given defect.

DISCLOSURE

No conflicts of interest to disclose.

REFERENCES

1. Steel BJ, Cope MR. A brief history of vascularized free flaps in the oral and maxillofacial region. J Oral Maxillofac Surg 2015;73(4):786.e1-11.
2. SEIDENBERG B, ROSENAK SS, HURWITT ES, et al. Immediate reconstruction of the cervical esophagus by a revascularized isolated jejunal segment. Ann Surg 1959;149(2):162–71.
3. Song YG, Chen GZ, Song YL. The free thigh flap: a new free flap concept based on the septocutaneous artery. Br J Plast Surg 1984;37(2):149–59.
4. Koshima I, Fukuda H, Utunomiya R, et al. The anterolateral thigh flap; variations in its vascular pedicle. Br J Plast Surg 1989;42(3):260–2.

5. Koshima I, Fukuda H, Yamamoto H, et al. Free anterolateral thigh flaps for reconstruction of head and neck defects. Plast Reconstr Surg 1993;92(3):421–8 [discussion: 429–30].

6. Kimata Y, Uchiyama K, Ebihara S, et al. Versatility of the free anterolateral thigh flap for reconstruction of head and neck defects. Arch Otolaryngol Head Neck Surg 1997;123(12):1325–31.

7. Gedebou TM, Wei FC, Lin CH. Clinical experience of 1284 free anterolateral thigh flaps. Handchir Mikrochir Plast Chir 2002;34(4):239–44.

8. Hayden RE, Deschler DG. Lateral thigh free flap for head and neck reconstruction. Laryngoscope 1999;109(9):1490–4.

9. Lin DT, Coppit GL, Burkey BB. Use of the anterolateral thigh flap for reconstruction of the head and neck. Curr Opin Otolaryngol Head Neck Surg 2004;12(4): 300–4.

10. Lueg EA. The anterolateral thigh flap: radial forearm's "big brother" for extensive soft tissue head and neck defects. Arch Otolaryngol Head Neck Surg 2004; 130(7):813–8.

11. Yu P. Characteristics of the anterolateral thigh flap in a Western population and its application in head and neck reconstruction. Head Neck 2004;26(9):759–69.

12. Agostini V, Dini M, Mori A, et al. Adipofascial anterolateral thigh free flap for tongue repair. Br J Plast Surg 2003;56(6):614–8.

13. De Virgilio A, Iocca O, Di Maio P, et al. Head and neck soft tissue reconstruction with anterolateral thigh flaps with various components: Development of an algorithm for flap selection in different clinical scenarios. Microsurgery 2019;39(7): 590–7.

14. Kimura N, Satoh K, Hasumi T, et al. Clinical application of the free thin anterolateral thigh flap in 31 consecutive patients. Plast Reconstr Surg 2001;108(5): 1197–208 [discussion: 1209–10].

15. Genden EM, Jacobson AS. The role of the anterolateral thigh flap for pharyngoesophageal reconstruction. Arch Otolaryngol Head Neck Surg 2005;131(9):796–9.

16. Ali RS, Bluebond-Langner R, Rodriguez ED, et al. The versatility of the anterolateral thigh flap. Plast Reconstr Surg 2009;124(6 Suppl):e395–407.

17. Murray DJ, Gilbert RW, Vesely MJ, et al. Functional outcomes and donor site morbidity following circumferential pharyngoesophageal reconstruction using an anterolateral thigh flap and salivary bypass tube. Head Neck 2007;29(2): 147–54.

18. Yildirim S, Gideroğlu K, Aydogdu E, et al. Composite anterolateral thigh-fascia lata flap: a good alternative to radial forearm-palmaris longus flap for total lower lip reconstruction. Plast Reconstr Surg 2006;117(6):2033–41.

19. Hanasono MM, Sacks JM, Goel N, et al. The anterolateral thigh free flap for skull base reconstruction. Otolaryngol Head Neck Surg 2009;140(6):855–60.

20. Lakhiani C, Lee MR, Saint-Cyr M. Vascular anatomy of the anterolateral thigh flap: a systematic review. Plast Reconstr Surg 2012;130(6):1254–68. https://doi.org/10.1097/PRS.0b013e31826d1662.

21. Yang GF, Chen PJ, Gao YZ, et al. Forearm free skin flap transplantation: a report of 56 cases. 1981. Br J Plast Surg 1997;50(3):162–5.

22. Cha YH, Nam W, Cha IH, et al. Revisiting radial forearm free flap for successful venous drainage. Maxillofac Plast Reconstr Surg 2017;39(1):14.

23. Demirkan F, Wei FC, Lutz BS, et al. Reliability of the venae comitantes in venous drainage of the free radial forearm flaps. Plast Reconstr Surg 1998;102(5): 1544–8.

24. Urken ML, Cheney ML, Blackwell KE, et al. Atlas of regional and free flaps for head and neck reconstruction: flap harvest and insetting. 2nd edition. Baltimore, MD: LWW; 2012.
25. Seikaly H, Rieger J, O'Connell D, et al. Beavertail modification of the radial forearm free flap in base of tongue reconstruction: technique and functional outcomes. Head Neck 2009;31(2):213–9.
26. Ismail TI. The free fascial forearm flap. Microsurgery 1989;10(3):155–60.
27. Azizzadeh B, Yafai S, Rawnsley JD, et al. Radial forearm free flap pharyngoesophageal reconstruction. Laryngoscope 2001;111(5):807–10.
28. Harii K, Ebihara S, Ono I, et al. Pharyngoesophageal reconstruction using a fabricated forearm free flap. Plast Reconstr Surg 1985;75(4):463–76.
29. Sadove RC, Luce EA, McGrath PC. Reconstruction of the lower lip and chin with the composite radial forearm-palmaris longus free flap. Plast Reconstr Surg 1991; 88(2):209–14.
30. Bruin LL, Hundepool CA, Duraku LS, et al. Higher incidences of neuropathic pain and altered sensation following radial forearm free flap: A systematic review. J Plast Reconstr Aesthet Surg 2022;75(1):1–9.
31. Jones BM, O'Brien CJ. Acute ischaemia of the hand resulting from elevation of a radial forearm flap. Br J Plast Surg 1985;38(3):396–7.
32. Soutar DS, Scheker LR, Tanner NS, et al. The radial forearm flap: a versatile method for intra-oral reconstruction. Br J Plast Surg 1983;36(1):1–8.
33. Swanson E, Boyd JB, Manktelow RT. The radial forearm flap: reconstructive applications and donor-site defects in 35 consecutive patients. Plast Reconstr Surg 1990;85(2):258–66.
34. Bollig CA, Walia A, Pipkorn P, et al. Perioperative Outcomes in Patients Who Underwent Fibula, Osteocutaneous Radial Forearm, and Scapula Free Flaps: A Multicenter Study. JAMA Otolaryngol Head Neck Surg 2022;148(10):965–72.
35. Gonzalez-Castro J, Petrisor D, Ballard D, et al. The double-barreled radial forearm osteocutaneous free flap. Laryngoscope 2016;126(2):340–4.
36. Silverman DA, Przylecki WH, Shnayder Y, et al. Expanding the Utilization of the Osteocutaneous Radial Forearm Free Flap beyond Mandibular Reconstruction. J Reconstr Microsurg 2016;32(5):361–5.
37. Werle AH, Tsue TT, Toby EB, et al. Osteocutaneous radial forearm free flap: its use without significant donor site morbidity. Otolaryngol Head Neck Surg 2000; 123(6):711–7.
38. Villaret DB, Futran NA. The indications and outcomes in the use of osteocutaneous radial forearm free flap. Head Neck 2003;25(6):475–81.
39. Shnayder Y, Tsue TT, Toby EB, et al. Safe osteocutaneous radial forearm flap harvest with prophylactic internal fixation. Craniomaxillofac Trauma Reconstr 2011; 4(3):129–36.
40. Arganbright JM, Tsue TT, Girod DA, et al. Outcomes of the osteocutaneous radial forearm free flap for mandibular reconstruction. JAMA Otolaryngol Head Neck Surg 2013;139(2):168–72.
41. Bardsley AF, Soutar DS, Elliot D, et al. Reducing morbidity in the radial forearm flap donor site. Plast Reconstr Surg 1990;86(2):287–92 [discussion: 293–4].
42. Lovie MJ, Duncan GM, Glasson DW. The ulnar artery forearm free flap. Br J Plast Surg 1984;37(4):486–92.
43. Wax MK, Rosenthal EL, Winslow CP, et al. The ulnar fasciocutaneous free flap in head and neck reconstruction. Laryngoscope 2002;112(12):2155–60.
44. Taylor GI, Miller GD, Ham FJ. The free vascularized bone graft. A clinical extension of microvascular techniques. Plast Reconstr Surg 1975;55(5):533–44.

45. Hidalgo DA. Fibula free flap: a new method of mandible reconstruction. Plast Reconstr Surg 1989;84(1):71–9.

46. Jones NF, Swartz WM, Mears DC, et al. The "double barrel" free vascularized fibular bone graft. Plast Reconstr Surg 1988;81(3):378–85.

47. Burgess M, Leung M, Chellapah A, et al. Osseointegrated implants into a variety of composite free flaps: A comparative analysis. Head Neck 2017;39(3):443–7.

48. Levine JP, Bae JS, Soares M, et al. Jaw in a day: total maxillofacial reconstruction using digital technology. Plast Reconstr Surg 2013;131(6):1386–91.

49. Patel A, Harrison P, Cheng A, et al. Fibular Reconstruction of the Maxilla and Mandible with Immediate Implant-Supported Prosthetic Rehabilitation: Jaw in a Day. Oral Maxillofac Surg Clin North Am 2019;31(3):369–86.

50. Runyan CM, Sharma V, Staffenberg DA, et al. Jaw in a Day: State of the Art in Maxillary Reconstruction. J Craniofac Surg 2016;27(8):2101–4.

51. Goodacre TE, Walker CJ, Jawad AS, et al. Donor site morbidity following osteocutaneous free fibula transfer. Br J Plast Surg 1990;43(4):410–2.

52. Katsaros J, Schusterman M, Beppu M, et al. The lateral upper arm flap: anatomy and clinical applications. Ann Plast Surg 1984;12(6):489–500.

53. Song R, Song Y, Yu Y. The upper arm free flap. Clin Plast Surg 1982;9(1):27–35.

54. Katsaros J, Tan E, Zoltie N, et al. Further experience with the lateral arm free flap. Plast Reconstr Surg 1991;87(5):902–10.

55. Kang SY, Eskander A, Patel K, et al. The unique and valuable soft tissue free flap in head and neck reconstruction: Lateral arm. Oral Oncol 2018;82:100–7.

56. Rivet D, Buffet M, Martin D, et al. The lateral arm flap: an anatomic study. J Reconstr Microsurg 1987;3(2):121–32.

57. Graham B, Adkins P, Scheker LR. Complications and morbidity of the donor and recipient sites in 123 lateral arm flaps. J Hand Surg Br 1992;17(2):189–92.

58. Fujino T, Maruyama Y, Inuyama I. Double-folded free myocutaneous flap to cover a total cheek defect. J Maxillofac Surg 1981;9(2):96–100.

59. Swartz WM, Banis JC, Newton ED, et al. The osteocutaneous scapular flap for mandibular and maxillary reconstruction. Plast Reconstr Surg 1986;77(4):530–45.

60. Harii K, Yamada A, Ishihara K, et al. A free transfer of both latissimus dorsi and serratus anterior flaps with thoracodorsal vessel anastomoses. Plast Reconstr Surg 1982;70(5):620–9.

61. Guerra AB, Metzinger SE, Lund KM, et al. The thoracodorsal artery perforator flap: clinical experience and anatomic study with emphasis on harvest techniques. Plast Reconstr Surg 2004;114(1):32–41 [discussion: 42–3].

62. Ugurlu K, Ozçelik D, Hacikerim S, et al. The combined use of flaps based on subscapular vascular system for unilateral facial deformities. Plast Reconstr Surg 2000;106(5):1079–89.

63. Patel KB, Low TH, Partridge A, et al. Assessment of shoulder function following scapular free flap. Head Neck 2020;42(2):224–9.

64. Harii K, Ohmori K, Torii S. Free gracilis muscle transplantation, with microneurovascular anastomoses for the treatment of facial paralysis. A preliminary report. Plast Reconstr Surg 1976;57(2):133–43.

65. Yousif NJ, Matloub HS, Kolachalam R, et al. The transverse gracilis musculocutaneous flap. Ann Plast Surg 1992;29(6):482–90.

66. Chiesa-Estomba CM, González-García J, Piazza C, et al. Gracilis free flap in head and neck reconstruction beyond facial palsy reanimation. Acta Otorrinolaringol Esp 2022;73(5):310–22.

67. Hasegawa K, Amagasa T, Araida T, et al. Oral and maxillofacial reconstruction using the free rectus abdominis myocutaneous flap. Various modifications for reconstruction sites. J Cranio-Maxillo-Fac Surg 1994;22(4):236–43.
68. Holmström H. The free abdominoplasty flap and its use in breast reconstruction. An experimental study and clinical case report. Scand J Plast Reconstr Surg 1979;13(3):423–7.
69. Boyd JB, Taylor GI, Corlett R. The vascular territories of the superior epigastric and the deep inferior epigastric systems. Plast Reconstr Surg 1984;73(1):1–16.
70. Mayo-Yáñez M, Rodríguez-Pérez E, Chiesa-Estomba CM, et al. Deep inferior epigastric artery perforator free flap in head and neck reconstruction: A systematic review. J Plast Reconstr Aesthet Surg 2021;74(4):718–29.
71. Urken ML, Turk JB, Weinberg H, et al. The rectus abdominis free flap in head and neck reconstruction. Arch Otolaryngol Head Neck Surg 1991;117(9):1031.
72. Chicarilli ZN, Davey LM. Rectus abdominis myocutaneous free-flap reconstruction following a cranio-orbital-maxillary resection for neurofibrosarcoma. Plast Reconstr Surg 1987;80(5):726–31.
73. Man LX, Selber JC, Serletti JM. Abdominal wall following free TRAM or DIEP flap reconstruction: a meta-analysis and critical review. Plast Reconstr Surg 2009;124(3):752–64.
74. Nakayama B, Hyodo I, Hasegawa Y, et al. Role of the anterolateral thigh flap in head and neck reconstruction: advantages of moderate skin and subcutaneous thickness. J Reconstr Microsurg 2002;18(3):141–6.
75. Hwang WY, Chen SZ, Han LY, et al. Medial leg skin flap: vascular anatomy and clinical applications. Ann Plast Surg 1985;15(6):489–91.
76. Chen HC, Tang YB, Noordhoff MS. Posterior tibial artery flap for reconstruction of the esophagus. Plast Reconstr Surg 1991;88(6):980–6.
77. Chan YW, Ng RWM, Wei WI. Anatomical study and clinical applications of free posterior tibial flap in the head and neck region. Plast Reconstr Surg 2011;128(3):131e–9e.
78. Taylor GI, Townsend P, Corlett R. Superiority of the deep circumflex iliac vessels as the supply for free groin flaps. Plast Reconstr Surg 1979;64(5):595–604.
79. Urken ML, Vickery C, Weinberg H, et al. The internal oblique-iliac crest osseomyocutaneous free flap in oromandibular reconstruction. Report of 20 cases. Arch Otolaryngol Head Neck Surg 1989;115(3):339–49.
80. Urken ML, Buchbinder D, Costantino PD, et al. Oromandibular reconstruction using microvascular composite flaps: report of 210 cases. Arch Otolaryngol Head Neck Surg 1998;124(1):46–55.
81. Wilkman T, Husso A, Lassus P. Clinical Comparison of Scapular, Fibular, and Iliac Crest Osseal Free Flaps in Maxillofacial Reconstructions. Scand J Surg 2019;108(1):76–82.
82. Buckspan GS, Newton ED, Franklin JD, et al. Split jejunal free-tissue transfer in oropharyngoesophageal reconstruction. Plast Reconstr Surg 1986;77(5):717–28.
83. McLean DH, Buncke HJ. Autotransplant of omentum to a large scalp defect, with microsurgical revascularization. Plast Reconstr Surg 1972;49(3):268–74.
84. Bayles SW, Hayden RE. Gastro-omental free flap reconstruction of the head and neck. Arch Facial Plast Surg 2008;10(4):255–9.
85. Mazzaferro D, Song P, Massand S, et al. The Omental Free Flap-A Review of Usage and Physiology. J Reconstr Microsurg 2018;34(3):151–69.

Regional Flap Donor Sites in Head and Neck Reconstruction

Andrew J. Holcomb, MD[a],*, Daniel G. Deschler, MD[b]

KEYWORDS

- Pectoralis major flap • Submental flap • Supraclavicular flap • Temporalis flap
- Temporoparietal fascia flap • Latissimus flap • Regional flap
- Head and neck reconstruction

KEY POINTS

- Regional flaps may be harvested from numerous sites from the head, neck, and torso for the reconstruction of head and neck defects.
- Regional flaps generally offer rapid harvest and favorable donor site morbidity.
- Regional flaps are highly reliable, and their utilization minimizes risk of reoperation due to pedicle compromise that accompanies free tissue transfer.

INTRODUCTION

Free tissue transfer has largely supplanted regional flaps for most indications within the head and neck, as free flaps are versatile, reliable, and offer donor sites outside the head and neck, which may improve cosmesis. However, regional flaps continue to serve important roles in head and neck reconstruction and in many circumstances may be preferable to free flaps. In this article, we highlight 4 of the most useful regional flaps in detail and comment briefly on 3 flaps that are used less often. These flaps are presented in decreasing order of usefulness.

BRIEF HISTORY OF REGIONAL FLAPS

The concept of regional tissue transfer dates back millennia, with descriptions of the midline vertical forehead flap in the Indian literature in approximately 700 BC.[1] The

The authors have no commercial or financial conflicts of interest or funding sources to disclose.
[a] Department of Head & Neck Surgical Oncology, Estabrook Cancer Center, Nebraska Methodist Hospital, 8303 Dodge Street Suite 304, Omaha, NE, USA; [b] Department of Otolaryngology Head & Neck Surgery, Massachusetts Eye and Ear, Harvard Medical School, 243 Charles Street, Boston, MA 02114, USA
* Corresponding author.
E-mail address: Andrew.holcomb@nmhs.org

Otolaryngol Clin N Am 56 (2023) 639–651
https://doi.org/10.1016/j.otc.2023.04.008
0030-6665/23/© 2023 Elsevier Inc. All rights reserved.

Tagliacozzi flap is a well-known early form of regional tissue transfer, used in the late sixteenth century predominately for nasal reconstruction.[2] This flap transferred a bridge of skin from the upper arm to the nose and required suspension of the arm for several weeks before pedicle division. The deltopectoral flap was perhaps the first "workhorse" flap of the head and neck. Although it was described initially in the early 1900s, Bakamjian is credited with popularization of the medially based version of this flap in the 1960s.[3] In 1979, Baek and Ariyan separately described the pectoralis major myocutaneous flap, which largely supplanted the deltopectoral flap due to its improved vascularity, greater length and bulk, as well as ability to be transferred in single stage reconstruction.[4,5] Although the first head and neck free tissue transfer was performed in 1957, and descriptions of several free flaps widely used in head and neck reconstruction were published in the 1970s and 1980s, microvascular training, especially among Otolaryngologists, remained limited.[6] Eventually, free flaps began to supplant regional flaps but newer regional flaps such as the submental island, which was described in 1993, continued to develop.[7] Today, regional flaps are the cornerstone of reconstruction in many areas of the world and retain an important role in head and neck reconstruction in the United States.

PECTORALIS MAJOR FLAP
Relevant Anatomy

- The pectoralis flap is based primarily on the pectoral branch of the thoracoacromial artery, which originates from the second portion of the axillary artery (**Fig. 1**A–C). Secondary contributions from internal mammary perforators originate medially, and the lateral thoracic artery (LTA) supplies variable aspects of the lateral portion of the muscle. The medial and lateral pectoral nerves travel with the pectoral branch of the thoracoacromial artery and the LTA, respectively, and each penetrates the muscle at its deep surface.
- The pectoralis muscle originates broadly from the medial half of the clavicle, the sternum, several costal cartilages, and the external oblique aponeurosis, and it insets onto the humerus, serving primarily to flex, adduct, and medially rotate the arm.

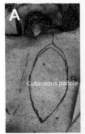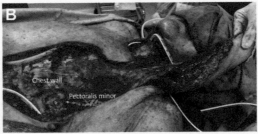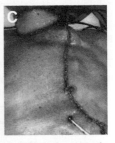

Fig. 1. (*A*) Pectoralis flap design. This very large skin paddle extends inferiorly over the rectus fascia but includes substantial skin overlying the pectoralis major muscle to incorporate cutaneous perforators in this region. (*B*) Pectoralis flap after elevation. In this case, the intervening skin between the flap harvest site and the head and neck has been divided to facilitate transfer of this large flap, although in many cases the flap may be tunneled beneath the skin bridge and delivered to the head and neck. (*C*) The flap is inset into the head and neck defect, and the chest is closed primarily after undermining despite the harvest of a large skin paddle.

Indications/Contraindications

- The pectoralis flap has been used as a myocutaneous or myofascial flap extensively for a wide variety pharyngeal, oral cavity, parotid, cutaneous, and oropharyngeal defects.
- The flap is generally considered to reach to the level of the zygomatic arch, although several techniques have been described to increase the arc of rotation, including the extension of the skin paddle inferiorly to cover the rectus sheath as well as the removal of a portion of the medial clavicle.[8,9]
- This may be harvested as a myofascial flap with no skin paddle, or a skin paddle may be included. Harvest of rib or sternal bone has also been described, as has prefabrication with skin grafts for composite defects.[10,11]
- The flap is reliable with very low rates of total flap loss, and the muscle is very well vascularized. Donor site morbidity can be greater than for other types of regional flaps but has not been extensively studied.
- Congenital absence of the pectoralis muscle (Poland syndrome) is rare. Chest wall trauma or surgery may compromise the vascular supply of the flap. Obesity may also render a myocutaneous flap too large for practical use. Defects that are too cephalad to be reached by the pectoralis flap without tension are at risk of dehiscence and may be better reconstructed with another method.

Pearls and Pitfalls

- Design of the skin paddle is ideally placed over the inferomedial chest within the distribution of cutaneous perforators of the pectoral branch of the thoracoacromial artery. The inferior placement allows for maximal reach of the pectoralis flap. The skin paddle may extend inferiorly to overlie the rectus fascia if 2 considerations are followed. First, the skin paddle should extend superiorly to sufficiently overlay the pectoralis muscle to allow incorporation of the muscle perforators from the main pectoral artery pedicle. Second, the rectus fascia deep to the skin paddle should be harvested with the flap to capture vessels lying superficial to the rectus sheath that aid in perfusion of the overlying skin.
- The lateral aspect of the skin paddle is incised first, followed by lateral dissection to identify the full extent of the pectoralis muscle. If the skin paddle is placed too inferiorly and predominately overlies the rectus fascia, an adjustment can be made at this time.
- An inframammary skin paddle can be designed in female patients to optimize donor site esthetics, and this approach is also ideal when a myofascial flap is used.
- Although the deep plane of dissection along the chest wall is developed readily, especially laterally, it is important medially to avoid injury to costal perichondrium while releasing the muscular attachments to the first to sixth ribs. Careful control of intercostal perforators when encountered is essential to reduce the risk of chest wall hematoma and to avoid conductive injury to cutaneous perforators. Finally, the avoidance of injury to the internal mammary perforators, especially the second and third perforators, is optimal to preserve a deltopectoral flap should one be necessary.
- The pedicle may be identified relatively early coursing along the deep surface of the flap, and the LTA may also be seen early in the dissection.
- The pectoral nerves and the lateral thoracic vessels typically require division to optimize the reach of the flap especially if the flap is rotated 180° to avoid constriction of the venous pedicle.

- Adequate hemostasis is essential during division of the humeral insertion of the flap to minimize the risk of axillary hematoma.
- Partial necrosis of the skin paddle may occur and is likely due in part to insufficient inclusion of muscular perforators if the skin paddle predominately overlies the rectus fascia and/or secondary to traction of the skin paddle during transfer. Ensuring an adequate subcutaneous tunnel width before transfer and consideration of using tacking sutures to secure the skin paddle to the muscle before transfer through the tunnel are beneficial.

SUBMENTAL ARTERY FLAP
Relevant Anatomy

- The submental flap is a soft tissue flap consisting of skin, subcutaneous tissue, and muscle inferior to the mandible near the midline (**Fig. 2**A–D). The flap is based on the submental artery and vein, which usually originate from the facial vessels. The submental vessels course superior to the submandibular gland and then pass superficial to the mylohyoid muscle before sending perforating branches through the platysma to the skin.

Indications/Contraindications

- The submental flap is ideally suited to moderate-sized soft tissue defects including cutaneous, parotid, oral cavity, and oropharynx. The flap has an excellent color match for cutaneous defects of the parotid bed or lateral temporal bone. The flap is also well suited to oral cavity reconstruction, especially of the lateral tongue, floor of mouth, and buccal mucosa.
- Concerns have been raised about oncologic safety in oral cavity reconstruction as level one nodal contents may be incorporated into the flap. However, multiple studies have demonstrated oncologic safety for this purpose, and complete removal of level one nodal contents can be achieved when harvesting this flap.[12,13]
- Excess submental laxity makes this flap ideal for older patients, although it can be successfully used in younger patients as well. Earlier neck dissection, especially of level one, is a contraindication to use of this flap. Need for a very large flap, anatomic site remote from the submentum, and inadequate submental laxity are also relative contraindications.

Pearls and Pitfalls

- Proper incision placement is key to successful harvest of this flap. A Doppler ultrasound may be used to identify the position of cutaneous perforators from the submental artery, which should be incorporated into the flap. These originate in the region overlying the mylohyoid muscle adjacent to the anterior belly of digastric, approximately one finger breath inferior to the mandible. The superior limb of the incision should lie at the inferior border of the mandible to optimize the esthetic outcome. The craniocaudal extent of the flap should allow for closure without substantial tension, which can be estimated using a "pinch test." The lateral aspect of the incision should naturally extend to a skin crease suitable for neck dissection.
- An important aspect of dissection is the removal of the submandibular gland, which is carefully dissected away from the overlying marginal mandibular nerve and from perforating branches of the facial artery, of which 2 to 4 are typically encountered, and which should be clipped and divided to release the gland.

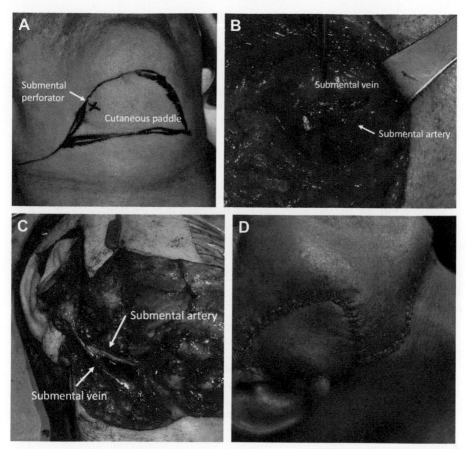

Fig. 2. (*A*) The submental artery flap is designed in the midline with a broad base and the superior limit resting just inferior to the mandible. Note the position of the cutaneous perforator as identified by Doppler ultrasound is marked and included within the flap design. (*B*) The submental artery and vein are identified after removal of the submandibular gland. Note that the vein typically drains into the facial vein as in this case but that variations in venous anatomy may exist. (*C*) The submental flap is rotated into position to reconstruct a preauricular defect. The vascular pedicle should be inspected to ensure that no tension or kinking is present. If necessary, the distal facial vessels may be ligated to increase length, or the vein may be divided and anastomosed to another recipient vein such as the external jugular vein if length is insufficient. (*D*) Submental flap after inset and closure. The flap provides an excellent color and texture match for facial defects in this region.

- The submental vessels will be encountered immediately superior to the gland and must not be injured during harvest. The facial vein also must be preserved because it is most often the primary venous drainage of the flap.
- Inclusion of the anterior belly of digastric and the mylohyoid in the flap protects the distal aspect of the submental vessels and cutaneous perforators and simplifies the harvest, in addition to increasing the bulk of the flap.[14]
- The mylohyoid has a broad attachment to the mandible, and complete release of the muscle is necessary to permit flap transfer.
- The key anatomic variation of this flap is the venous drainage, which may be primarily into external or anterior jugular venous systems in some cases.

Preservation of all venous structures near the flap is critical until venous drainage of the submental vein into the facial vein is visually confirmed.

- If the flap cannot reach its intended recipient site due to vascular stretch, the facial vessels may be divided distal to the takeoff of the submental vessels. Alternatively, the vein may be transected and anastomosed to a recipient vein as a "hybrid flap," or the flap may be harvested as a free flap.[15]
- One should avoid undermining of the skin of the chin so as not to pull the lip downward. By contrast, the inferior skin flap of the secondary defect is widely undermined for tension-free closure.

SUPRACLAVICULAR FLAP
Relevant Anatomy

- The supraclavicular flap is a fasciocutaneous flap based on the supraclavicular artery (**Fig. 3**A, B). This artery typically branches from the transverse cervical artery and is identified in a triangle bounded by the clavicle inferiorly, the external jugular vein laterally, and the sternocleidomastoid muscle anteriorly. The artery is typically found approximately 2 cm posterior to the sternocleidomastoid and 2 to 4 cm superior to the clavicle. The flap is designed over the pectoralis major and deltoid muscles.

Indications/Contraindications

- The supraclavicular flap is well suited to a variety of defects within the head and neck, including pharyngoesophageal, cervicofacial cutaneous, parotid, and oral cavity defects.[16]
- The flap is thin, pliable, and may be folded or tubed as desired to meet reconstructive needs. The flap is reliable, easily harvested, and poses minimal donor site morbidity.
- The primary contraindication for this flap is previous neck dissection, especially level-5 neck dissection.

Pearls and Pitfalls

- Design of the skin paddle is of key importance in harvest of this flap. A Doppler ultrasound may be used to verify the patency and position of the transverse cervical artery in the supraclavicular fossa, especially in cases of prior neck

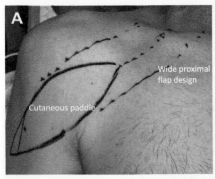 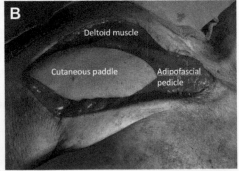

Fig. 3. (*A*) Supraclavicular flap is designed over the anterior deltoid and pectoralis major. Note the wide proximal flap design. (*B*) Supraclavicular flap after harvest. The flap is raised in the subfascial plane over the deltoid and pectoralis muscles. The proximal adipofascial pedicle may be deepithelialized at the outset of harvest, after harvest, or a peninsular flap may be used.

dissection. CT angiography and fluorescence imaging are other options for pedicle identification.[17,18] The flap is then designed with its base extending from the lateral aspect of the sternocleidomastoid attachment to the clavicle to a point 7 to 8 cm lateral to this, allowing for the inclusion of anterior branches of the supraclavicular artery. The skin island is then planned to overlie the anterior deltoid and pectoralis major, maintaining the same width from the base to the distal flap. The flap may be harvested as a peninsular interpolated flap but single stage transfer is permitted through harvest as an island flap with tunneling to the recipient site or through inset of the proximal peninsula into the cervical skin between the harvest site and the defect.

- The proximal adipofascial bridge may be deepithelialized, or it may be simpler to elevate the skin off the underlying tissue at the onset of harvest. Maintain a wide proximal flap to maximize vascularity of the distal tissues.
- The superior skin flap should be sufficiently wide to allow passage of the flap without compression. This is often elevated in the supraplatysmal plane for 2 to 3 cm initially before entering the subplatysmal plane to minimize the risk of injury to the pedicle.
- Any perforating vessel encountered distal to the clavicle can safely be divided without compromising the vascular supply to the flap.
- As the harvest progresses medially, the clavicular periosteum may be harvested with the pedicle to further protect the pedicle.
- Blunt release of the deep cervical fascia may improve upward rotation of the flap in a safe manner. Note that the pedicle may not be directly visualized during this method of harvest.

TEMPORALIS FLAP/TEMPOROPARIETAL FASCIA FLAP
Relevant Anatomy

- The temporalis muscle flap is an axial muscle flap based on the deep temporal branches of the maxillary artery, which penetrates the deep muscle surface (**Fig. 4**A–C). A secondary blood supply originates from the middle temporal vessels, which branch from the superficial temporal artery (STA) and enter the muscle superficially. This muscle overlies the temporal fossa originating from the superior temporal line and lies deep to the TPFF. The muscle inserts onto the coronoid process and serves to elevate and retract the mandible during mastication. The muscle is enveloped by the temporalis fascia, which divides inferiorly into deep and superficial layers approximately 2 cm cephalad to the zygomatic arch. The superficial temporal fat pad resides between these 2 layers. The temporalis muscle receives innervation from the mandibular nerve (V3).
- The temporoparietal fascia (TPF) flap is an axial flap harvested based on the STA. This fascia is also known as superficial temporal fascia and is part of a musculofascial system including the superficial musculoaponeurotic system in the face and the galea aponeurosis. The TPF is found in the temporal fossa deep to the dermis and subcutaneous fat and superficial to the deep temporal fascia and temporalis muscle. The STA is a terminal branch of the external carotid artery that enters the TPF at the level of the zygomatic arch.
- The temporal branch of the facial nerve crosses the zygomatic arch along a line extending from 0.5 cm inferior to the tragus to a point 1.5 cm superior and lateral to the brow. It lies just deep to the TPF and superficial to the deep temporal fascia. This is the critical neural structure to avoid injuring during harvest of either flap.

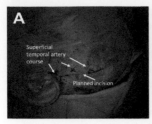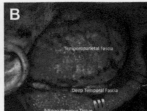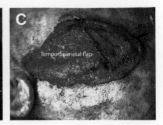

Fig. 4. (*A*) Design of the cutaneous incision for temporoparietal flap. The course of the superficial temporal artery is followed with a Doppler ultrasound and marked on the skin. Planning the incision 2 mm posterior to the course of this vessel can reduce the risk of inadvertent injury. The superior extension can be designed in a number of ways and was designed linearly in this case. (*B*) TPF flap in situ after superficial elevation of the adipocutaneous tissues and incision of the flap margins. The superficial plane is quite tedious to harvest, whereas a loose areolar plane permits rapid elevation of the deep plane off the deep temporal fascia. (*C*) Complete harvest of the TPF flap. Note that the proximal pedicle can be carefully narrowed to increase the arc of rotation. Superiorly, galea was included in the flap to increase bulk and reach.

Indications/Contraindications

- The temporalis flap may be used for a variety of indications, including reconstruction of orbital, temporal bone, skull base, maxillofacial, and oral cavity defects in addition to use in facial reanimation.
- The TPFF flap is highly versatile, being used for many of the same defects as the temporalis flap. The TPFF may also be used for microtia repair and to reconstruct the secondary defect after temporalis flap transfer.
- The TPFF may be harvested as a fasciocutaneous flap including the overlying scalp, or it may be harvested in combination with the deep temporal fascia and temporalis muscle if the middle temporal artery is included in the dissection.
- Extensive history of trauma, cranial base surgery, extended neck dissection, or parotidectomy may compromise vascularity to either of these flaps and should be considered a relative contraindication to flap harvest, although the integrity of the STA can reliably be assessed with ultrasound. Radiation to this area may also render flap harvest more challenging. Finally, the recipient site should be sufficiently close to the donor site to allow for transfer without vascular tension.

Technical Pearls/Pitfalls

- Both the TPF flap and the temporalis flap may be harvested using a variety of incisional orientations depending on the site of planned transferal and patient hairline. In most cases, a preauricular incision is extended superiorly to a point at least 2 cm superior to the temporal line.
- During harvest of the temporalis flap, preservation of the TPFF for secondary defect reconstruction may help minimize contour irregularity.[19] Fat grafting may alternatively be used for this purpose.
- The entire temporalis muscle may be harvested, or a central 2 to 3 cm strip may be used for facial reanimation.
- Incision of the superficial layer of the deep temporal fascia is safest near the root of the zygomatic arch near the ear, posterior to the position of the temporal branch of the facial nerve. Extending this incision anteriorly allows for broad

access to the zygomatic arch and for elevation of the superficial layer of the deep temporal fascia with the temporoparietal facial, which will protect the facial nerve.

- Intraoral transfer of the temporalis flap may require osteotomies of the zygomatic arch, which can be gently elevated away from the infratemporal fossa while maintaining its inferior vascular attachments. The bone can then be replaced, and low-profile titanium plates or absorbable plating may be used to replace the mobilized arch segment.

- The TPF flap may be designed based on the position of the STA, which is identifiable using a handheld Doppler probe. In cases of previous surgery in this area, this step is essential to confirm the viability of the artery before proceeding.

- Elevation of the overlying skin and subcutaneous fat from the superficial surface of the TPFF is the most challenging aspect of harvest of this flap. This is a tedious process as no loose areolar layer is present between these tissue layers. The dermis becomes more adherent to the underlying TPF as the flap progresses superiorly, so starting this process inferiorly may be beneficial.

- The cranial galea is continuous with the TPFF, and inclusion of galea in the TPFF flap may extend the reach or improve bulk of this flap.

LATISSIMUS DORSI PEDICLED FLAP

More often used as a free flap, the latissimus dorsi pedicled flap remains a useful option in head and neck reconstruction (**Fig. 5**A–C). The latissimus dorsi spans a large portion of the lower back and adducts, extends, and internally rotates the arm. The thoracodorsal artery and vein provide the primary blood supply to the flap. The flap may be designed as a myofascial or musculocutaneous flap. When transferred as a pedicled flap, it is tunneled between the pectoralis major and minor muscles through the axilla. Methods to increase reach of the flap include exteriorization of the pedicle with delayed transection, division of the serratus anterior branches of the thoracodorsal pedicle, division of the circumflex scapular vessels, and division of the latissimus dorsi tendon.[20–22] The flap can reach numerous sites in the head and neck and is ideal for the reconstruction of cervical, temporal bone, and scalp defect. It is also useful for the management of pharyngocutaneous fistula after laryngectomy. Donor site morbidity after transfer of this flap is generally favorable when compared with other large myofascial flaps such as the pectoralis and trapezius. Harvest may be accomplished in a decubitus or supine position, the latter allowing for a 2-team approach.[23] Avoidance of injury to neurovascular structures during transfer and injury to the brachial plexus from arm positioning is critical, and avoidance of kinking or compression of the pedicle is necessary for flap survival. Partial flap necrosis is not uncommon, especially if the skin paddle is designed over caudal aspects of the muscle where perforator density is lower.

DELTOPECTORAL FLAP

A workhorse flap in head and neck reconstruction for 2 decades, the deltopectoral flap has limited usefulness in modern reconstruction. A fasciocutaneous flap is based on the second and third perforating branches of the internal mammary artery; this flap may be used to resurface cervicofacial cutaneous, pharyngeal, and oral cavity defects. This flap is limited by distal necrosis, which may be substantially minimized by limiting lateral extension of the flap over the deltoid or by raising the distal portion in an initial procedure and then performing delayed transfer.[24] In addition, when raised as a peninsular flap, a staged second operation is usually necessary unless the

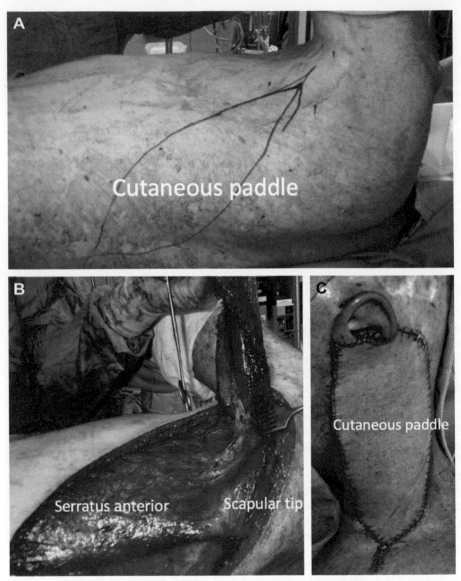

Fig. 5. (*A*) Design of latissimus dorsi pedicled flap. Very large skin paddles can be harvested with this flap and makes it ideally suited to resurface large defects in the head and neck. (*B*) The latissimus flap is harvested. The flap is tunneled through the axilla between the pectoralis major and minor muscles. (*C*) Latissimus dorsi flap inset into a lateral neck wound. This flap easily reaches defects in this area and can extend further to the scalp if needed.

intervening skin bridge excised. Elevation of an island flap is a useful to alternative to eliminate this limitation and allow single-stage transfer.[25] The internal mammary artery perforator flap is a modified version of the deltopectoral flap that is based on a single perforator, allowing for greater arc of rotation and a smaller secondary defect, thereby potentially limiting donor site morbidity.

TRAPEZIUS FLAP

The trapezius covers large portions of the upper back and posterior neck and serves distinct functions from the upper, mid, and lower portions of the muscle (**Fig. 6**). Similarly, 3 different flaps can be harvested from this muscle based on different blood supplies. The superior trapezius flap is based on paraspinous perforators and the occipital artery. This highly reliable flap is typically transferred as a peninsular flap to resurface cutaneous defects of the posterolateral neck.[26] The flap is superiorly based, which mitigates effects of gravity that may worsen outcomes of other regional flaps. Earlier transection of the transverse cervical vessels from radical neck dissection may improve the reliability of this flap through a delay phenomenon. A lower island trapezius flap offers an excellent arc of rotation to reach numerous sites in the head and neck.[27] This flap is based on the transverse cervical artery and is designed as an island over the paraspinous skin medial to the lower aspect of the scapula. The primary disadvantage of this flap is the need to harvest in the lateral decubitus position. The lateral island trapezius flap requires meticulous dissection of the transverse cervical vessels and has a limited arc of rotation, making it less useful than the other flaps based on this muscle.

ROLE OF REGIONAL FLAPS IN MODERN HEAD AND NECK RECONSTRUCTION

Regional flaps continue to hold an important place in the current reconstructive armamentarium even in settings where free tissue transfer is widely available. In heavily treated patients with vascular depletion, regional flaps may prove more reliable and minimize risk of reoperation.[28] In many cases, regional flap transfer is more rapid than free tissue transfer given the lack of need for microvascular anastomosis and may be better suited to frail patients in which minimizing operative time is to be prioritized. Although some regional flaps such as the pectoralis flap may carry major morbidity relative to comparable free flaps, in most cases the donor site morbidity of regional flaps is minimal. Finally, in settings of diminished resources, where microvascular training or equipment are lacking, regional flaps can successfully reconstruct a large portion of defects within the head and neck.

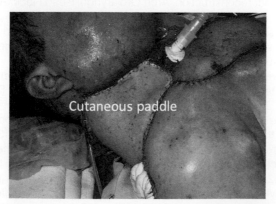

Fig. 6. Superiorly based trapezius flap is used for closure after a radical neck dissection with cutaneous excision. This flap resists negative effects of gravity due to its superior base, and its vascular supply is robust.

CLINICS CARE POINTS

- Design of the pectoralis flap skin paddle over the inferomedial aspect of the muscle optimizes superior reach of the flap with maximum perforator density.

- Inclusion of the anterior belly of digastric and the mylohyoid muscles protects the vascular pedicle of the submental flap and increases flap bulk.

- The anterior branches of the supraclavicular artery course over the anterior shoulder adjacent to the deltopectoral groove, and an anterior design allows for recruitment of this vascularity and improves flap reliability.

REFERENCES

1. Conley JJ, Price JC. The midline vertical forehead flap. Otolaryngol Head Neck Surg 1981;89(1):38–44.
2. Miller TA. The Tagliacozzi flap as a method of nasal and palatal reconstruction. Plast Reconstr Surg 1985;76(6):870–4.
3. Bakamjian VY, Long M, Rigg B. Experience with the medially based deltopectoral flap in reconstructive surgery of the head and neck. Br J Plast Surg 1971;24: 174–83.
4. Ariyan S. The pectoralis major myocutaneous flap. A versatile flap for reconstruction in the head and neck. Plast Reconstr Surg 1979;63(1):73–81.
5. Baek S, Biller HF, Krespi YP, et al. The pectoralis major myocutaneous island flap for reconstruction of the head and neck. Head Neck Surg 1979;1(4):293–300.
6. Rickard RF, Hudson DA. A history of vascular and microvascular surgery. Ann Plast Surg 2014;73(4):465–72.
7. Martin D, Pascal JF, Baudet J, et al. The submental island flap: a new donor site. Anatomy and clinical applications as a free or pedicled flap. Plast Reconstr Surg 1993;92(5):867–73.
8. Fabian RL. Pectoralis major myocutaneous flap reconstruction of the laryngopharynx and cervical esophagus. Laryngoscope 1988;98(11):1227–31.
9. Resto VA, McKenna MJ, Deschler DG. Pectoralis major flap in composite lateral skull base defect reconstruction. Arch Otolaryngol Head Neck Surg 2007;133(5): 490–4.
10. Dennis D, Kashima H. Introduction of the Janus flap: a modified pectoralis major myocutaneous flap for cervical esophageal and pharyngeal reconstruction. Arch Otolaryngol 1981;107(7):431–5.
11. Cuono CB, Ariyan S. Immediate reconstruction of a composite mandibular defect with a regional osteomusculocutaneous flap. Plast Reconstr Surg 1980;65(4): 477–83.
12. Patel UA. The submental flap for head and neck reconstruction: comparison of outcomes to the radial forearm free flap. Laryngoscope 2020;130:S1–10.
13. Howard BE, Nagel TH, Donald CB, et al. Oncologic safety of the submental flap for reconstruction in oral cavity malignancies. Otolaryngol Head Neck Surg 2014; 150(4):558–62.
14. Patel UA, Bayles SW, Hayden RE. The submental flap: a modified technique for resident training. Laryngoscope 2007;117(1):186–9.
15. Hayden RE, Nagel TH, Donald CB. Hybrid submental flaps for reconstruction in the head and neck: part pedicled, part free. Laryngoscope 2014;124(3):637–41.

16. Herr MW, Emerick KS, Deschler DG. The supraclavicular artery flap for head and neck reconstruction. JAMA Facial Plast Surg 2014;16(2):127–32.
17. Bigcas JLM, DeBiase CA, Ho T. Indocyanine green angiography as the principal design and perfusion assessment tool for the supraclavicular artery island flap in head and neck reconstruction. Cureus 2022;14(9):e29007.
18. Adams AS, Wright MJ, Johnston S, et al. The use of multislice CT angiography preoperative study for supraclavicular artery island flap harvesting. Ann Plast Surg 2012;69(3):312–5.
19. Cheney ML, Mckenna MJ, Megerian CA, et al. Early temporalis muscle transposition for the management of facial paralysis. Laryngoscope 1995;105(9): 993–1000.
20. Friedrich W, Herberhold C, Lierse W. Vascularization of the myocutaneous latissimus dorsi flap. Cells Tissues Organs 1988;131(2):97–102.
21. Maves MD, Panje WR, Shagets FW. Extended latissimus dorsi myocutaneous flap reconstruction of major head and neck defects. Otolaryngol Head Neck Surg 1984;92(5):551–8.
22. Hayden RE, Kirby SD, Deschler DG. Technical modifications of the latissimus dorsi pedicled flap to increase versatility and viability. Laryngoscope 2000; 110(3):352–7.
23. Feng AL, Nasser HB, Rosko AJ, et al. Revisiting pedicled latissimus dorsi flaps in head and neck reconstruction: contrasting shoulder morbidities across mysofascial flaps. Plast Aesthet Res 2021;8. https://doi.org/10.20517/2347-9264.2021.03.
24. McGregor IA, Morgan G. Axial and random pattern flaps. Br J Plast Surg 1973; 26(3):202–13.
25. Jacksox IANT, Lang W. Secondary esophagoplasty after pharyngolaryngectomy, using a modified deltopectoral flap. Plast Reconstr Surg 1971;48(2):155–9.
26. Aviv JE, Urken ML, Lawson W, et al. The superior trapezius myocutaneous flap in head and neck reconstruction. Arch Otolaryngol Head Neck Surg 1992;118(7): 702–6.
27. Zenga J, Sharon JD, Santiago P, et al. Lower trapezius flap for reconstruction of posterior scalp and neck defects after complex occipital-cervical surgeries. J Neurol Surg B Skull Base 2015;76(05):397–408.
28. Chang BA, Asarkar AA, Horwich PM, et al. Regional pedicled flap salvage options for large head and neck defects: the old, the new, and the forgotten. Laryngoscope Investig Otolaryngol 2022;8(1):63–75.

Tenants of Mandibular Reconstruction in Segmental Defects

Scott Bevans, MD[a,b,*], Daniel Hammer, DDS, FACS[b,c]

KEYWORDS

• Mandible • Defect • Reconstruction

KEY POINTS

- Mandibular reconstruction of benign segmental defects of less than 6 cm can be safely performed of using non-vascularized bone grafting, particularly using tissue engineering (BMP-2, bone marrow aspirates, etc.). Water-tight oral cavity closure is paramount. Success rates are higher with lateral vs anterior defects.
- Reconstruction of composite defects is most reliably performed with free tissue transfer. Fibula, Iliac Crest and Scapula free flaps are most common. The choice may be dictated by quantity of soft tissue, lenght of necessary bone, pedicle length, and patient co-morbidities.
- Planning for the occlusive restoration (placing reconstructed mandible more superior and lingual) is critical in ability to achieve return to normal chewing function.
- VSP, CAD and CAM are increasingly popular options to help improve accuracy, plan for dental implant placement, and decrease operative time.

INTRODUCTION

The aesthetic form (facial width and projection) created by the mandibular contour contributes to its functions of preserving the oropharyngeal and hypopharyngeal airway, masticating, swallowing, and articulating. Therefore, reconstruction, whether from traumatic or oncologic etiologies must consider both form and function. One of the most complex functional end goals is to achieve a functional occlusion which bears the force of chewing. The variables in achieving this are numerous: preventing the malposition of the mandibular condyles, preservation of temporomandibular joint

Financial disclosures: None.
[a] Department of Otolaryngology, Tripler Army Medical Center, 1 Jarrett White Road, TAMC, HI 96818, USA; [b] Uniformed Services University, 4301 Jones Bridge Road, Bethesda, MD 20814, USA; [c] Department of Oral Maxillofacial Surgery, Naval Medical Center San Diego, 34800 Bob Wilson Drive, San Diego, CA 92134, USA
* Corresponding author.
E-mail address: scott.e.bevans.mil@health.mil

function, osseous reconstruction of the mandibular arch in a way that restores contour and preserves remaining occlusion, soft tissue coverage that recreates a gingivobuccal sulcus, and (potentially) the ability to directly load the reconstructed segment of mandible with an implant-retained dental prosthetic.

The methods by which surgeons reconstruct segmental defects of the mandible include: soft tissue only with reconstruction plate (no bone), alloplastic material reconstruction (ie, titanium) with or without non-vascularized bone grafting (autogenous cortical strut, morselized autogenous cancellous bone, and/or tissue engineering), and vascularized bone grafting (fibula and iliac crest free flaps being the most common) with or without immediate dental implant placement and/or dental prosthetic. The selection of strategy for reconstruction is based on the location of the mandibular defect and several patient and facility-specific factors.

In this summary, we will review data from the last decade and discuss current and future considerations influencing choice in the method of mandibular reconstruction in continuity defects.

Anatomy

The U-shaped mandible is considered a closed arch from a biomechanical perspective. The unique nature of the temporomandibular joint allows both rotational and translational vectors of opening providing 20 and 30 mm, respectively, to achieve a maximal incisive opening (MIO) of approximately 50 mm.[1] Mandibular opening is driven by the depressor action of the mylohyoid and anterior belly of the digastric as well as the anterior translation function of the lateral pterygoid muscle. Mandibular closure that allows for mastication is the function of the masseter, medial pterygoid, and temporalis muscles. The functional housing of the mandible resides in bilateral temporomandibular joints, the body's only ginglymoarthrodial joint, allowing both rotational and translational movement. This architecture facilitates narrowing and widening of the mandible during function to enhance speech and swallow function.

The mandible has an superior alveolar segment that holds 16 teeth and an inferior load-bearing segment with a higher cortical to cancellous ratio. This alveolar segment of the mandible is lingual when compared with the location of the mandibular body and inferior border of the mandible, which sits in a relatively buccal position. Therefore, it is critical, regardless of reconstruction technique, to restore the mandible's alveolar, dentate segment in its natural lingualized position in relation to the inferior border of the mandible. By doing so, the surgeon ensures definitive dental restoration and patient function are feasible. If the facial contour of the patient is prioritized instead by placing bony reconstruction at the inferior border of the mandible (therefore not restoring the lingualized alveolar segment), the patient will have a crossbite and it may be impossible to achieve definitive and functional dental restoration (**Fig. 1**).

Classification of Mandibular Defects

There are several different classification systems of mandibular defects. In 1989, Jewer and colleagues described mandibular continuity defects as lateral (not involving the condyle or canine), central (involving the central sextant of tooth-bearing mandible), and hemi mandibulectomy (involving the condyle). These were abbreviated L, C, and H, respectively, and could be used in isolation or combined to describe the bony defect in question; for example, HC would describe a hemi-mandibulectomy defect extending into the central sextant, or HCL would describe a defect extending from one condyle through the contralateral mandibular body.[2] As each of these regions carries different reconstructive considerations, it has remained an effective description scheme. Boyd added descriptors for the soft tissue defect, differentiating

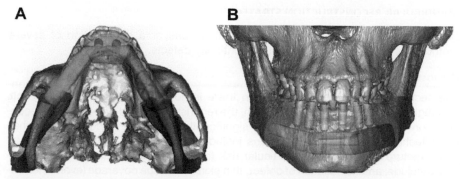

Fig. 1. Refining placement of mandibular reconstruction grafts to align the alveolar (dental segment) with inferior load-bearing segment. (*A*). Inferior view of a native mandible with planned resection demonstrates the inferior basal bone position which is buccal to the tooth-bearing alveolar segment. Notice to optimize rehabilitation, the reconstructed mandible sits lingual to the "ideal" more buccal position of the native bone. (*B*). The anterior view of native and reconstructed mandible demonstrates the superior position of the reconstruction relative to the pre-operative inferior projection of the mandible. This allows for more effective occlusal restoration and the difference is easily camouflaged with the additional soft tissue accompanying free flap reconstruction.

skin (s), mucosal (m), and tongue (t) soft tissue components.[3] Brown submits another classification based on the number of corners that a defect crosses, from I to IV, which often lends to the length of the defect and number of osteotomies that will be required for reconstruction.[4]

Clinically the Jewer-Boyd defect classification correlates with several of the challenges surrounding reconstruction, specifically, the length of segment, condylar involvement, number of osteotomies required, tooth-bearing segmentation, and soft tissue reconstruction required.

Etiology of Defect

Etiology and treatment of that etiology (surgical and nonsurgical) may affect the vascularity and volume of the surrounding soft tissue is critical to consider. In cases of trauma, was the soft tissue envelope maintained via external fixation or additional methods to prevent contraction? For patient with malignancies who will undergo radiation, is it predicable to offer a soft tissue only or avascular osseous reconstruction? For large composite mandibular defects, it may be more difficult to reconstruct with a single vascularized osteocutaneous free flap. In these cases, greater consideration may be given to nonosseous free flaps in addition to osteocutaneous flaps for mandibular reconstruction.[5]

specifically in considering the need for vascularized tissue reconstruction in cases of osteoradionecrosis, several factors must be considered. Studies of the pattern of bone necrosis show that cortical necrosis (particularly at the densest inferior portion of the mandible) is more prevalent than cancellous necrosis.[6] Absence of necrosis at the margins of resected bone do not necessarily assure the prevention of progression.[7] MRI may be more sensitive and specific, but CT scan evidence of cortical irregularity likely warrants at least a 1 cm margin and guided resection. After the resection of the affected bone, the clinical examination should confirm the presence of bleeding bone at the margins.[8] Some authors advocate for using fluorescent intraoperative visualization with preoperative administration of tetracycline (which will only fluoresce viable bone that has blood flow).[9–12]

MANDIBULAR RECONSTRUCTION STRATEGIES

Based on these factors, surgeons may choose one or a combination of several methods for reconstructing mandibular continuity defects.

Reconstruction Plate

This technique can only be used when there is no associated soft tissue deficit. Although it is an option for reconstruction, the reconstructive plate alone for the reconstruction of the mandibular arch has a significantly higher rate of complication than other techniques. These complications include plate exposure (20%–37%) and/or plate fracture (5%–18%).[13–15] Particular risk factors for complications in recent reviews include: anterior location of defect, thin skin/soft tissue coverage (even when using a pedicled skin/soft tissue flap for coverage) and radiation.[16–18] Recent specialized locking "bridging plates" may reduce the risk of plate exposure to closer to 10% when covered by vascularized soft tissue flaps.[19,20] While certainly a consideration in patients with poor prognosis and severe medical comorbidities, surgeons should be wary of the risk of plate related complications and consider robust soft tissue coverage and bicortical fixation on the densest portion the mandibular construct (**Fig. 2**).

Nonvascularized Bone Grafts (Autogenous and/or Tissue Engineering)

Well-vascularized mandible defects (without a history of radiation or vascular compromise) with adequate soft tissue envelope and posterior or lateral defects of 6 cm or less have been successfully reconstructed with nonvascularized bone grafts and reconstruction plate with or without titanium mesh bone tray.[21,22] Traditionally, these autografts come from the anterior iliac crest (less commonly from other areas). Success rates in non-radiated patients in achieving bony union that allows for dental implantation can be as high as 77% to 87% in patients with benign etiologies and lateral segmental defects.[23,24] Proponents point to lower operative time and hospitalization

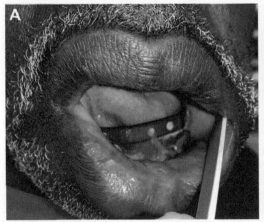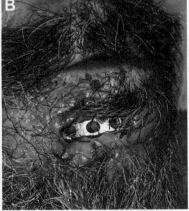

Fig. 2. Exposed mandibular reconstruction plates. (*A*). Male patient with the history of resection of benign anterior mandibular tumor reconstructed with PSI titanium reconstruction bar without autologous or free tissue augmentation. Exposed intra-orally at 6 weeks postoperatively. (*B*). Male patient with a shattered mandible and segmental defect from drug-related blunt trauma reconstructed with reconstruction bar, exposed at 3 months postoperatively.

period, although more operative interventions may be required and the use of autogenous bone requires a second surgical site. These autografts rarely accommodate primary endosseous implantation, as watertight closure and prevention of bacterial contamination are thought to be significant risk factors for failures.[24–26] A more recent meta-analysis suggests that anterior defects and defects larger than 6 cm may be still reconstructed with nonvascularized bone grafting.[27] These recent analysis suggests there may be several factors at play for the increased success using nonvascularized grafts, including: the ability for water-tight closure, use of bone morphogenic protein, platelet rich plasma, biomolecules, and hyperbaric oxygen. Unfortunately, this meta-analysis was unable to differentiate the etiology of mandibular defect and radiation as risk factors for failure. Most authors agree that cases with malignant etiologies, significant soft tissue deficits or those with compromised blood flow (or need for post operative radiation) , free tissue transfer has a higher success rate.[27–29]

Recent literature advocates that advancement of clinical tissue engineering using bone allograft with Bone Morphogenic Protein-2, and bone marrow aspirate concentrate, has resulted success rates that rival non-vascularized autograft, even in complex head and neck defects, and carries less (or zero) donor site morbidity **(Fig. 3)**.[30] These advancements and high bone restoration rates have challenged the 6 cm limitation on non-vascularized reconstruction.

Vascularized Bone Grafts (Free Tissue Transfer)

Among microvascular osteocutaneous flaps, three types are most commonly used: the fibula, iliac crest, and scapula free flaps. Less commonly used is the osteocutaneous radial forearm free flap (as the bone volume is generally not adequate for later dental implant placement and dental restoration). Important considerations in selecting which flap to use are: the location and length of osseous defect, need for osteotomies, presence of ipsilateral versus contralateral donor vessels, and volume of soft tissue reconstruction necessary. Rodriguez and Schultz and colleagues nicely summarize many of these factors in their 2015 publication providing an algorithm to consider in approaching reconstruction. Relative to the 70% to 80% success rate of nonvascularized bone grafting, microsurgical reconstruction rates are reported at 87% to 97%.[22,31–34] In one retrospective study from India, microsurgical success rate with fibular free flaps was considerably lower (72%) in very large hemimandibulectomy reconstructions that crossed midline (as noted by earlier authors),

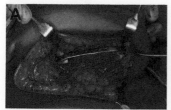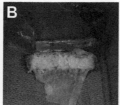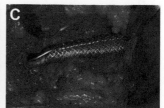

Fig. 3. Teenage male with benign mandibular tumor resected resulting in segmental defect reconstructed with particulate bone and custom titanium recon bar and standard mesh tray. (A). Right lateral mandibular body defect, approximately 7.5 cm in length. (B). Cortical/cancellous allograft particulate substrate wrapped with bone morphogenic protein 2. (Not shown is the instillation of mesenchymal stem cells in the form of autologous bone marrow aspirate which act as a signaler.) Construct is wrapped in collagen bilayer to stabilize during implantation. (C) The titanium mesh around the engineered graft is adapted to the reconstruction bar. Watertight oral cavity closure was achieved prior to implantation.

need for a skin paddle greater than 6 × 10 cm, and/or use of additional flaps (pectoralis major, deltopectoral or supraclavicular artery island flap).[35] Important in patient counseling is the caveat that, while surgery may be considered "successful" and quality of life improvements are noted in greater than 75% of patients, return to presurgical speech and swallow function is less common.[35–38] The additional donor site does carry some morbidity, which varies based on type and extent of free flap chosen.[39] More recently the ability for the primary implantation of reconstructed bone with the potential for early dental rehabilitation has further accelerated the use of free flap reconstruction of segmental defects. The advantages and considerations of the three most commonly used flaps are discussed later in discussion, including recent data on postoperative morbidity associated with each. Key features of these flaps are summarized in **Fig. 4** and with additional considerations in choosing surgical approach listed in **Table 1**. Notably absent are less commonly employed osseous flaps such as the osteocutaneous radial forearm, medial femoral condyle, and serratus rib free flaps.

Fibula Free Flap

For the past three decades, the fibula-free flap has been the most used osteocutaneous free tissue option in many institutions. The flap is based on the peroneal artery and accompanying venae, which branches off the tibioperoneal trunk. While it is the longest osseous graft and the graft of choice for angle-to-angle reconstructions, it may still be insufficient to reach from condyle to condyle.[40–42] Total or near-total mandibular reconstructions that cross midline carry an increased rate of complications. Possibly because of the peripheral location of this flap, smoking has also been linked to a higher risk of vascular compromise.[33] Preoperative evaluation to confirm normal three vessel runoff can be performed using doppler or CT angiography. CT is additionally helpful when planning to use virtual surgical planning (VSP). In cases of questionable vascular narrowing, ankle-brachial indices should be performed.

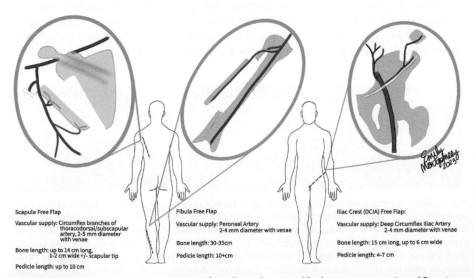

Scapula Free Flap

Vascular supply: Circumflex branches of
thoracodorsal/subscapular
artery, 2-5 mm diameter
with venae
Bone length: up to 14 cm long,
1-2 cm wide +/- scapular tip
Pedicle length: up to 10 cm

Fibula Free Flap

Vascular supply: Peroneal Artery
2-4 mm diameter with venae
Bone length: 30-35cm
Pedicle length: 10+cm

Iliac Crest (DCIA) Free Flap:

Vascular supply: Deep Circumflex Iliac Artery
2-4 mm diameter with venae
Bone length: 15 cm long, up to 6 cm wide
Pedicle length: 4-7 cm

Fig. 4. Illustration of common osseous free flaps for mandibular reconstruction. (*Courtesy:* Emily Montgomery.)

Table 1
Considerations in osseous free flap selection

Type of Flap	Fibula Flap	Iliac Crest (DCIA) Flap	Scapula Flap
Advantages	• Supine (simultaneous) two team harvest • Longest osseous component (25+ cm) • Long pedicle, often allowing for contralateral anastomosis • Multiple soft tissue paddle options • High Cortical to cancellous ratio, able to accommodate implants • Periosteal blood supply allows multiple osteotomies	• No preop vascular screening • Supine (simultaneous) two team harvest • Excellent height of bone stock • High ratio of cancellous to cortical • Multiple soft tissue paddle options • Natural curvature matches mandibular contour • Favorable scar healing	• No preop vascular screening • Multiple soft tissue paddle options, significant soft tissue bulk • Favorable scar healing • No gait disturbance postoperatively
Disadvantages	• Reduced height of bone stock (can be "double barreled") • Requires vascular screening (vascular disease, anomalous arterial supply) • Risk of compartment syndrome postop • Risk of Hallux dorsiflexion disability, ankle instability long-term	• Limited bone length • Short pedicle length • Risk of hernia postop • Limited ability for osteotomies • Significant risk of gait disturbance and pain postoperatively	• Limited bone length • Limited ability for osteotomies • Less favorable for simultaneous harvest • Less robust bone quality
Ideal use	Long segment, multiple osteotomies, limited soft tissue deficit, two team, dental implantation	Lateral/ramus defect, moderate soft tissue defect with short pedicle length	Short segment, lateral defect, significant chimeric soft tissue reconstruction

Critics of the fibula flap cite the relatively low bone height relative to the native mandible or iliac crest free flap. The largely septocutaneous perforators may also be musculocutaneous perforators in a minority of patients. And perforators may be insufficient to drive a large skin paddle (prior annotations of skin paddles greater than 6 × 10 cm are at risk of inadequate vascular supply).[35]

It has generally been found to have a relatively low donor site morbidity, although wound healing and lower rate of functional deficit in some studies may favor iliac crest.[39,43] As additional extremity specific disability testing has been studied post operatively , hallux dorsiflexion (55%), hallux flexion (32%), ankle instability, and lateral leg numbness (32%) have been found with surprising frequency which has the potential for neagitve on quality of life.[44,45] These deficits were decreased when distal residual fibula length increased.[44] Gait analysis confirmed these changes and demonstrated valgus deformities, likely associated with imbalance between agonist and antagonist muscles.[46–48] While significant improvement is seen within 6 months of surgery, multi-disciplinary care with targeted rehabilitation programs may be beneficial in addressing these deficits.[45,49] Life or limb-threatening complications, such as compartment syndrome and tibial fracture from osteomyelitis are rare, however strict attention should be paid to avoid closing the wound under excessive tension.[48,50,51]

Iliac Crest (Deep Circumflex Iliac Artery) Free Flap

The deep circumflex iliac artery bone flap has become increasingly popular since the initial description by Taylor with subsequent clarifications by Urken and colleagues, particularly for lateral or purely anterior mandibular defect.[52–54] The arterial supply for this flap is based on the external iliac system with accompanying (often larger) venous outflow. The bone length can be up to 15 cm. Height is typically 2.5 cm. Overlying soft tissue can be harvest in the form of an osteocutaneous flap based on the superficial branch of the circumflex artery. Alternatively, the adjacent superior epigastric artery groin flap and or the internal oblique muscle can be harvested on a common pedicle.[54–56] The contour of the ipsilateral iliac crest is favorable for mandibular replacement.[57,58] Owing to its generous width and height, successful oral rehabilitation with osseous implantation has been widely successful.[1,54,55,59–61] Disadvantages may be the flap's soft tissue is very bulky when harvesting an osteocutaneous flap that can hinder dental rehabilitation. The nature of the periosteal supply limits the ability for osteotomy without significantly risking blood flow to the distal bone (care must be taken to preserve the periosteum and iliacus muscle on the medial surface of the graft).[1] Thus, the use of the bone flap is often reserved for single segment reconstructions and surgeons may need to use vein grafting to lengthen the pedicle in cases of contralateral neck vasculature.[62]

In evaluations of donor site morbidity, some authors have suggested favorable scar healing.[63] Thorough evaluations of postoperative functional limitations are variable, some note gait disturbances in 59% and persistent pain in 11% of postoperative patients.[47] Conversely, retrospective comparisons published by other institutions have shown lower rates of complication relative to fibula-free flap.[60] Intuitively, the disruption of the muscular attachments on the iliac crest leads to potential for incidence of hernia, which can be reduced with the use of mesh at the time of donor site closure.[59]

Scapular Free Flap

The scapular free flap is based on the circumflex scapular system. The osseous portion of this flap can be harvested from the lateral border of the scapula (branches of the circumflex scapular) or the scapular tip (angular branch) and reach 14 cm in total bone length.[1,64] Proponents for using the scapular system note the variety of skin, subcutaneous and muscular components that allow for the design of a complex chimeric flap with varying options for bulk.[65,66] The pedicle length can be extended to nearly 10 cm in many circumstances. While typically there is not thought to be segmental blood supply that allows for multiple osteotomies, several authors have described multiple osseous subunits in a single flap.[64,67] Because of the complexity of exposing the scapula system, simultaneous harvest may not be possible in all institutions.

While the surgical site allows for early ambulation, nearly all patients will have at least early deficit elevating the arm above the head.[66] Long-term analysis shows significant improvement and often complete resolution in the first 3 to 6 months postoperatively.[67]

SPECIAL CONSIDERATIONS
Condylar Reconstruction (Rib, Temporomandibular Joint Arthroplasty, or Fibula-Free Flap)

As previously discussed, the restoration at least the rotational function of the temporomandibular joint in mandibular reconstruction is required for the patient to masticate postoperatively. In segmental mandibular defects that include removal of the condyle, preoperative planning is exceptionally helpful be completed to ensure an optimal outcome is possible for the patient. There are several reconstructive options cited in the literature, most commonly including :avascular rib graft, TMJ arthroplasty, and fibula-free flap. When determining indications for each option, the patient's age and the etiology that caused condylar defect are most critical. In the growing patient, the most employed technique is the avascular rib graft given the patient's growing facial skeleton. Both TMJ arthroplasty and fibula-free flap are well tolerated for reconstruction following trauma or benign tumor extirpation (as the patient is unlikely to have radiation treatment). For condylar reconstruction in patients who will undergo radiation therapy, a vascularized tissue-free flap is preferred over the other options, as an alloplastic joint (with a higher volume of titanium in particular) may cause dosage scatter and an avascular graft would not be viable postradiation (**Fig. 5**).

Advances in Mandibular Reconstruction

There has been a paradigm shift to using virtual surgical planning to achieve the desired outcome (occlusive result) and then reerse engineer the reconstrutive process

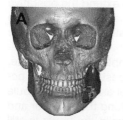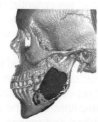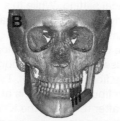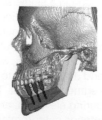

Fig. 5. Condylar reconstruction with fibula-free flap. (*A*). Pre-resection demostration of benign left ramus tumor, resection including condyle, but preserving TMJ disc. (*B*). Virtually planned fibula reconstruction with the immediate restoration of anterior dentition. Not shown is the custom reduction guide allows for the creation of a rounded neo-condyle to restore functiontal rotational movement insetting the end of the fibula into the residual TMJ disc. This is secured with an absorbable suture from the plate on the fibula to the temporalis fascia in a vertical vector.

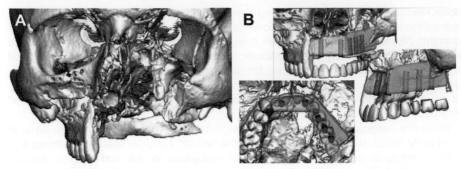

Fig. 6. Occlusion based reconstruction. (*A*). Left hemi-maxillary defect. Traditional approaches in facial reconstruction would dictate beginning planning with bone reconstruction at the inferior border of the native position, which is often not ideal for occlusive reconstruction. (*B*). Virtual surgical planning allows for the consideration of the position of necessary dental reconstruction first, then placing bone reconstruction in the ideal location to facilitate this restoration.

(**Fig. 6**). Several advances in the past decade have contributed to the surgical team's ability to accurately predict and achieve bone placement with useable implants for prosthetic rehabilitation. In our facilities, surgical teams have accelerated this process from an 18 month multi-stage process to a single day surgical effort; the so called "Jaw in a Day."

Computer-Aided Design and Computer-Aided Manufacturing
The application of digital planning, printing, milling has revolutionized mandibular reconstruction. Numerous studies have demonstrated improved accuracy in mandibular reconstruction with decreased displacement of the condyle, improved contour and angulation as well as improved capacity for implantation. By some analysis, there are both cost and time savings in surgical care as well as potential reductions in postoperative stay.[68–77]

Immediate Dental Rehabilitation in Free Tissue Transfer
The use of these technologies in combination (CAD/CAM) allows for the completion of the entire surgical process from extirpation to reconstruction including dental rehabilitation in a single surgical setting. While this has the potential to extend the operative intervention, particularly during the initial learning curve, it dramatically improves the rate of dental rehabilitation, speeds molding of the soft tissue structures, and saves several potential future operative interventions.[78–81]

In our facilities, we use CAD/CAM to incorporate the dental implant locations, size, and angulation into the fibula cut guides. Typically we plan at least two implants per segment of fibula. The fibula cut guide is attached to the lateral aspect of the fibula during elevation, and after releasing the IO membrane and making the superior and inferior osteotomies, the implants are predrilled and placed while the fibula is still perfusing and prior to the egmental osteotomies (which can make the bone less stable relative to the cut guide). Last, the dental prosthesis is indexed to the fibula and dental implants to ensure proper occlusion at the time of inset. The enormous advantage is that (at least using fibula-free flaps) this entire process can be completed after flap elevation, but before harvest, having no significant effect on ischemia time (**Fig. 7**).

Various portions of this process can be performed without manufacturer involvement. Premade dental prosthetic can be printed, reconstruction bars can be prebent to 3D printed models, occlusal splints can guide free-handed placement of implants at the time of surgery.[82]

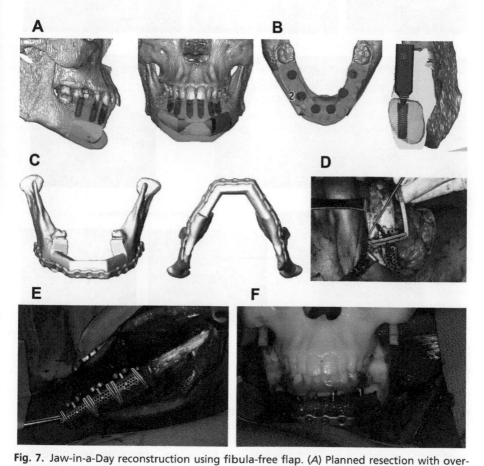

Fig. 7. Jaw-in-a-Day reconstruction using fibula-free flap. (*A*) Planned resection with overlaying planned fibula reconstruction and implants. (*B*) VSP allows for placement of 6 implants in the most appropriate regions of the fibula-free flap with controlled angulation. (*C*) Patient-specific implant-titanium reconstruction bar manufactured (printed or milled) with screw holes to accommodate placement of implants. (*D*) Based on VSP, titanium cut guides secure to the native mandible and allow for precise resection. (*E*) Corresponding cut guides for the fibula-free flap allow for simultaneous harvest with high degree of accuracy. (*F*) Using 3D model of the maxilla and bite registration guides, the ostoeotomies, application of reconstruction bar, placement of implants, and provisional "pick up" of the prosthetic can all be achieved while the fibula-free flap is perfusing. (*G*) The graft is then harvested and transposed to the oral cavity defect (*H*) Planned dental prosthetic (*I*) Intraoral sutures are placed, but not secured, which allows for delivery of the recon bar and fibula with implants. (*J*). After inset, the prosthesis re-affixed. (*K*). 4 month post-operative. (*L*) 15 months postoperative, the final prosthesis is completely healed and allowing functional occlusion. (*M*) Notice the minor difference in mandibular projection allowing for high stable and functional occlusive restoration.

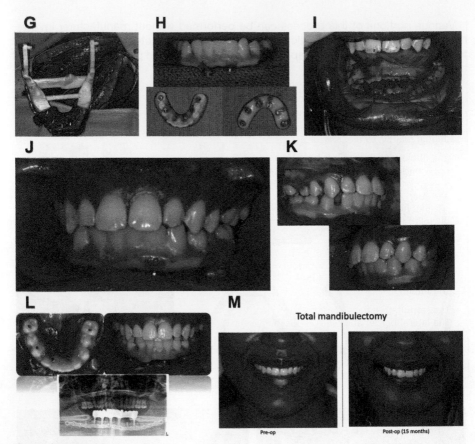

Fig. 7. (*continued*).

SUMMARY

The primary tenant of all mandibular reconstruction (whether complex trauma reconstruction, treating ablative segmental defects, or resecting incompetent mandibular bone) is achieving functional maxillomandibular occlusion. While reconstruction plates and non-vascularized bone grafts have great utility in some circumstances, for significant multi-unit defects and/or those with soft tissue loss, composite reconstruction using microvascular techniques provides an optimal outcome. Particularly with the trend toward single-operative stage reconstruction including osseous implantation with dental prosthetic placement, patient recovery, maintenance of function, and return to the pre-lesional quality of life can be optimized. Further research into effects of early loading of mandibular reconstructions and the long-term effects on implant viability, tolerance of radiation, and long-term health care costs are ongoing and hope to provide further evidence to guide treatment teams.

CLINICS CLINICAL PEARLS

- Segmental defects for benign disease of 6 cm or less may be reconstructed with tissue-engineered products which have low morbidity but do not allow for immediate dental rehabilitation.

- Reconstruction bar alone without osseous reconstruction has a high degree of failure.
- For longer segmental defects, particularly with a significant soft tissue component, vascularized osseous reconstruction has become the method of choice for reconstruction.
- Computer-Aided Design (CAD) and Computer-Aided Manufacturing (CAM) is increasingly used for planning reconstruction to allow for the consideration of dental prosthetics.
- Reconstruction should ideally focus on placing bone capable of load bearing near the position of the native alveolar segment of the mandible (which is more superior and lingual relative to the inferior border of the native mandible).
- The fibula-free flap, which is based on the peroneal system, is the most common free flap, allowing for the long osseous reconstructive segment, multiple osteotomies, 2 team harvest, long pedicle length, and immediate dental restoration. Alterations in techniques for elevation allow for variable soft tissue components. Some studies suggest moderate donor site mobility which can be mitigated with slight alterations in flap elevation and multi-disciplinary rehabilitation.
- The iliac crest (deep circumflex iliac artery) free flap, is based on the external iliac system. The bone stock is excellent, although shorter than the fibula. Harvest allows for the elevation of significant soft tissue flaps, although pedicle length is shorter and multiple osteotomies may be tenuous. Donor site morbidity with potential for gait disturbance and hernia must be considered.
- The scapula-free flap is based on the circumflex scapular branch of the subscapular system. The lateral border and tip of the scapula can be harvested with various chimeric soft tissue components which allow for so called "mega flap" reconstruction. Donor site morbidity is low; however, the bone stock is less robust than fibula (and possibly iliac) if endosseous dental restoration is being considered.

ACKNOWLEDGMENTS

The authors wish to thank Emily A Montgomery, MS for her illustration adding clarity and visual interest to the manuscript.

DISCLOSURE

Drs S. Bevans and D. Hammer are members of the US Military. Reference herein to any specific commercial products, process, or service by trade name, trademark, manufacturer, or otherwise, does not necessarily constitute or imply its endorsement, recommendation, or favoring by the United States Government. The views expressed here are those of the authors and do not reflect the official policy or position of the Department of the Army, Navy, Department of Defense, or the U.S. Government.

REFERENCES

1. Chim H, Salgado CJ, Mardini S, et al. Reconstruction of mandibular defects. Semin Plast Surg 2010;24(2):188–97.
2. Jewer DD, Boyd JB, Manktelow RT, et al. Orofacial and mandibular reconstruction with the iliac crest free flap: a review of 60 cases and a new method of classification. Plast Reconstr Surg 1989;84(3):391–403 [discussion: 404-395].
3. Boyd JB, Gullane PJ, Rotstein LE, et al. Classification of mandibular defects. Plast Reconstr Surg 1993;92(7):1266–75.
4. Brown JS, Barry C, Ho M, et al. A new classification for mandibular defects after oncological resection. Lancet Oncol 2016;17(1):e23–30.

5. Cordeiro PG, Henderson PW, Matros E. A 20-Year Experience with 202 Segmental Mandibulectomy Defects: A Defect Classification System, Algorithm for Flap Selection, and Surgical Outcomes. Plast Reconstr Surg 2018;141(4):571e–81e.

6. Akashi M, Hashikawa K, Wanifuchi S, et al. Heterogeneity of Necrotic Changes between Cortical and Cancellous Bone in Mandibular Osteoradionecrosis: A Histopathological Analysis of Resection Margin after Segmental Mandibulectomy. BioMed Res Int 2017;2017:3125842.

7. Zaghi S, Miller M, Blackwell K, et al. Analysis of surgical margins in cases of mandibular osteoradionecrosis that progress despite extensive mandible resection and free tissue transfer. Am J Otolaryngol 2012;33(5):576–80.

8. Qaisi M, Montague L. Bone Margin Analysis for Osteonecrosis and Osteomyelitis of the Jaws. Oral Maxillofac Surg Clin North Am 2017;29(3):301–13.

9. Pautke C, Tischer T, Neff A, et al. In vivo tetracycline labeling of bone: an intraoperative aid in the surgical therapy of osteoradionecrosis of the mandible. Oral Surg Oral Med Oral Pathol Oral Radiol Endod 2006;102(6):e10–3.

10. Pautke C, Bauer F, Bissinger O, et al. Tetracycline bone fluorescence: a valuable marker for osteonecrosis characterization and therapy. J Oral Maxillofac Surg 2010;68(1):125–9.

11. Lang K, Held T, Meixner E, et al. Frequency of osteoradionecrosis of the lower jaw after radiotherapy of oral cancer patients correlated with dosimetric parameters and other risk factors. Head Face Med 2022;18(1):7.

12. Ristow O, Birgel JL, Ruckschloss T, et al. Osteoradionecrosis of the Jaw-Comparison between Bone and Soft Tissue Injury and Their Influence on Surgical Outcomes-A Retrospective Cohort Study. Diagnostics 2023;13(3).

13. Chepeha DB, Teknos TN, Fung K, et al. Lateral oromandibular defect: when is it appropriate to use a bridging reconstruction plate combined with a soft tissue revascularized flap? Head Neck 2008;30(6):709–17.

14. Fanzio PM, Chang KP, Chen HH, et al. Plate exposure after anterolateral thigh free-flap reconstruction in head and neck cancer patients with composite mandibular defects. Ann Surg Oncol 2015;22(9):3055–60.

15. Sadr-Eshkevari P, Rashad A, Vahdati SA, et al. Alloplastic mandibular reconstruction: a systematic review and meta-analysis of the current century case series. Plast Reconstr Surg 2013;132(3):413e–27e.

16. Kawasaki G, Imayama N, Yoshitomi I, et al. Clinical Study of Reconstruction Plates Used in the Surgery for Mandibular Discontinuity Defect. In Vivo 2019; 33(1):191–4.

17. Sakakibara A, Hashikawa K, Yokoo S, et al. Risk factors and surgical refinements of postresective mandibular reconstruction: a retrospective study. Plast Surg Int 2014;2014:893746.

18. Haroun F, Benmoussa N, Bidault F, et al. Outcomes of mandibular reconstruction using three-dimensional custom-made porous titanium prostheses. J Stomatol Oral Maxillofac Surg 2023;124(1S):101281.

19. Schwaiger M, Wallner J, Pau M, et al. Clinical experience with a novel structure designed bridging plate system for segmental mandibular reconstruction: The TriLock bridging plate. J Cranio-Maxillo-Fac Surg 2018;46(9):1679–90.

20. Peters F, Kniha K, Mohlhenrich SC, et al. Evaluation of a novel osteosynthesis plate system for mandibular defects. Br J Oral Maxillofac Surg 2020;58(9): e109–14.

21. Anthony JP, Foster RD, Kaplan MJ, et al. Fibular free flap reconstruction of the "true" lateral mandibular defect. Ann Plast Surg 1997;38(2):137–46.

22. Foster RD, Anthony JP, Sharma A, et al. Vascularized bone flaps versus nonvascularized bone grafts for mandibular reconstruction: an outcome analysis of primary bony union and endosseous implant success. Head Neck 1999;21(1): 66–71.

23. Handschel J, Hassanyar H, Depprich RA, et al. Nonvascularized iliac bone grafts for mandibular reconstruction–requirements and limitations. In Vivo 2011;25(5): 795–9.

24. Ren ZH, Fan TF, Zhang S, et al. Nonvascularized Iliac Bone Reconstruction for the Mandible Without Maxillofacial Skin Scarring. J Oral Maxillofac Surg 2020;78(2): 288–94.

25. Pogrel MA, Podlesh S, Anthony JP, et al. A comparison of vascularized and nonvascularized bone grafts for reconstruction of mandibular continuity defects. J Oral Maxillofac Surg 1997;55(11):1200–6.

26. Okoturo E. Non-vascularised iliac crest bone graft for immediate reconstruction of lateral mandibular defect. Oral Maxillofac Surg 2016;20(4):425–9.

27. Shin JY, Chun JY, Chang SC, et al. Association between non-vascularised bone graft failure and compartment of the defect in mandibular reconstruction: a systematic review and meta-analysis. Br J Oral Maxillofac Surg 2022;60(2):128–33.

28. Wang W, Yeung KWK. Bone grafts and biomaterials substitutes for bone defect repair: A review. Bioact Mater 2017;2(4):224–47.

29. Zhang D, Wu X, Chen J, et al. The development of collagen based composite scaffolds for bone regeneration. Bioact Mater 2018;3(1):129–38.

30. Melville JC, Tran HQ, Bhatti AK, et al. Is Reconstruction of Large Mandibular Defects Using Bioengineering Materials Effective? J Oral Maxillofac Surg 2020; 78(4):661 e661–e661 e629.

31. Fatani B, Fatani JA, Fatani OA. Approach for Mandibular Reconstruction Using Vascularized Free Fibula Flap: A Review of the Literature. Cureus 2022;14(10): e30161.

32. Bak M, Jacobson AS, Buchbinder D, et al. Contemporary reconstruction of the mandible. Oral Oncol 2010;46(2):71–6.

33. van Gemert JTM, Abbink JH, van Es RJJ, et al. Early and late complications in the reconstructed mandible with free fibula flaps. J Surg Oncol 2018;117(4):773–80.

34. Mashrah MA, Aldhohrah T, Abdelrehem A, et al. Survival of vascularized osseous flaps in mandibular reconstruction: A network meta-analysis. PLoS One 2021; 16(10):e0257457.

35. Qayyum Z, Khan ZA, Maqsood A, et al. Outcome Assessment after Reconstruction of Tumor-Related Mandibular Defects Using Free Vascularized Fibular Flap-A Clinical Study. Healthcare (Basel) 2023;11(2).

36. Tassone P, Clookey S, Topf M, et al. Quality of life after segmental mandibulectomy and free flap for mandibular osteonecrosis: Systematic review. Am J Otolaryngol 2022;43(5):103586.

37. Jenkins GW, Kennedy MP, Ellabban I, et al. Functional outcomes following mandibulectomy and fibular free-flap reconstruction. Br J Oral Maxillofac Surg 2023; 61(2):158–64.

38. Ferreira JJ, Zagalo CM, Oliveira ML, et al. Mandible reconstruction: History, state of the art and persistent problems. Prosthet Orthot Int 2015;39(3):182–9.

39. Russell J, Volker G, McGarvey D, et al. An objective analysis of composite free flap donor site morbidity in head and neck surgery: Prospective series. Head Neck 2023;45(2):398–408.

40. Vittayakittipong P, Jarudejkajon J, Kirirat P, et al. Feasibility of the vascularized fibula bone graft for reconstruction of the mandible: a cadaveric study. Int J Oral Maxillofac Surg 2016;45(8):960–3.
41. Fan S, Wang YY, Lin ZY, et al. Synchronous reconstruction of bilateral osteoradionecrosis of the mandible using a single fibular osteocutaneous flap in patients with nasopharyngeal carcinoma. Head Neck 2016;38(Suppl 1):E607–12.
42. Gholami M, Hedjazi A, Kiamarz Milani A. Evaluation of Anatomic Variations of Fibula Free Flap in Human Fresh Cadavers. World J Plast Surg 2019;8(2):229–36.
43. Russell J, Pateman K, Batstone M. Donor site morbidity of composite free flaps in head and neck surgery: a systematic review of the prospective literature. Int J Oral Maxillofac Surg 2021;50(9):1147–55.
44. Wu H, Mao J, Zhai Z, et al. Analysis of related factors of long-term complications after vascularized fibular transplantation. Clin Oral Investig 2022;26(12):6961–71.
45. Hatchell AC, Schrag CH, Temple-Oberle CF, et al. Patient-Reported Outcomes after Fibula Free Flap Harvest: A Pilot Study. Plast Reconstr Surg 2021;148(6):1007e–11e.
46. Hadouiri N, Feuvrier D, Pauchot J, et al. Donor site morbidity after vascularized fibula free flap: gait analysis during prolonged walk conditions. Int J Oral Maxillofac Surg 2018;47(3):309–15.
47. Schardt C, Schmid A, Bodem J, et al. Donor site morbidity and quality of life after microvascular head and neck reconstruction with free fibula and deep-circumflex iliac artery flaps. J Cranio-Maxillo-Fac Surg 2017;45(2):304–11.
48. Durst A, Clibbon J, Davis B. Distal tibial fractures are a poorly recognised complication with fibula free flaps. Ann R Coll Surg Engl 2015;97(6):409–13.
49. Maben D, Anehosur V, Kumar N. Assessment of Donor Site Morbidity Following Fibula Flap Transfer. J Maxillofac Oral Surg 2021;20(2):258–63.
50. Li P, Fang Q, Qi J, et al. Risk Factors for Early and Late Donor-Site Morbidity After Free Fibula Flap Harvest. J Oral Maxillofac Surg 2015;73(8):1637–40.
51. Ling XF, Peng X. What is the price to pay for a free fibula flap? A systematic review of donor-site morbidity following free fibula flap surgery. Plast Reconstr Surg 2012;129(3):657–74.
52. Taylor GI. Reconstruction of the mandible with free composite iliac bone grafts. Ann Plast Surg 1982;9(5):361–76.
53. Urken ML, Buchbinder D, Costantino PD, et al. Oromandibular reconstruction using microvascular composite flaps: report of 210 cases. Arch Otolaryngol Head Neck Surg 1998;124(1):46–55.
54. Urken ML, Vickery C, Weinberg H, et al. The internal oblique-iliac crest osseomyocutaneous free flap in oromandibular reconstruction. Report of 20 cases. Arch Otolaryngol Head Neck Surg 1989;115(3):339–49.
55. Jung HD, Nam W, Cha IH, et al. Reconstruction of combined oral mucosa-mandibular defects using the vascularized myoosseous iliac crest free flap. Asian Pac J Cancer Prev 2012;13(8):4137–40.
56. Kim HS, Kim BC, Kim HJ, et al. Anatomical basis of the deep circumflex iliac artery flap. J Craniofac Surg 2013;24(2):605–9.
57. Rana M, Warraich R, Kokemuller H, et al. Reconstruction of mandibular defects - clinical retrospective research over a 10-year period. Head Neck Oncol 2011;3:23.
58. Essig H, Rana M, Kokemueller H, et al. Pre-operative planning for mandibular reconstruction - a full digital planning workflow resulting in a patient specific reconstruction. Head Neck Oncol 2011;3:45.

59. Cariati P, Farhat MC, Dyalram D, et al. The deep circumflex iliac artery free flap in maxillofacial reconstruction: a comparative institutional analysis. Oral Maxillofac Surg 2021;25(3):395–400.

60. Lonie S, Herle P, Paddle A, et al. Mandibular reconstruction: meta-analysis of iliac- versus fibula-free flaps. ANZ J Surg 2016;86(5):337–42.

61. van Gemert JT, van Es RJ, Rosenberg AJ, et al. Free vascularized flaps for reconstruction of the mandible: complications, success, and dental rehabilitation. J Oral Maxillofac Surg 2012;70(7):1692–8.

62. Schultz BD, Sosin M, Nam A, et al. Classification of mandible defects and algorithm for microvascular reconstruction. Plast Reconstr Surg 2015;135(4): 743e–54e.

63. Garajei A, Kheradmand AA, Miri SR, et al. A retrospective study on mandibular reconstruction using iliac crest free flap. Ann Med Surg (Lond). 2021;66:102354.

64. Choi N, Cho JK, Jang JY, et al. Scapular Tip Free Flap for Head and Neck Reconstruction. Clin Exp Otorhinolaryngol 2015;8(4):422–9.

65. Fujiki M, Miyamoto S, Sakuraba M, et al. A comparison of perioperative complications following transfer of fibular and scapular flaps for immediate mandibular reconstruction. J Plast Reconstr Aesthet Surg 2013;66(3):372–5.

66. Bianchi B, Ferri A, Ferrari S, et al. Reconstruction of mandibular defects using the scapular tip free flap. Microsurgery 2015;35(2):101–6.

67. Coleman SC, Burkey BB, Day TA, et al. Increasing use of the scapula osteocutaneous free flap. Laryngoscope 2000;110(9):1419–24.

68. Benlidayi ME, Gaggl A, Burger H, et al. Comparative study of the osseointegration of dental implants after different bone augmentation techniques: vascularized femur flap, non-vascularized femur graft and mandibular bone graft. Clin Oral Implants Res 2011;22(6):594–9.

69. Tarsitano A, Del Corso G, Ciocca L, et al. Mandibular reconstructions using computer-aided design/computer-aided manufacturing: A systematic review of a defect-based reconstructive algorithm. J Cranio-Maxillo-Fac Surg 2015;43(9): 1785–91.

70. Cercenelli L, Babini F, Badiali G, et al. Augmented Reality to Assist Skin Paddle Harvesting in Osteomyocutaneous Fibular Flap Reconstructive Surgery: A Pilot Evaluation on a 3D-Printed Leg Phantom. Front Oncol 2021;11:804748.

71. Darwich K, Ismail MB, Al-Mozaiek MYA, et al. Reconstruction of mandible using a computer-designed 3D-printed patient-specific titanium implant: a case report. Oral Maxillofac Surg 2021;25(1):103–11.

72. Yang C, Shen S, Wu J, et al. A New Modified Method for Accurate Mandibular Reconstruction. J Oral Maxillofac Surg 2018;76(8):1816–22.

73. van Baar GJC, Liberton N, Forouzanfar T, et al. Accuracy of computer-assisted surgery in mandibular reconstruction: A postoperative evaluation guideline. Oral Oncol 2019;88:1–8.

74. Mahendru S, Jain R, Aggarwal A, et al. CAD-CAM vs conventional technique for mandibular reconstruction with free fibula flap: A comparison of outcomes. Surg Oncol 2020;34:284–91.

75. Ince B, Ismayilzade M, Dadaci M, et al. Computer-Assisted versus Conventional Freehand Mandibular Reconstruction with Fibula Free Flap: A Systematic Review and Meta-Analysis. Plast Reconstr Surg 2020;146(5):686e–7e.

76. Yang WF, Powcharoen W, Su YX. Computer-Assisted Surgery Increases Efficiency of Mandibular Reconstruction with Fibula Free Flap. Plast Reconstr Surg 2020;146(5):687e–8e.

77. Weyh AM, Quimby A, Fernandes RP. Three-Dimensional Computer-Assisted Surgical Planning and Manufacturing in Complex Mandibular Reconstruction. Atlas Oral Maxillofac Surg Clin North Am 2020;28(2):145–50.
78. Runyan CM, Sharma V, Staffenberg DA, et al. Jaw in a Day: State of the Art in Maxillary Reconstruction. J Craniofac Surg 2016;27(8):2101–4.
79. Sukato DC, Hammer D, Wang W, et al. Experience With "Jaw in a Day" Technique. J Craniofac Surg 2020;31(5):1212–7.
80. Pu JJ, Hakim SG, Melville JC, et al. Current Trends in the Reconstruction and Rehabilitation of Jaw following Ablative Surgery. Cancers 2022;14(14).
81. Ong A, Williams F, Tokarz E, et al. Jaw in a Day: Immediate Dental Rehabilitation during Fibula Reconstruction of the Mandible. Facial Plast Surg 2021;37(6):722–7.
82. Chang YM, Wei FC. Fibula Jaw-in-a-Day with Minimal Computer-Aided Design and Manufacturing: Maximizing Efficiency, Cost-Effectiveness, Intraoperative Flexibility, and Quality. Plast Reconstr Surg 2021;147(2):476–9.

Oral Cavity Reconstruction

Pablo Quadri, MD[a], Caitlin McMullen, MD[a],*

KEYWORDS

- Free tissue flaps • Surgical flaps • Reconstructive surgery • Mandible • Maxilla
- Oral cancer • Tongue cancer • Oral cavity reconstruction

KEY POINTS

- There are numerous options with acceptable outcomes for soft tissue and osseous reconstruction of minor and major oral cavity defects.
- The selection of reconstructive modality should be based on patient factors, defect considerations, and surgeon experience.
- For small oral cavity defects, primary closure, secondary intention, skin grafts, dermal substitute grafts, and locoregional flaps can provide very good functional outcomes depending on the defect site.
- For defects involving the ventral tongue or floor of mouth, a lower threshold should be held for using regional or free tissue transfer to prevent tethering of the tongue.
- With thorough preoperative assessment and planning, osteocutaneous free flaps can reconstruct large composite oral cavity defects with good outcomes.

INTRODUCTION

Surgical resection has remained standard of care for initial treatment of oral cavity squamous cell cancers.[1–4] Surgery can result in significant cosmetic deformity, and it can affect oral functions such as mastication, deglutition, and speech.[1,3] To obtain clear half centimeter (cm) microscopic margins, an additional 1 to 1.5 cm of normal tissue from the gross tumor border is recommended; therefore, reconstruction of the defect ends up being significantly larger than the tumor size itself.[2] The volume of the remnant structures in the oral cavity significantly affects functional outcomes.

One of the most important improvements in the surgical management of oral cavity tumors has been the development of a wide variety of reconstructive options to improve quality of life and functionality after ablative surgery.[5] For the appropriate patient and defect, primary closure (PC), secondary intention (SI), obturator, dermal substitutes, and locoregional flaps can be excellent options with acceptable functional

[a] Department of Head and Neck-Endocrine Oncology, Moffitt Cancer Center, 12902 Magnolia Drive, CSB – 6 Floor, Tampa, FL 33612, USA
* Corresponding author.
E-mail address: caitlin.mcmullen@moffitt.org

Otolaryngol Clin N Am 56 (2023) 671–686
https://doi.org/10.1016/j.otc.2023.04.002
0030-6665/23/© 2023 Elsevier Inc. All rights reserved.

outcomes. Existing evidence shows that there is variability in what surgeons may select to reconstruct similar defects, based on the surgeon's experience, training, and institutional support.[6] This variability highlights the lack of solid evidence to support reconstructive choices in oral cavity defects.

The goals of reconstruction for optimal function and recovery are to recreate volume and to seal the oral cavity from the neck or sinuses. For medium to large size defects, microvascular free tissue transfer plays a critical role in oral cavity and has shown successful outcomes achieving preservation of function.[1,4,7,8] This article reviews the options in the "reconstructive ladder" for oral cavity surgical defects, discusses specific reconstructive choices for commonly encountered tumor locations, and reviews the evidence to support those options. A useful algorithm for selecting reconstruction modalities for soft tissue defects of the oral cavity is depicted in **Fig. 1.**

The "Reconstructive Ladder" for Oral Cavity Defects

Primary closure

PC involves the direct approximation of the defect edges with suture. Few sites in the oral cavity are truly amenable to PC, but it can be a good option for small to medium defects of the oral tongue that spare the floor of mouth. For anterior lateral tongue defects, rather than a craniocaudal closure, an anterior-posterior rotational closure of the defect may minimize tethering of the ventral tongue to the floor of mouth. PC, for selected patients, can have very good functional and quality of life outcomes with only minor speech deficits.[9] For larger defects such as those involving about 40% of the oral tongue, PC may result in inferior quality of life outcomes.[10] PC is typically not an appropriate choice for most other defects of the oral cavity, including composite mandible resections, medium-sized defects involving the floor of mouth or ventral tongue, palatal defects, or most buccal defects.

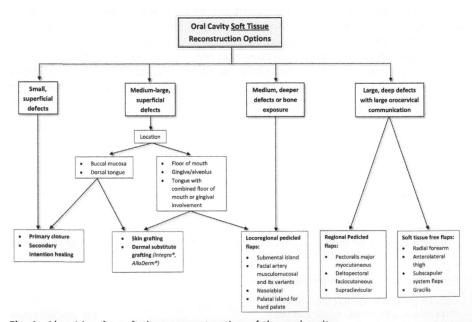

Fig. 1. Algorithm for soft tissue reconstruction of the oral cavity.

Secondary intention healing
SI that involves allowing defects to heal in without coverage or tissue approximation may be an excellent option for small oral tongue defects. Although some surgeons hesitate to pursue SI due to fears of increased surgical complications, there is little evidence to support that concern. Evidence suggests that SI may have better speech outcomes compared with PC and compared with flap reconstruction for defects less than 50% of the tongue.[11,12] There does not seem to be a significant increase in complications with SI, though minor secondary hemorrhage has been reported.[11] SI may also be appropriate for mucosal-only defects of the hard palate.

Skin and dermal substitute grafting
Skin grafts, typically split thickness, and acellular dermal matrix (ADM) materials are options to resurface a surgically created oral cavity defect. ADM materials, such as AlloDerm (Lifecell Corporation, Branchburg, NJ, USA), can either be from cadaveric or xenogeneic sources. These materials provide a scaffold for mucosalization/epithelialization by providing a basement membrane and collagen layer, promoting host cell infiltration and neovascularization.[3] Newer materials composed of chemically cross-linked bovine collagen type I, and shark chondroitin-6-sulfate glycosaminoglycan with a nonabsorbable silicone layer, such as Integra (LifeSciences, Plainsboro, NJ, USA), similarly can provide a scaffold for regrowth. Typically, a bolster is secured over the grafted material to improve tissue approximation and incorporation for anywhere from 5 days to 3 weeks.

Skin grafts may be selected due to the ease of harvest from a distant donor site, usually the thigh, and large/variable qualities of skin for grafting. Skin grafting may have a higher success rate than ADM, possibly due to the thin nature of the graft, though success rates with ADMs are also high[3,13,14] for various sites in the oral cavity. When directly compared, the failure rate was greater with ADM (14% vs 0%) with similar rates of contraction.[3] Although these investigators found that despite the commercial price of ADM, overall costs were higher with skin grafting with increased morbidity to the patient due to a second surgical site.[3] Some benefits of ADMs include surgical time reduction and absence of donor site morbidity. Functional measures seem to favor ADMs.[3] Excessive thickness of the ADM graft material may result in poor graft success rates, suggesting caution in ADM material selection.[3]

Integra has been described in oral cavity reconstruction, but studies are generally limited to case reports or series.[15–17] These reports describe successful remucosalization in most cases with minimal contraction.

Locoregional pedicled flaps
Medium size oral defects represent a challenge as they can be too large for a PC and yet too small for a free flap.[2] Smaller defects that involve the ventral tongue or floor of mouth risk tethering with PC, but free flaps would result in excessive bulk. Locoregional pedicled flaps may achieve appropriate reconstruction of soft tissue defects in these situations to optimize functional outcomes.

Acceptable outcomes have been described with various regional pedicled flaps, including submental artery island flap (SMAIF), the supraclavicular flap (SCF), palatal island, facial artery musculomucosal (FAMM) flap, buccal myomucosal flap, as well as nasolabial, infrahyoid, pedicled buccal fat, and platysma flaps.[18–25] Accumulating evidence shows reliable outcomes with certain locoregional pedicled flaps including shorter operative times, lower costs, and good functional outcomes.[2,18,20,23,26–29] The FAMM flap and SMAIF seem to be the most applicable for small to medium oral cavity defects, as the other flaps mentioned above have limited reach (nasolabial, pedicled buccal fat) or have higher partial/total necrosis rates such as platysma[30] and SCF.[31]

The FAMM flap, first described in 1992,[32] is a reliable method of resurfacing small oral tongue, ventral tongue, floor of mouth, and retromolar or lateral palate defects with acceptable functional outcomes.[28,33] This can be harvested as a pedicled flap or island flap with reliable vascularity and low partial/total necrosis rates.[34] Compared with the radial forearm free flap (RFFF) for oral cavity defects, FAMM flaps had significantly lower operative time, fewer complications that did not require take back to the operating room (OR), lower costs, and fewer donor site issues with equivalent functional outcomes.[18] The buccinator myomucosal flap, a superiorly based variant supplied by the buccal branch of the internal maxillary artery, has also shown favorable functional outcomes with minimal morbidity without compromising oncological outcomes and can serve as a good reconstructive option for more posterior small and medium defects.[2,35]

The SMAIF, based on the submental branches of the facial artery and vein,[36] is an excellent, reliable option with variable size that can reach to cover floor of mouth, oral tongue, buccal, and even palatal defects. A significant benefit of the flap is that the donor site can be primarily closed based on a "pinch test,"[36] and the incisions can be incorporated into neck dissection incisions without difficulty. Compared with RFFF, the SMAIF has a shorter operative time and shorter hospitalization but has a higher rate of partial flap necrosis and less soft tissue available, though this is controversial.[20,37–39] Although dissection of the SMAIF involves traversing lymph node level 1, it does not seem to be any compromise in oncologic outcomes with this flap choice with concurrent nodal dissection.[37,40] Overall, it is generally a reliable and versatile oral reconstruction option in experienced hands. **Fig. 2**B demonstrates the use of a submental artery island flap for coverage of a marginal mandibulectomy and floor of mouth medium size defect.

SCFs have been described in oral cavity reconstruction, but they may have a higher partial and complete necrosis rate which can result in fistula and other downstream complications when used in the oral cavity. Although some investigators report lower costs, shorter operative time, similar complication rates, and acceptable functional outcomes with SCF compared with RFFF reconstruction,[40] others report high necrosis rates, including one study citing a 28% complete necrosis rate.[31]

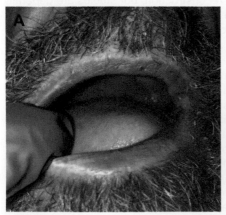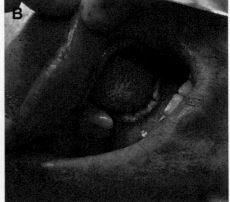

Fig. 2. Examples of soft tissue options for oral reconstruction. (A) Latissimus musculocutaneous flap for total glossectomy defect. (B) Submental artery island flap for coverage of a marginal mandibulectomy and floor of mouth defect.

The pectoralis major myocutaneous flap (PMMF), based on the thoracoacromial artery, is one of the most important reconstructive methods in head and neck due to its simple technical aspects, versatility, anatomic proximity to the head and neck region, and reliable vascular supply. Pectoralis flaps are limited by unnecessary bulk, neck deformity due to the pedicle, possible shoulder dysfunction, and limited cranial reach. When compared with free flap reconstruction in the oral cavity, PMMF seems to result in inferior speech, shoulder function, and quality of life.[4] PMMF with rib has been described for composite mandibular and maxillofacial reconstruction, but outcomes with the addition of rib are reportedly unsatisfactory.[41] Because the functional outcomes with PMMF are not optimal while the vascular supply is reliable, the PMMF can be an acceptable salvage option for medium to large oral cavity defects if needed.

Microvascular free flaps
Free flap reconstruction has evolved to play a critical role in the care of patients with oral cancer, allowing for safe, reliable closure of a range of oral cavity surgical wounds. Free flap reconstruction is indicated for medium to large defects, particularly for defects that involve the mandible or create a large fistula into the neck. Small soft tissue free flaps can also be helpful in smaller defects that involve the ventral tongue or floor of mouth to minimize tethering of the mobile tongue.

Soft tissue microvascular free flaps. The most common choices for soft tissue free flap reconstruction of the oral cavity are the RFFF and the anterolateral thigh free flap (ALTFF). The RFFF, due its thickness, reliable donor site anatomy, long pedicle, and pliability, has become the true workhorse for oral cavity soft tissue reconstruction.[1,18] Neurotization of the RFFF has been described with anastomosis of the antebrachial cutaneous nerve to the lingual nerve.[42–44] The RFFF has notable donor site morbidity, both in terms of function and appearance.[1] Typically, the donor site is closed with a split thickness skin graft, but variations of donor site closure including full thickness grafts,[45] local flaps[46,47] and negative pressure devices[48,49] have been described with variable results. RFFF donor site can present complications as seen in **Fig. 3**A and B with partial loss of skin graft and tendon exposure respectively.

As an alternative to the RFFF, ALTFF has been proposed. This flap can provide a great deal of bulk for the oral cavity depending on the patient's habitus.[18] ALTFF has emerged as a favorable and versatile alternative, providing pliable tissue, availability of muscle, and potential for chimeric reconstruction with multiple paddles or bone incorporating a portion of femur with the anterolateral thigh osteocutaneous flap.[1,50–52] This flap is based on musculocutaneous or septocutaneous perforators supplied by the descending branch of the lateral femoral circumflex artery. Anatomic

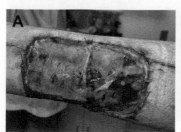
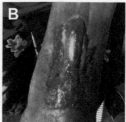
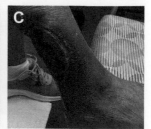

Fig. 3. Common complications encountered for radial forearm and fibula donor sites include: (A) partial loss of skin graft; (B) tendon exposure; (C) cellulitis and delayed wound healing.

variations with no useable perforator are encountered in approximately 1% to 5% of cases.[53–55] The ALTFF can be harvested with comparatively less morbidity than the RFFF, as the defect can typically be closed primarily.[1] The ALTFF can be significantly bulkier than an RFFF, but variations exist such as fascia-only harvest and perforator dissection including minimal vastus lateralis muscle, which can reduce flap thickness.

When directly compared, ALTFF and RFFF for soft tissue oral cavity reconstruction showed no significant difference in flap survival, partial necrosis, vascular crises, or hematoma.[1] When comparing donor site complications, ALTFF had significantly less hypertrophic scar, tendon exposure (see **Fig. 3**B), paresthesia and movement impairment at the donor site, social stigma associated with the donor site and more satisfaction with donor site appearance compared with than RFFF.[1] When comparing quality of life, there was no difference in all the domains evaluated including: pain, appearance, activity, recreation, swallowing, chewing, speech, shoulder, saliva, mood, and anxiety except for taste where RFFF showed significantly higher scores.[1] The decision where to use RFFF or ALTFF depends on the surgeon's familiarity, defect characteristics, and patient factors such as comorbidities and body habitus.[1] For patients with equivalent thickness and pliability of both the ALTFF and RFFF with low concern for pedicle length, the ALTFF has lower donor site morbidity.[1]

Latissimus dorsi free flap is a useful flap for large defects including total glossectomy for its relative ease of harvest, significant bulk, ability to innervate, and low donor site morbidity. It is a versatile and reliable flap that can be modified to accommodate various defects, including musculocutaneous or muscle only flaps, the addition of scapular bone for composite defects, adding serratus anterior muscle for additional size, or including additional skin paddles based on the circumflex artery for full thickness defects. **Fig. 2**A illustrates a reconstruction with a latissimus musculocutaneous flap for total glossectomy defect. **Fig. 4** shows a large through-and-through buccal cancer reconstructed with an angular tip of scapula bone graft and folded latissimus musculocutaneous chimeric flap with two skin paddles covering oral cavity and facial skin defects. The thoracodorsal nerve can be included to innervate the flap.[56,57] A thinner modification of this donor site can be harvested as a perforator only flap called the thoracodorsal artery perforator flap (TDAP). This TDAP can be harvested with bone as well for versatile

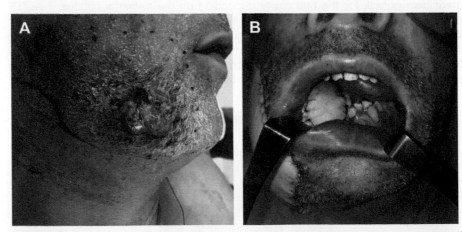

Fig. 4. A large through-and-through buccal cancer reconstructed with an angular tip of scapula bone graft and folded latissimus musculocutaneous chimeric flap. Soft tissue was later debulked with excellent esthetic and functional results. (*A*) Primary buccal tumor extending through skin. (*B*) Folded latissimus for intraoral and cutaneous reconstruction.

applications.[5,58–60] Innervated gracilis muscle free flap has also been described in limited case series for dynamic reconstruction of total glossectomy defects.[61]

Osseous and osteocutaneous microvascular free flaps. Numerous options exist for composite oral cavity defects requiring osseous reconstruction. Fibular bone, angular tip and lateral border scapula, iliac crest, and osteocutaneous radial forearm are the most commonly used and described in the literature. The most suitable flap choice is selected based on careful consideration of patient factors such as habitus and profession/hobbies, defect components, and surgeon's experience.

The fibula osteocutaneous free flap (FFF) has historically been the workhouse of mandibular and maxilla reconstruction. First described in 1989 for oral cavity defects,[62] the FFF is based on the peroneal artery and its cutaneous perforators. Large areas of bone and skin can be harvested, allowing for versatile applications. The preoperative assessment of acceptable collateral blood supply should be performed to ensure adequate vascular supply to the distal extremity with harvest. Imaging is very helpful, but the use of imaging is supported by overall low-quality evidence, and some investigators advocate that physical examination alone is adequate.[63,64] Computed tomography with angiography (CTA) is helpful because the vascular and perforator anatomy can be seen clearly, and the bone component can be used for patient-specific virtual surgical planning (VSP). Alternatives to CTA include ultrasound with Doppler vascular assessment and magnetic resonance angiography. Advantages of the FFF include a thin and pliable skin flap, long bone, and solid bone stock for potential dental implantation. Disadvantages of the FFF include significant donor site morbidities including prolonged wound healing, ankle swelling, chronic pain, limited ankle dorsiflexion, risk of vascular compromise to the distal extremity, and potential reduced mobility due to pain during healing.[65,66] **Fig. 3C** represents an FFF donor site complication with a cellulitis and delayed wound healing surrounding the skin graft in the lower leg.

Scapular bone free flaps are highly versatile options for the reconstruction of osseous oral defects with multiple chimeric bone and soft tissue options based of the subscapular artery system. Lateral border of the scapula is based on the periosteal perforators of the circumflex scapular artery, and angular tip bone is based on the angular branch of the thoracodorsal artery. These flaps can be harvested with various soft tissue and muscle flaps for complex defects including latissimus muscle, TDAP, serratus, scapular, and parascapular fasciocutaneous flaps. This investigator prefers angular tip of scapula with thoracodorsal-based muscle or cutaneous flaps to allow for a slightly longer pedicle. Angular tip scapula is an excellent choice due to the flap shape and attached muscle for reconstruction of large or total hard palate defects.[67] A two-team approach with scapular donor sites compared with iliac crest or FFF can be challenging but is feasible. Another major advantage of the scapula is the relatively lower rate of donor site complications including no risk of extremity vascular compromise.[67–69] Most donor site defects can be primarily closed. When directly compared in retrospective study, scapula seems to have fewer complications such as hardware issues.[70]

Iliac crest can be harvested as an osteocutaneous or osteomusculocutaneous free flap based on the deep circumflex iliac artery. The bone can be harvested in variable shapes to facilitate a more natural contour for mandible or maxilla reconstruction with or without internal oblique muscle. Limited studies show good functional outcomes with an esthetic donor site scar.[71] Meta-analysis showed similar rates of flap failure, donor site complications, recipient site complications, dental outcomes for fibula, and iliac crest free flaps.[72,73] Complications can include hernia development, denervation of the rectus abdominis, pain limiting postoperative mobility, damage to intraperitoneal contents, and the femoral nerve.

Osteocutaneous radial forearm flap can be useful for reconstruction of certain oral composite defects, such as premaxilla or smaller mandible defects with reliable results.[74] A significant disadvantage is the donor site morbidity, thinner bone stock, high rates of fracture of the donor radius (~15%), decreased range of motion, and bone exposure are described in the literature.[75,76] Internal fixation of the radius at the time of harvest may reduce the rate of fracture.[77]

The use of VSP has become an essential tool for preplanning complex oromandibular reconstructions, allowing for customized, predictable, and reliable outcomes that expedite operative cases, now used by a majority of head and neck reconstructive surgeons.[5,78,79] Democratization of technology and increased accessibility to 3D printing devices have allowed some surgeons to access preplanned materials at a relatively lower cost. The investigators have shown, in a case matched series, which using VSP results in shorter length of stay, shorter procedure times, and similar overall costs compared with non-VSP cases.[78] VSP may allow for better bone contact and anatomically correct segmentation.[80] However, studies so far are case series and are not standardized by application or outcomes.[81] For institutions and patients with available resources, VSP has assisted "jaw in a day" procedures with immediate osseointegrated implant placement in fibula bone mandible and maxilla reconstructions.[82,83] This option may be ideal for patients with benign pathology who have not being radiated. **Fig. 5** provides the examples of cases of mandible reconstruction with generic fibula cutting guides how they would translate into the patient's reconstruction.

Defect-Driven Reconstruction Key Points

Lip

- The goals of reconstruction are restoration of oral competence with adequate aperture and provision of an acceptable esthetic outcome.[84,85] Constant motion and wound contraction contribute to reconstructive challenges.[84]
- Local flaps generally provide the best match for quality of the skin and mucosa of the lips (**Fig. 6**).[84]
- For smaller defects, a fusiform excision with PC is the preferred method.[84]
- Mucosal lip: labial mucosal advancement flap. Mucosal incisions are made toward the gingivobuccal, and mucosa is elevated off the orbicularis muscle.[84]
- Full-thickness defects: small defects that involve less than 30% of the width of the lip can be closed primarily. Medium size defects (30%–60%) can be repaired with an Abbe or Estlander flap where a rotational pedicled flap is created from the non-affected lip and.[84,85] For defects affecting 70% to 80% of the lip, Gillies fan flap or Karapandzic flap can be used.
- Total lip: The RFFF can be transferred with the palmaris longus tendon, which anchors to the orbicularis muscle and/or modiolus to function as a sling between two commissures and to provide static support and oral competence.[85,86]

Buccal mucosa

- The main reconstructive goal is maintenance of optimal mouth opening.
- For small, superficial defects, PC or dermal substitute grafts are acceptable.
- For larger defects, thin pliable flaps such as RFFF or ALTFF are optimal depending on the patient habitus. These can be folded or designed with a chimeric paddle (ALTFF) for through-and-through defects.
- SMAIF and SCF may be acceptable options in experienced hands for medium and large mucosal defects.

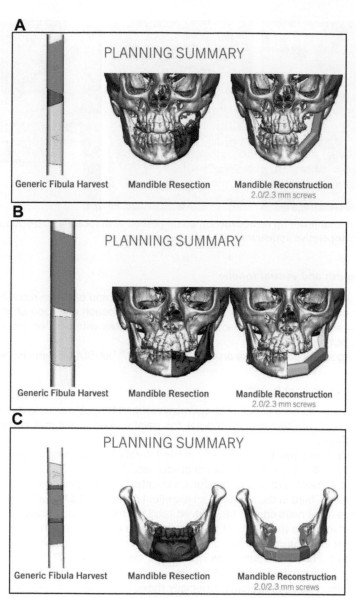

Fig. 5. Virtual surgical planning (VSP) is a useful tool to prefabricate hardware and plan osteotomies. The provided examples are cases of mandible reconstruction with generic fibula cutting guides. (*A*) Mandible reconstruction for osteoradionecrosis. (*B*) Mandible reconstruction including a vertical segment for malignancy. (*C*) Anterior composite reconstruction for benign disease.

Mandibular alveolus

- Coverage of alveolar bone is important for minimizing chronic bone exposure and osteonecrosis.
- SMAIF, nasolabial flaps, and FAMM flaps are acceptable options.

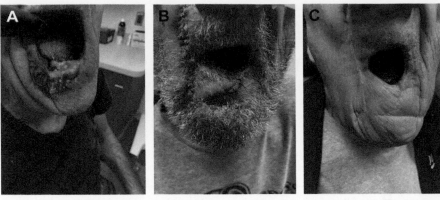

Fig. 6. Near-total lower lip reconstruction accomplished with local flaps. (*A*) Tumor. (*B*) Immediate postoperative appearance. (*C*) Long-term outcome.

Floor of mouth and ventral tongue

- The goal for reconstruction is to minimize tethering and optimize mobility, specifically protrusion and elevation of the tongue for speech and food control.[5]
- For smaller, superficial defects, dermal substitutes with bolster and FAMM as good options.
- For larger defects, RFFF is an excellent choice,[5] but SMAIF can also work well.

Partial glossectomy up to 50%

- The goal of reconstruction is to optimize residual tongue movement and replace the volume of the resected tongue for palatal contact without compromising movement.[5]
- Resection of small lesions mostly in the lateral or dorsal tongue can be closed primarily with very good functional outcomes.[9,87]
- Anterior-posterior rotational flap for small defects (<4 cm) involving the anterior or middle one-third of the tongue is an excellent option.[87] The limitation of this flap is that the tip or base cannot be involved, and the tumor cannot pass the midline.[87]
- For defects less than 50% of the tongue, there does not seem to be significant differences in functional outcomes for local tissue flap versus free flap reconstruction. Functional outcomes may hinge on the tumor (T) stage, rather than the reconstruction choice to fill the defect.[88]
- For medium to larger defects especially those involving ventral tongue or floor of mouth, soft tissue reconstruction with RFFF or SMAIF provides similar acceptable outcomes.[20,24]

Glossectomy greater than 50%

- Large tissue volumes are required to create, allow for palatal contact.[5]
- Free flap options include latissimus, TDAP, gracilis, ALTFF, and rectus abdominis flaps.
- To prevent inferior migration of the flap into the inframandibular defect, techniques such as retromolar trigone suspension, mounded flap contouring, use of fascia or bone to recreate the diaphragm of the oral cavity, and hyoid suspension to the mandible have been described with variable results.[5]

Composite oromandibular defects

- Anterior: Multisegment FFF is an excellent option for this type of reconstruction.
- Resuspending the hyoid bone should be considered when the anterior mandible is resected and soft tissue of the floor of mouth is detached from the bone.
- Lateral body and vertical ramus: Soft tissue only may be acceptable for lateral/posterior defects with excellent functional outcomes especially on edentulous patients. If osseous reconstruction is chosen, bone should be suspended from the residual joint capsule if possible. Temporary postoperative mandibulomaxillary fixation may assist with occlusion.

Hard palate

- Obturator can provide acceptable functional outcomes avoiding the morbidity and prolonged OR time of a free flap. Obturators are ideal for lateral/posterior defects in patients with teeth to anchor the device. Large defects can limit the use of the obturator due to inability to anchor the prosthesis.
- For small to medium defects, soft tissue locoregional flaps (buccal fat, greater palatine island, or nasolabial flap) can be used. For larger defects posterior to the canine, RFFFs are an excellent reconstruction option. OCRFF can be useful for smaller anterior defects.
- For larger defects with significant bone loss and lack of support, bone free flaps should be considered including angular tip scapular flap or multisegmented FFF.

SUMMARY

Oral cavity reconstruction represents one of the most significant challenges for head and neck surgeons due to the multiple functional and esthetic aspects that need to be considered. The ideal reconstructive strategy will depend on multiple factors such as defect considerations, patient factors, and surgeon experience/training. Free tissue transfer has opened a whole new variety of reconstructive options which helped improve significantly functional and esthetic outcomes. New technology including virtual planning has optimized the use of this tissue transfer improving outcomes and efficiency.

CLINICS CARE POINTS

- Secondary intention and skin and dermal substitute grafts are useful for small, superficial oral cavity defects.
- For moderate sized soft tissue defects, submental artery island flaps, facial artery myomucosal flaps, and radial forearm free flaps are useful tools.
- Total glossectomy defects require bulk such as latissimus or anterolateral thigh free flaps. Augmenting suspension with retromolar/hyoid/inframnadibular suspension tools is helpful.
- Virtual surgical planning is a useful tool for osseous reconstruction.

DISCLOSURE

The authors have no relevant commercial, financial conflicts of interest or funding sources.

REFERENCES

1. Ranganath K, Jalisi SM, Naples JG, et al. Comparing outcomes of radial forearm free flaps and anterolateral thigh free flaps in oral cavity reconstruction: A systematic review and meta-analysis. Oral Oncol 2022;135:106214.
2. Ahn D, Lee GJ, Sohn JH. Reconstruction of oral cavity defect using versatile buccinator myomucosal flaps in the treatment of cT2-3, N0 oral cavity squamous cell carcinoma: Feasibility, morbidity, and functional/oncological outcomes. Oral Oncol 2017;75:95–9.
3. Girod DA, Sykes K, Jorgensen J, et al. Acellular dermis compared to skin grafts in oral cavity reconstruction. Laryngoscope 2009;119(11):2141–9.
4. Hsing CY, Wong YK, Wang CP, et al. Comparison between free flap and pectoralis major pedicled flap for reconstruction in oral cavity cancer patients–a quality of life analysis. Oral Oncol 2011;47(6):522–7.
5. Gilbert RW. Reconstruction of the oral cavity; past, present and future. Oral Oncol 2020;108:104683.
6. Akakpo KE, Varvares MA, Richmon JD, et al. The tipping point in oral cavity reconstruction: A multi-institutional survey of choice between flap and non-flap reconstruction. Oral Oncol 2021;120:105267.
7. González-García R, Rodríguez-Campo FJ, Naval-Gías L, et al. Radial forearm free flap for reconstruction of the oral cavity: clinical experience in 55 cases. Oral Surg Oral Med Oral Pathol Oral Radiol Endod 2007;104(1):29–37.
8. Vega C, León X, Cervelli D, et al. Total or subtotal glossectomy with microsurgical reconstruction: functional and oncological results. Microsurgery 2011;31(7):517–23.
9. Ochoa E, Larson AR, Han M, et al. Patient-Reported Quality of Life After Resection With Primary Closure for Oral Tongue Carcinoma. Laryngoscope 2021;131(2):312–8.
10. Canis M, Weiss BG, Ihler F, et al. Quality of life in patients after resection of pT3 lateral tongue carcinoma: Microvascular reconstruction versus primary closure. Head Neck 2016;38(1):89–94.
11. Pai P, Tuljapurkar V, Balaji A, et al. Comparative study of functional outcomes following surgical treatment of early tongue cancer. Head Neck 2021;43(10):3142–52.
12. Ji YB, Cho YH, Song CM, et al. Long-term functional outcomes after resection of tongue cancer: determining the optimal reconstruction method. Eur Arch Oto-Rhino-Laryngol 2017;274(10):3751–6.
13. Rhee PH, Friedman CD, Ridge JA, et al. The use of processed allograft dermal matrix for intraoral resurfacing: an alternative to split-thickness skin grafts. Arch Otolaryngol Head Neck Surg 1998;124(11):1201–4.
14. Shi LJ, Wang Y, Yang C, et al. Application of acellular dermal matrix in reconstruction of oral mucosal defects in 36 cases. J Oral Maxillofac Surg 2012;70(11):e586–91.
15. Mumtaz S, Patel H, Singh M. Use of Integra® dermal regeneration template and flowable matrix to reconstruct an oral cavity defect involving the nasal floor. Br J Oral Maxillofac Surg 2020;58(10):e343–4.
16. Beech A, Farrier J. Use of the Integra skin regeneration system in an intraoral mandibular defect in osteoradionecrosis. Int J Oral Maxillofac Surg 2016;45(9):1159–61.

17. Srivastava A, Maniakas A, Myers J, et al. Reconstruction of intraoral oncologic surgical defects with Integra(®) bilayer wound matrix. Clin Case Rep 2021; 9(1):213–9.

18. Ibrahim B, Rahal A, Bissada E, et al. Reconstruction of medium-size defects of the oral cavity: radial forearm free flap vs facial artery musculo-mucosal flap. J Otolaryngol Head Neck Surg 2021;50(1):67.

19. Dean A, Alamillos F, García-López A, et al. The buccal fat pad flap in oral reconstruction. Head Neck 2001;23(5):383–8.

20. Paydarfar JA, Patel UA. Submental island pedicled flap vs radial forearm free flap for oral reconstruction: comparison of outcomes. Arch Otolaryngol Head Neck Surg 2011;137(1):82–7.

21. Varghese BT, Sebastian P, Cherian T, et al. Nasolabial flaps in oral reconstruction: an analysis of 224 cases. Br J Plast Surg 2001;54(6):499–503.

22. Szudek J, Taylor SM. Systematic review of the platysma myocutaneous flap for head and neck reconstruction. Arch Otolaryngol Head Neck Surg 2007;133(7): 655–61.

23. Kozin ED, Sethi RK, Herr M, et al. Comparison of Perioperative Outcomes between the Supraclavicular Artery Island Flap and Fasciocutaneous Free Flap. Otolaryngol Head Neck Surg 2016;154(1):66–72.

24. Sittitrai P, Reunmakkaew D, Srivanitchapoom C. Submental island flap versus radial forearm free flap for oral tongue reconstruction: a comparison of complications and functional outcomes. J Laryngol Otol 2019;133(5):413–8.

25. Gao Q, Yang Z, Ma N, et al. Buccal Myomucosal Flap for Reconstruction of Red Lip Defects Close to Mouth Angle. J Craniofac Surg 2022;34(2):e175–8.

26. Rigby MH, Hayden RE. Regional flaps: a move to simpler reconstructive options in the head and neck. Curr Opin Otolaryngol Head Neck Surg 2014;22(5):401–6.

27. Zhang S, Chen W, Cao G, et al. Pedicled Supraclavicular Artery Island Flap Versus Free Radial Forearm Flap for Tongue Reconstruction Following Hemiglossectomy. J Craniofac Surg 2015;26(6):e527–30.

28. Ayad T, Xie L. Facial artery musculomucosal flap in head and neck reconstruction: A systematic review. Head Neck 2015;37(9):1375–86.

29. Deganello A, Gitti G, Parrinello G, et al. Cost analysis in oral cavity and oropharyngeal reconstructions with microvascular and pedicled flaps. Acta Otorhinolaryngol Ital 2013;33(6):380–7.

30. Mazzola RF, Benazzo M. Platysma flap for oral reconstruction. Clin Plast Surg 2001;28(2):411–9.

31. Padiyar BV, Azeem Mohiyuddin SM, Sagayaraj A, et al. Usefulness of supraclavicular flap in reconstruction following resection of oral cancer. World J Otorhinolaryngol Head Neck Surg 2018;4(2):148–52.

32. Pribaz J, Stephens W, Crespo L, et al. A new intraoral flap: facial artery musculomucosal (FAMM) flap. Plast Reconstr Surg 1992;90(3):421–9.

33. Benjamin M, Aliano K, Davenport T, et al. Functional Outcomes Regarding Facial Artery Musculomucosal Flap for Reconstruction of Partial Glossectomy Defects. Ann Plast Surg 2020;85(S1 Suppl 1):S76–9.

34. Giudice G, Fragola R, Nicoletti G, et al. Facial Artery Myomucosal Flap vs. Islanded Facial Artery Myomucosal Flap Viability: A Systematic Review. Appl Sci 2021;11(9):4202.

35. Bozola AR, Gasques JA, Carriquiry CE, et al. The buccinator musculomucosal flap: anatomic study and clinical application. Plast Reconstr Surg 1989;84(2): 250–7.

36. Martin D, Pascal JF, Baudet J, et al. The submental island flap: a new donor site. Anatomy and clinical applications as a free or pedicled flap. Plast Reconstr Surg 1993;92(5):867–73.

37. Kramer FJ, Böhrnsen F, Moser N, et al. The submental island flap for the treatment of intraoral tumor-related defects: No effect on recurrence rates. Oral Oncol 2015;51(7):668–73.

38. Mooney SM, Sukato DC, Azoulay O, et al. Systematic review of submental artery island flap versus free flap in head and neck reconstruction. Am J Otolaryngol 2021;42(6):103142.

39. Jørgensen MG, Tabatabaeifar S, Toyserkani NM, et al. Submental Island Flap versus Free Flap Reconstruction for Complex Head and Neck Defects. Otolaryngol Head Neck Surg 2019;161(6):946–53.

40. Howard BE, Nagel TH, Donald CB, et al. Oncologic safety of the submental flap for reconstruction in oral cavity malignancies. Otolaryngol Head Neck Surg 2014; 150(4):558–62.

41. Ord RA. The pectoralis major myocutaneous flap in oral and maxillofacial reconstruction: a retrospective analysis of 50 cases. J Oral Maxillofac Surg 1996; 54(11):1292–5, discussion 5-6.

42. Urken ML. The restoration or preservation of sensation in the oral cavity following ablative surgery. Arch Otolaryngol Head Neck Surg 1995;121(6):607–12.

43. Marchiano E, Kana L, Bellile E, et al. Neurotization of the radial forearm free flap improves swallowing outcomes in hemiglossectomy defects. Head Neck 2022; 45(4):798–805.

44. Kuriakose MA, Loree TR, Spies A, et al. Sensate radial forearm free flaps in tongue reconstruction. Arch Otolaryngol Head Neck Surg 2001;127(12):1463–6.

45. Shimbo K, Osaki T, Koshima I. An Ideal Choice for Closure of Large Free Radial Forearm Flap Donor Site Using a Local Full-Thickness Skin Graft. J Craniofac Surg 2022;33(6):1897–8.

46. Mashrah MA, Lingjian Y, Handley TP, et al. Novel technique for the direct closure of the radial forearm flap donor site defect with a local bilobed flap. Head Neck 2019;41(9):3282–9.

47. Gessert TG, Pflum ZE, Thompson JD, et al. The radial forearm snake flap: An underutilized technique for fasciocutaneous and osteocutaneous forearm flaps with primary closure. Head Neck 2022;44(5):1106–13.

48. Halama D, Dreilich R, Lethaus B, et al. Donor-site morbidity after harvesting of radial forearm free flaps-comparison of vacuum-assisted closure with conventional wound care: A randomized controlled trial. J Cranio-Maxillo-Fac Surg 2019;47(12):1980–5.

49. Shimada K, Ojima Y, Ida Y, et al. Negative-pressure wound therapy for donor-site closure in radial forearm free flap: A systematic review and meta-analysis. Int Wound J 2022;19(2):316–25.

50. Shanti RM, Choi J, Thomas WW, et al. Reconstruction of Through-and-Through Composite Segmental Mandibulectomy Defect in a Patient With a Dominant Peroneal Artery Using an Anterior Lateral Thigh Osteomyocutaneous Free Flap: A Case Report and Description of Flap. J Oral Maxillofac Surg 2020;78(8): 1436.e1–7.

51. Graboyes EM, Hornig JD. Evolution of the anterolateral thigh free flap. Curr Opin Otolaryngol Head Neck Surg 2017;25(5):416–21.

52. Cannady SB, Mady LJ, Brody RM, et al. Anterolateral thigh osteomyocutaneous flap in head and neck: Lessons learned. Microsurgery 2022;42(2):117–24.

53. Kimata Y, Uchiyama K, Ebihara S, et al. Anatomic variations and technical problems of the anterolateral thigh flap: a report of 74 cases. Plast Reconstr Surg 1998;102(5):1517–23.

54. Celik N, Wei FC, Lin CH, et al. Technique and strategy in anterolateral thigh perforator flap surgery, based on an analysis of 15 complete and partial failures in 439 cases. Plast Reconstr Surg 2002;109(7):2211–6, discussion 7-8.

55. Luo S, Raffoul W, Luo J, et al. Anterolateral thigh flap: A review of 168 cases. Microsurgery 1999;19(5):232–8.

56. Polyakov AP, Mordovskiy AV, Ratushnyy MV, et al. Functional tongue and floor of mouth reconstruction with a chimeric flap after total glossectomy. Oral Maxillofac Surg 2021;25(2):271–7.

57. Bin C, Yu S, Koh K. Total Tongue Reconstruction with Innervated Latissimus Dorsi Free Flap. Journal of the Korean Society of Plastic and Reconstructive Surgeons 2003;109–13.

58. Pau M, Wallner J, Feichtinger M, et al. Free thoracodorsal, perforator-scapular flap based on the angular artery (TDAP-Scap-aa): Clinical experiences and description of a novel technique for single flap reconstruction of extensive oromandibular defects. J Cranio-Maxillo-Fac Surg 2019;47(10):1617–25.

59. Wallner J, Rieder M, Schwaiger M, et al. Donor Site Morbidity and Quality of Life after Microvascular Head and Neck Reconstruction with a Chimeric, Thoracodorsal, Perforator-Scapular Flap Based on the Angular Artery (TDAP-Scap-aa Flap). J Clin Med 2022;11(16):4876.

60. Ferrari M, Sahovaler A, Chan HHL, et al. Scapular tip-thoracodorsal artery perforator free flap for total/subtotal glossectomy defects: Case series and conformance study. Oral Oncol 2020;105:104660.

61. Righini S, Festa BM, Bonanno MC, et al. Dynamic tongue reconstruction with innervated gracilis musculocutaneos flap after total glossectomy. Laryngoscope 2019;129(1):76–81.

62. Hidalgo DA. Fibula free flap: a new method of mandible reconstruction. Plast Reconstr Surg 1989;84(1):71–9.

63. Alolabi N, Dickson L, Coroneos CJ, et al. Preoperative Angiography for Free Fibula Flap Harvest: A Meta-Analysis. J Reconstr Microsurg 2019;35(5):362–71.

64. Lutz BS, Wei FC, Ng SH, et al. Routine donor leg angiography before vascularized free fibula transplantation is not necessary: a prospective study in 120 clinical cases. Plast Reconstr Surg 1999;103(1):121–7.

65. Kearns M, Ermogenous P, Myers S, et al. Osteocutaneous flaps for head and neck reconstruction: A focused evaluation of donor site morbidity and patient reported outcome measures in different reconstruction options. Arch Plast Surg 2018;45(6):495–503.

66. Russell J, Pateman K, Batstone M. Donor site morbidity of composite free flaps in head and neck surgery: a systematic review of the prospective literature. Int J Oral Maxillofac Surg 2021;50(9):1147–55.

67. Clark JR, McCluskey SA, Hall F, et al. Predictors of morbidity following free flap reconstruction for cancer of the head and neck. Head Neck 2007;29(12):1090–101.

68. Miles BA, Gilbert RW. Maxillary reconstruction with the scapular angle osteomyogenous free flap. Arch Otolaryngol Head Neck Surg 2011;137(11):1130–5.

69. Blumberg JM, Walker P, Johnson S, et al. Mandibular reconstruction with the scapula tip free flap. Head Neck 2019;41(7):2353–8.

70. Tsang GFZ, Zhang H, Yao C, et al. Hardware complications in oromandibular defects: Comparing scapular and fibular based free flap reconstructions. Oral Oncol 2017;71:163–8.
71. Ma H, Van Dessel J, Shujaat S, et al. Long-term functional outcomes of vascularized fibular and iliac flap for mandibular reconstruction: A systematic review and meta-analysis. J Plast Reconstr Aesthet Surg 2021;74(2):247–58.
72. Han J, Guo Z, Wang Z, et al. Comparison of the complications of mandibular reconstruction using fibula versus iliac crest flaps: an updated systematic review and meta-analysis. Int J Oral Maxillofac Surg 2022;51(9):1149–56.
73. Gu Y, Ma H, Shujaat S, et al. Donor- and recipient-site morbidity of vascularized fibular and iliac flaps for mandibular reconstruction: A systematic review and meta-analysis. J Plast Reconstr Aesthet Surg 2021;74(7):1470–9.
74. Militsakh ON, Werle A, Mohyuddin N, et al. Comparison of radial forearm with fibula and scapula osteocutaneous free flaps for oromandibular reconstruction. Arch Otolaryngol Head Neck Surg 2005;131(7):571–5.
75. Thoma A, Khadaroo R, Grigenas O, et al. Oromandibular reconstruction with the radial-forearm osteocutaneous flap: experience with 60 consecutive cases. Plast Reconstr Surg 1999;104(2):368–78, discussion 79-80.
76. Smith AA, Bowen CV, Rabczak T, et al. Donor site deficit of the osteocutaneous radial forearm flap. Ann Plast Surg 1994;32(4):372–6.
77. Werle AH, Tsue TT, Toby EB, et al. Osteocutaneous radial forearm free flap: its use without significant donor site morbidity. Otolaryngol Head Neck Surg 2000; 123(6):711–7.
78. Mazzola F, Smithers F, Cheng K, et al. Time and cost-analysis of virtual surgical planning for head and neck reconstruction: A matched pair analysis. Oral Oncol 2020;100:104491.
79. Miles BA, McMullen CP, Sweeny L, et al. Practice patterns of virtual surgical planning: Survey of the reconstructive section of the American Head and Neck Society. Am J Otolaryngol 2022;43(1):103225.
80. Swendseid BP, Roden DF, Vimawala S, et al. Virtual Surgical Planning in Subscapular System Free Flap Reconstruction of Midface Defects. Oral Oncol 2020;101:104508.
81. Chan TJ, Long C, Wang E, et al. The state of virtual surgical planning in maxillary Reconstruction: A systematic review. Oral Oncol 2022;133:106058.
82. Patel A, Harrison P, Cheng A, et al. Fibular Reconstruction of the Maxilla and Mandible with Immediate Implant-Supported Prosthetic Rehabilitation: Jaw in a Day. Oral Maxillofac Surg Clin North Am 2019;31(3):369–86.
83. Chang YM, Santamaria E, Wei FC, et al. Primary insertion of osseointegrated dental implants into fibula osteoseptocutaneous free flap for mandible reconstruction. Plast Reconstr Surg 1998;102(3):680–8.
84. Larrabee YC, Moyer JS. Reconstruction of Mohs Defects of the Lips and Chin. Facial Plast Surg Clin North Am 2017;25(3):427–42.
85. Matin MB, Dillon J. Lip reconstruction. Oral Maxillofac Surg Clin North Am 2014; 26(3):335–57.
86. Neligan PC. Strategies in lip reconstruction. Clin Plast Surg 2009;36(3):477–85.
87. Lu J, Chen Y, Xia RH, et al. Modification of the anterior-posterior tongue rotation flap for oral tongue reconstruction. Head Neck 2020;42(12):3769–75.
88. Sun J, Weng Y, Li J, et al. Analysis of determinants on speech function after glossectomy. J Oral Maxillofac Surg 2007;65(10):1944–50.

Pharyngeaoesophageal Reconstruction

Z-Hye Lee, MD, Matthew M. Hanasono, MD*

KEYWORDS

- Pharyngoesophageal reconstruction • Total laryngopharyngectomy
- Anterolateral thigh flap • Tracheoesophageal speech • Supercharged jejunum

KEY POINTS

- Goals of pharyngoesophageal reconstruction include re-establishing alimentary continuity, restoring speech, and protecting the neck vessels.
- Fasciocutaneous flaps, most commonly the alanine transaminase or forearm-based flaps, are the preferred reconstructive option for pharyngoesophageal reconstructions involving the cervical esophagus.
- Fasciocutaneous flaps have lower donor site morbidity and better speech outcomes compared with free jejunal flaps.
- Supercharged jejunal flaps are indicated for patients who require thoracic esophageal reconstruction and are not candidates for the gastric pull-up procedure.
- Proper management of postoperative complications is critical to prevent life-threatening sequelae and maximize function.

INTRODUCTION

Pharyngoesophageal reconstruction poses some of the greatest challenges in head and neck surgery and requires meticulous surgical execution and timely management of postoperative complications. Defects in this region are most commonly caused by total laryngopharyngectomy for treatment of laryngeal and hypopharyngeal malignancies. Other etiologies include pharyngocutaneous fistulas, benign strictures, and thyroid cancer involving the pharynx and esophagus. The goals of pharyngoesophageal reconstruction are to provide alimentary continuity, restore speech and swallowing, and protect critical blood vessels of the neck.

With the evolution of microsurgical techniques and the advent of perforator flaps, morbidity and mortality in pharyngoesophageal reconstruction have decreased dramatically. The earliest reconstructions in the late 1800s utilized random pattern skin flaps that carried exceedingly high rates of wound complications and fistula

The University of Texas MD Anderson Cancer Center, 1515 Holcombe Boulevard, Houston, TX 77030, USA
* Corresponding author.
E-mail address: mhanasono@mdanderson.org

Otolaryngol Clin N Am 56 (2023) 687–702
https://doi.org/10.1016/j.otc.2023.04.005
0030-6665/23/© 2023 Elsevier Inc. All rights reserved.

formation.[1,2] With the development of muscle and myocutaneous flaps, the pedicled pectoralis major muscle flap emerged as a workhorse option in the 1980s.[3] In the era of microsurgery, the jejunal free flaps offered a superior reconstructive option and, now, fasciocutaneous perforator flaps have become the gold standard in most centers.

ANATOMY

The pharynx is anatomically divided into 3 regions: the nasopharynx, oropharynx, and hypopharynx. The nasopharynx consists of structures in the nasal cavity and above the soft palate. The oropharynx is surrounded by the oral cavity anteriorly, the nasopharynx superiorly, and the hypopharynx and larynx inferiorly. The superior border of the oropharynx is at the plane of the soft palate, and the inferior border is at the level of the hyoid bone. The main structures of the oropharynx are tonsillar pillars, the base of tongue, soft palate, and lateral and posterior oropharyngeal walls. The superior border of the hypopharynx is at the level of hyoid bone, and its inferior border is at the lower border of the cricoid cartilage. Then, the hypopharynx continues inferiorly as the cervical esophagus. The hypopharynx lies immediately posterior to the larynx, which is the organ responsible for phonation and protecting the trachea against aspiration of foods and liquids.

Commonly, defects of the hypopharynx and cervical esophagus are the result of surgical resection of cancers in the hypopharynx and larynx, advanced thyroid cancers, radiation strictures, and chemical injuries. Isolated tumors in the cervical esophagus are rare, but may also require esophagectomy and reconstruction. It is important to note that given the paradigm shift toward organ-sparing nonsurgical treatment for laryngeal and hypopharyngeal cancers, most patients who require pharyngoesophageal reconstruction present with prior history of radiation, which places them at significantly increased risk for complications.[4,5]

PREOPERATIVE EVALUATION
Patient Optimization

Performing a thorough medical evaluation is critical in order to identify and optimize risk factors before surgery. Cardiovascular and pulmonary complications such as respiratory failure, pneumonia, prolonged ventilator support, pulmonary embolism, arrhythmia, myocardial infarction, and stroke remain the most serious and debilitating medical complications after major head and neck surgery and microvascular reconstruction. A thorough pulmonary and cardiovascular workup should be performed before surgery. In addition, carotid disease is elevated in this population, and carotid artery imaging should be performed as indicated, especially in patients with history of cerebrovascular disease. Head and neck computed tomography (CT) with intravenous contrast can usually reveal the status of the carotid arteries and can also delineate the availability of recipient vessels in the neck. In addition, most patients with head and neck cancers have extensive history of alcohol and tobacco abuse, and many present at an advanced age. Patients are encouraged at the time of presentation to stop smoking and drinking and are referred to smoking cessation clinics as needed. Nutritional optimization is critical prior to undergoing major pharyngoesophageal ablative and reconstructive surgery. Significant weight loss upon presentation is not uncommon, and a gastrostomy feeding tube should be placed in these patients preoperatively. Delay of surgery for nutritional optimization is not unreasonable in cases of severe malnutrition.

Understanding the Defect

Indications for the various reconstructive options for pharyngoesophageal defects are based on the degree of esophageal involvement and whether the defect is partial or circumferential. Laryngopharyngectomy defects involving only the hypopharynx and the cervical esophagus can be reconstructed using a fasciocutaneous flap or a free jejunal flap as there is adequate access in the neck for flap inset (**Fig. 1**). The gastric pull-up technique is the preferred method of reconstruction after total esophagectomy, as there is only 1 mucosal anastomosis, and no microvascular anastomosis is required. The reconstructive surgeon is not typically involved at this stage but in cases of failed gastric pull-up, disease involvement of the stomach, previous stomach surgery, or history of radiation to the stomach, the supercharged jejunal flap is the reconstructive method of choice.

Many patients undergoing pharyngoesophageal reconstruction have a hostile neck because of radiation and, occasionally, prior surgery. Challenges associated with a previously irradiated neck include lack of recipient vessels, risk of carotid artery rupture during dissection, and external neck skin defects.[6] The transverse cervical vessels that arise from the thyrocervical trunk are a good choice for recipient vessels in patients in whom the external carotid arterial system and internal jugular vein are not readily available as recipients, as the transverse cervical vessels are typically at the margin of the radiation zone and not damaged from prior neck surgery.[7] Furthermore, when the carotid artery and internal jugular vein are encased in fibrotic tissue, they are

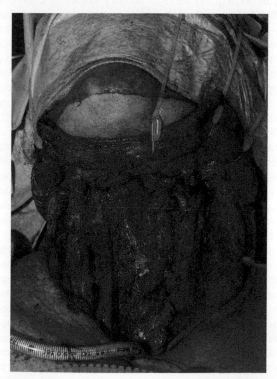

Fig. 1. Typical partial circumference pharyngoesophageal defect following laryngopharyngectomy in a patient undergoing salvage surgery following prior combined chemotherapy and radiation treatment for laryngeal cancer.

at high risk for rupture during dissection, and the best way to avoid this is to utilize vessels that are distant from these structures. Aside from the transverse cervical vessels, other options include the internal mammary vessels, thoracoacromial vessels, and cephalic vein.[8]

Pharyngoesophageal resection is often performed through a visor type neck incision, and the radiated anterior neck skin in these cases can have unreliable blood supply, resulting in necrosis. Releasing the scarred neck skin and removing fibrotic tissue further can result in a large neck skin defect. A second skin paddle or muscle component from a chimeric flap design or a second free or pedicled flap may be necessary for external resurfacing and should be factored into the reconstructive plan.

RECONSTRUCTIVE OPTIONS
Locoregional Flaps

Local and regional flaps are usually reserved for salvage surgeries when the primary free flap reconstruction has failed, for complications such as fistula and strictures, or for medically high-risk patients when free tissue transfer cannot be performed. The pectoralis major myocutaneous flap is the most commonly used regional flap.[9,10] The pectoralis muscle-only flap can also be used to cover a primary pharyngeal closure in a previously radiated patient to mitigate the risk of fistula formation as was demonstrated by a multicenter study involving 486 patients with cancer of the larynx or hypopharynx undergoing salvage surgery following chemoradiotherapy.[11] A third use of this flap is to resurface the neck in cases where radiation fibrosis and contracture make tension-free closure of the neck wound impossible. Reach of the flap can be increased, and bulk in the neck secondary to the proximal muscle can be minimized by islandizing the flap on the thoracoacromial pedicle (**Fig. 2**).

The latissimus dorsi myocutaneous flap is a second-line option for salvage reconstruction when large soft tissue/muscle coverage is needed. The flap is harvested in its usual fashion, but the skin paddle is designed distally to ensure reach into the neck. Major drawbacks to using the latissimus dorsi as a pedicled flap are limited reach and the bulky pedicle that must cross the axilla and chest.

Local fasciocutaneous flaps include the supraclavicular artery island flap (SCAIF) based on cutaneous perforators of the transverse cervical artery (93% of the time) or the suprascapular artery (7% of the time).[12] This flap has a good reach and minimal bulk, which are favorable attributes for pharyngoesophageal reconstruction. The area reliably supplied by the pedicle includes a mean length of 24.2 cm and mean width of 8.7 cm. The perforator is usually identified with a Doppler probe in the supraclavicular fossa, and dissection is distal to proximal parallel to the clavicle.

The internal mammary artery perforator flap is a modification of the deltopectoral flap, which was first described in 2006, and may also be used for pharyngocutaneous reconstruction, although the authors primarily use it for tracheostoma and lower neck skin reconstruction.[13] The flap is designed horizontally parallel to the corresponding intercostal space, usually over the second or third intercostal perforators, which tend to be the largest, with the medial edge at the midline of the sternum and the lateral edge extending as far as the anterior axillary fold. The flap is harvested in subfascial fashion from lateral to medial, and the medial edge can be incised and the flap rotated on its pedicle like a propeller for improved cosmesis. When used for pharyngocutaneous reconstruction, the flap is inset in 2 stages, with the superior end of the pharyngeal defect closed first, leaving a spit fistula, followed by division of the pedicle and closure of the inferior end of the pharyngeal defect several weeks later.

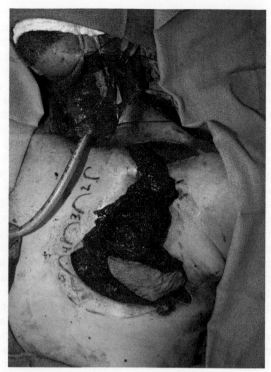

Fig. 2. The pectoralis major myocutaneous pedicled flap is used for neck reconstruction following laryngopharyngectomy and fasciocutaneous free flap pharyngoesophageal reconstruction. The skin paddle is designed over the interspace between the fourth and fifth ribs as the cutaneous perforator blood supply is dense in this area. The flap is islandized proximally to minimize bulk in the lower neck and increase the reach of the flap and its arc of rotation.

Thigh-Based Flaps

The anterolateral thigh (ALT) flap is based on perforators of the lateral circumflex femoral artery (LCFA) system and can be designed as a chimeric flap with multiple skin paddles or with the vastus lateralis muscle to use for neck resurfacing and to protect the great vessels. Because of its flexibility and low donor site morbidity, the ALT free flap is the authors' reconstructive flap of choice for the majority of partial and circumferential reconstructions involving the hypopharynx and cervical esophagus. Based on previous studies on ALT perforator mapping, the most consistent perforator is located near the midpoint of the line connecting the anterior superior iliac spine (ASIS) and the supralateral corner of the patella and 1.4 cm lateral to this line.[14] Commonly, there are 2 additional perforators approximately 5 cm proximal and distal to this perforator. In 96% of the thighs, these perforators originate from the descending branch, while the rest come from the transverse branch or the rectus femoris branch.[14,15]

Flap design is tailored based on whether defect is partial or circumferential. For a circumferential reconstruction, a neoesophagus with a diameter of approximately 3 cm requires a flap width of 9.4 cm (3 x π) to create a tube (**Fig. 3**). For partial defects, the width of the flap is calculated by subtracting the width of the remaining pharyngeal mucosa from 9.4 cm. Flap design is centered on the dominant perforator. When more than one perforator is present, a second skin paddle can be designed to allow for skin resurfacing and flap monitoring (**Figs. 4** and **5**). If only a single perforator is present but additional tissue is needed, a segment of the vastus lateralis muscle is included in the ALT flap as a chimeric flap to support skin grafting for neck resurfacing.[16]

Regarding the flap inset, the proximal anastomosis of the flap with the base of tongue and posterior pharyngeal mucosa is typically performed first. The longitudinal seam of the tubed flap is completed toward the distal end with simple, interrupted sutures. For the distal anastomosis, the anterior wall of the cervical esophagus is split longitudinally for approximately 1.5 cm to spatulate and enlarge the opening to minimize the risk of circumferential stricture. To complete the spatulation, a triangular lip is created on the flap and inserted into the longitudinal split of the esophagus. After completion of the distal anastomosis, the fascia of the flap or the included muscle is used to cover the suture lines. If available, the second skin paddle is then turned outward for neck resurfacing, trachea reconstruction, or flap monitoring (**Fig. 6**).

Although the ALT flap is available in most cases, 1 study found that approximately 5% of patients had no ALT perforator.[17] These patients typically have anteromedial thigh (AMT) perforators that supply this region. These perforators come from the rectus femoris branch, and originate from the proximal part of the descending branch of the LCFA. Septocutaneous perforators take a course within the septum between the rectus femoris and sartorius muscles, whereas musculocutaneous ones take a course through a thin layer of the rectus femoris muscle but never travel through the sartorius muscle.[18–21] The AMT flap harvest begins with a longitudinal incision similar to one that is made is during ALT flap harvest. Studies have demonstrated that the AMT flap is possible in only about 50% of patients, so this flap mainly serves as a secondary option when there are limited or unfavorable ALT perforators. Notably, there is a perfect reciprocal relationship between the ALT and AMT perforators.[22] Therefore, in cases when no ALT perforators are present, or only 1 ALT perforator is present but 2 independent skin islands are required for reconstruction, the chances of being able to harvest an AMT flap through the same incision in the same thigh as the primary flap or as a second fasciocutaneous flap in addition to an ALT flap are excellent.[23] Conveniently, because the pedicles of the AMT and ALT flaps share a common trunk above the bifurcation, surgeons can design and harvest chimeric flaps off the same common pedicle to include an ALT skin paddle, an AMT skin paddle, the vastus lateralis, or rectus femoris muscle.

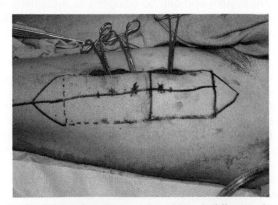

Fig. 3. Skin markings demonstrating design of a 2-skin paddle ALT free flap for simultaneous pharyngoesophageal and cutaneous neck reconstruction.

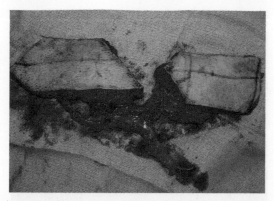

Fig. 4. Completed dissection of a 2-skin paddle ALT free flap. Note the triangular dart in the more superior skin paddle intended to widen the connection of the free flap to the remnant of the cervical esophagus.

Forearm-Based Flaps

The radial forearm flap is a time-honored, reliable flap that is familiar to all reconstructive surgeons. In the authors' practice, this flap is mostly reserved for partial circumference defects, although it is occasionally used for total circumference defects in

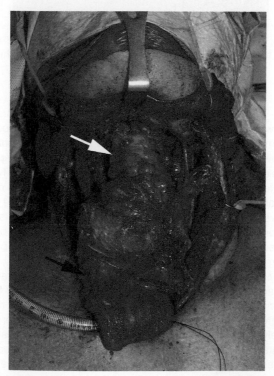

Fig. 5. One of the ALT free flap skin paddles has been tubed and re-establishes continuity between the oropharynx and the cervical esophagus (*white arrow*). The other skin paddle has not been inset yet and will be used to reconstruct the neck skin superior to the tracheostoma (*black arrow*).

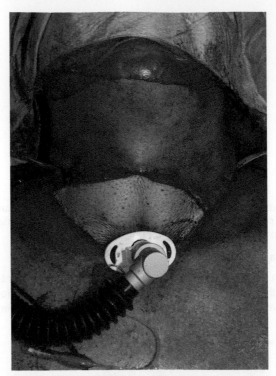

Fig. 6. Insetting of the distal ALT skin paddle to reconstruct the skin of the neck superior to the tracheostoma.

obese patients in whom the ALT flap is too thick to use as a tubed reconstruction. Flap elevation is performed in a similar fashion to those previously described in the literature with the following considerations.[24] Flap elevation is typically performed under tourniquet control and in suprafascial dissection over the tendons.[25] Need for cephalic vein harvest is determined by first exploring and examining the size of the vena comitantes of the radial vessels distally at the wrist. If the vein is at least 1 mm in diameter, cephalic vein harvest is not required.[26] If necessary, a second skin island based on a proximal perforator can be included as a part of flap design and can be externalized to resurface small neck skin defects or serve as a flap monitor. The flap dimensions and insetting considerations are identical to the thigh-based flaps.

The ulnar artery perforator (UAP) flap is the complement to the radial forearm and has potential advantages, including: a less conspicuous scar in the forearm, minimal sensory deficit distal to the flap, less hair on the skin, and minimal or no risk for tendon exposure with better skin graft take. Disadvantages include a shorter vascular pedicle that travels closely with the ulnar nerve requiring meticulous dissection, and less robust vascular anatomy because of its small perforators compared with the axially based radial forearm flap.[27] Perforators are found in a straight line drawn between the pisiform at the wrist and the epicondyle of the humerus at approximately 7 cm, 11 cm, and 16 cm, respectively from the pisiform.[28] All patients have at least 2 perforators, and nearly all the perforators are septocutaneous. The distal end of the flap is designed 5 cm above the pisiform. The lateral (radial) incision of the flap is made first and suprafascial dissection proceeds medially until perforators are seen between the flexor digitorum superficialis (FDS) and flexor carpi ulnaris (FCU) tendon. The fascia radial to the perforators is incised, and the FDS muscle and tendons are retracted radially, revealing the ulnar neurovascular bundle. The distal ulnar artery and vein are ligated, and the vascular pedicle is then carefully separated from the ulnar nerve. The vascular pedicle is traced toward the takeoff of the common interosseous artery, and the anterior interosseous nerve overlying the FDP and the median nerve should be protected in this region. The flap can be divided into 2 skin islands based on separate perforators as needed, and flap insetting is similar to ALT and radial forearm flap reconstruction.

Free Jejunal Flap

The free jejunal flap was first proposed in 1959 by Seidenberg for reconstruction of the cervical esophagus in an animal model. Following popularization of microvascular free flap surgery in human clinical use, the free jejunum became state of the art for pharyngoesophageal reconstruction in the 1980s and 1990s.[29–31] The jejunal flap is harvested through an upper midline abdominal incision. The desired jejunal segment, approximately 10 to 15 cm, is usually based on the second mesenteric vessels, and these are isolated to their origin at the superior mesenteric artery and vein. The mesentery between the adjacent arcade vessels is divided to the serosal border to unfurl the jejunal segment. The jejunum is divided using a linear cutting stapler, and the proximal segment is marked to maintain isoperistaltic orientation during inset.

To minimize the size discrepancy between the proximal pharyngeal defect and the jejunal opening, a 2 to 3 cm incision is made in the proximal end of the jejunum to widen the opening and allow for near end-to-side anastomosis. The anastomosis is typically performed in 2 layers using interrupted sutures followed by second layer Lempert serosal closure. The anastomoses are performed with the neck in neutral position to avoid redundancy and elongation over time, which can lead to dysphagia. The cervical esophagus is opened longitudinally to spatulate the distal anastomosis similar to insetting with the ALT flap. A monitoring jejunal segment approximately 3 cm in length can be created from the remaining jejunum based on branches of the pedicle vessels and externalized through the lateral neck incision. A 2-0 silk tie is placed loosely around the vascular pedicle, and this is later ligated at the beside when the segment is ready to be removed.

Supercharged Jejunal Flap

As mentioned previously, the supercharged jejunum is reserved for total esophageal reconstruction when the gastric pull-up procedure is deemed inadequate or unsafe.[32] This flap requires close coordination between plastic surgery, surgical oncology, and thoracic surgery. A similar upper midline abdominal incision is needed for harvest. The mesentery arcade of the jejunum is examined using transillumination. The first branch of the superior mesenteric vessels is identified and preserved. The second mesenteric vessels are typically dissected and divided for supercharging of the flap in the neck. The third mesenteric branch is divided, and the fourth branch serves as the blood supply for the pedicled portion of the flap (**Fig. 7**). The mesentery between the second and third branches is divided to the serosal border to unfurl the small bowel. The distal arcade vessels between the third and fourth branches must be preserved so that the fourth branch can perfuse the bowel normally perfused by the third branch while the bowel over the second branch is supercharged.

While the flap dissection is being performed, the thoracic surgery team continues with esophagectomy in the neck and widening the thoracic inlet. The left manubrium, first rib, and clavicular head are removed. A substernal tunnel is then created. Once this is done, the recipient vessels, usually the left internal mammary vessels, are dissected by the reconstructive team. The left transverse cervical vessels are the second choice. Turn down of the external jugular vein can serve as an excellent recipient vein when the internal mammary vein or transverse cervical vein is too small or absent.

Next, a sterile laparoscopic camera bag placed in the substernal tunnel is used to transfer the jejunal flap and its mesentery. Atraumatic transfer of the bowel flap to the neck is a critical part of the procedure, because improper transfer can disrupt the distal arcade vessels leaving the middle segment of the jejunal flap behind the sternum ischemic. The substernal transfer of the jejunal flap is preferred by most surgeons because of the excellent exposure in the lower neck and easy access to the internal mammary recipient vessels. The alternative route of transfer is the retrocardiac route, the native esophageal route that is only available in immediate reconstruction. The retrocardiac transfer does not offer access to the internal mammary vessels, and therefore, vein grafts are often needed to reach the neck recipient vessels.

Once the flap and the second mesentery branch are in the neck, microvascular anastomosis of the second branch of the superior mesenteric vessels and then esophagojejunostomy are performed while the thoracic and general surgery team restores bowel continuity in the abdomen, usually via a Roux-en-Y jejunojejunostomy (**Fig. 8**). The jejunum is secured to the diaphragm to minimize gravity pull on the flap. Similar to the free jejunal flap, a proximal segment of the jejunum can be used as a monitoring segment, and it can be removed around postoperative day 7 or before discharge.

POSTOPERATIVE CARE
Oral Diet

A modified barium swallow (MBS) study is performed postoperatively after pharyngoesophageal reconstruction to evaluate the swallowing function and healing process (**Fig. 9**). Timing of MBS study varies from 1 to 6 weeks after reconstruction, depending on the type of flaps used and history of radiotherapy, and oral feeding is held until the MBS study is complete. In the authors' practice, an MBS study for fasciocutaneous flaps is performed at 2 weeks postoperatively if there has been no prior radiation

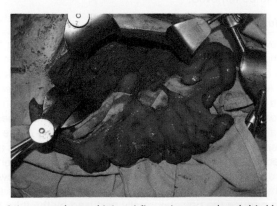

Fig. 7. Dissection of the supercharged jejunal flap. The second and third branches of the superior mesenteric artery and vein have been dissected and will be divided and ligated. The second branch artery and vein will be reanastomosed in the neck after transfer of the jejunum through the chest to maintain segmental blood supply to the flap.

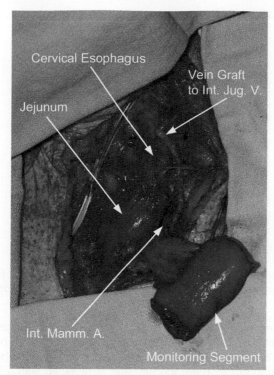

Fig. 8. Supercharged jejunal flap inset in the neck. Arterial anastomosis was performed to the internal mammary artery, and the venous anastomosis was completed to the internal jugular vein using a vein graft. The monitoring segment is externalized through the neck incision.

and at 6 weeks postoperatively if there has been prior radiation. In patients with no evidence of leaks or fistula, a liquid diet is started and then advanced to a soft diet 3 days later if no complications have occurred. Diet can then be advanced to regular diet as tolerated. In patients with a leak or fistula, oral intake is withheld, tube feeding is continued, and an MBS study is repeated in 2 weeks or longer, based on clinical judgment. Most asymptomatic leaks heal spontaneously within 2 weeks.

Voice Rehabilitation

Traditionally, tracheoesophageal puncture (TEP) is the preferred method of voice rehabilitation for a total laryngectomy. Primary TEP can be performed at the time of surgery or as a delayed secondary procedure. The authors' experience suggests that the rate of TEP failure is increased in both the ALT and jejunal flaps when performed at the time of laryngectomy and flap reconstruction. Therefore, patient selection for primary TEP should be carefully evaluated. Patients with good quality of tissue and adequate length of cervical esophagus remaining, who are compliant, have a good insufflation test, and more likely can manage the prosthesis postoperatively can be considered for primary TEP. Secondary TEP is usually performed 3 months after surgery in patients with few complications.

TEP is performed by puncturing the common wall between the trachea and esophagus about 1.5 cm or 2 cm below the rim of the tracheostoma. In patients who have

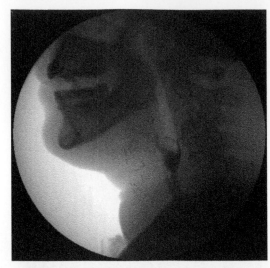

Fig. 9. Radiographic image from an MBS study taken 6 weeks after ALT free flap pharyng-oesophageal reconstruction showing a patent conduit and no leakage of barium.

had a very low resection of the cervical esophagus below the tracheostoma, the puncture is more challenging, as it needs to go through the flap and the posterior tracheal wall. Initially, a 14 F red rubber catheter is inserted through the trachea to the esophagus and secured in place. Then, the catheter is replaced with a voice prosthesis about 2 to 4 weeks after by speech pathologists. The prosthesis will be adjusted and fitted as the patients follow-up regularly with speech pathologists.

As speech rehabilitation requires significant patient motivation and commitment, careful patient selection is critical. Common TEP complications include widening of the puncture site with leakage around the voice prosthesis, fungal infections, and mucus plug formation inside the prosthesis. Studies have demonstrated better TEP voice quality and higher success rates with a fasciocutaneous flap than with a jejunal flap. In patients with a jejunal flap reconstruction, speech is often wet and labored because of flap redundancy, mucus production, and softness of the bowel wall that prevents adequate vibration.

OUTCOMES AND COMPLICATIONS
Outcomes

The largest single-center outcome study of pharyngoesophageal reconstruction included 349 cases, most of which involved laryngopharyngectomies, followed by total esophagectomy.[33,34] Following the trend of resection, the anterolateral thigh flap was the most commonly used flap (60%), followed by the supercharged jejunum (15%), the radial forearm flap (12%), the pectoralis major flap (6%), and the free jejunal transfer (4%). Of 349 patients, 55% of patients had circumferential defects, and 45% had partial defects. The rates of fistula (10.9 vs 6%), stricture (9.3 vs 3.8%), and overall complication (43.5 vs 34%) were higher in patients with circumferential defects than those of patients with partial defects.

A previous study directly comparing the ALT flaps versus the free jejunal flap demonstrated slightly higher fistula rates in the ALT group compared with the jejunal flap group (15% vs 8%).[35] Higher rates of successful tracheoesophageal speech and oral diet tolerance were seen in the ALT patients. The improvement in speech and swallowing outcomes and the decreased systemic morbidity for the ALT flap patients compared to the free jejunal transfer patients has established the ALT and other fasciocutaneous flaps as the preferred method for reconstruction at most centers.

POSTOPERATIVE COMPLICATIONS

Pharyngocutaneous fistulae can occur as a result of the disruption of the suture lines. Common risk factors for fistula formation are previous radiotherapy, technical errors, poor tissue quality at the anastomosis site, and nonroutine postoperative course. Typically, fistulae develop between 1 and 4 weeks postoperatively and can manifest as a leakage of saliva/liquids/solids or a subtle neck infection. Therefore, any type of neck infection or abscess that occurs after a pharyngoesophageal reconstruction should raise suspicion for an anastomotic leakage. To prevent possible fistula formation, any questionable tissue in the proximal pharynx and cervical esophagus should be excised prior to reconstruction until only well-vascularized tissue is seen. Meticulous flap inset is mandatory. The authors usually test for a water-tight closure following inset by flushing the oral cavity with saline and observing for leakage along the entire suture line.

Once a fistula is identified, oral intake is withheld, and local wound care is initiated. Patients with small asymptomatic fistulae without tumor recurrence or distal obstruction usually heal spontaneously within 2 weeks with conservative management. In patients with larger fistulas resulting in cellulitis of the neck, CT is usually performed to rule out abscess and assess the proximity of the fistula/abscess to the carotid arteries and flap pedicle. If an abscess around the carotid artery or flap pedicle is identified, early intervention with prompt irrigation and debridement is necessary to avoid carotid rupture. In some cases, primary repair of the fistula is possible. In others, efforts are made to direct the drainage away from the great vessels of the neck and the flap pedicle. Consideration is given to filling dead space and reinforcing fistula repairs with a pedicled pectoralis major muscle flap.

With the proper management, as described previously, persistent fistulas are rare. However, if a fistula does persist, then the patient should be evaluated for distal obstruction or tumor recurrence. As longstanding fistulas will eventually cause stricture because of scar tissue formation, reconstruction with a radial forearm free flap may be warranted in selected patients to prevent chronic, nonhealing fistulas.

Anastomotic strictures occur most commonly in circumferential defects and usually at the distal anastomosis. Distal anastomotic strictures can occur several months or years following reconstruction. In patients who develop dysphagia several months after reconstruction, an MBS study should be performed to rule out anastomotic strictures. Endoscopic balloon dilatation by a gastroenterologist is often effective, although this may need to be repeated periodically. Patients with refractory cases may require secondary reconstruction involving excision of the stricture and repair of a partial or total circumference defect with another free flap.

CLINICS CARE POINTS

- Keep in mind during the planning phase that neck skin reconstruction is often needed in radiated patients even if the quality and laxity of neck skin appears normal preoperatively.

- Avoid use of two narrow of a flap, otherwise, stenosis of the pharyngoesophageal conduit is likely. A 9.4 cm width is the ideal size, even if it means that the donor site cannot be closed primarily but needs a skin graft closure instead.

- A triangular dart in the distal closure of a tubed fasciocutaneous flap into the proximal cervical esophagus helps avoid stricture at this site.

- Closure of all suture lines must be meticulous to avoid a fistula. A water test is often helpful for identifying leaks.

DISCLOSURES

The authors have nothing to disclose.

REFERENCES

1. Wookey H. The surgical treatment of carcinoma of the hypopharynx and the oesophagus. Br J Surg 1948;35(139):249–66.
2. Bakamjian VY. A two-stage method for pharyngoesophageal reconstruction with a primary pectoral skin flap. Plast Reconstr Surg 1965;36:173–84.
3. Patel UA, Hartig GK, Hanasono MM, et al. Locoregional flaps for oral cavity reconstruction: a review of modern options. Otolaryngol Head Neck Surg 2017; 157(2):201–9.
4. Wolf GT, Fisher SG, Hong WK, et al. Induction chemotherapy plus radiation compared with surgery plus radiation in patients with advanced laryngeal cancer. N Engl J Med 1991;324(24):1685–90.
5. Weber RS, Berkey BA, Forastiere A, et al. Outcome of salvage total laryngectomy following organ preservation therapy: the Radiation Therapy Oncology Group trial 91-11. Arch Otolaryngol Head Neck Surg 2003;129(1):44–9.
6. Hanasono MM, Lin D, Wax MK, et al. Closure of laryngectomy defects in the age of chemoradiation therapy. Head Neck 2012;34:580–8.
7. Yu P. The transverse cervical vessels as recipient vessels for previously treated head and neck cancer patients. Plas Reconstr Surg 2005;115(5):1253–8.
8. Hanasono MM, Barnea Y, Skoracki RJ. Microvascular surgery in the previously operated and irradiated neck. Microsurgery 2009;29:1–7.
9. Baek SM, Lawson W, Biller HF. Reconstruction of hypopharynx and cervical esophagus with pectoralis major island myocutaneous flap. Ann Plast Surg 1981;7:18–24.
10. Schneider DS, Wu V, Wax MK. Indications for pedicled pectoralis major flap in a free tissue transfer practice. Head Neck 2012;34(8):1106–10.
11. Microvascular Committee of the American Academy of Otolaryngology-Head & Neck Surgery. Salvage laryngectomy and laryngopharyngectomy: multicancer review of outcomes associated with a reconstructive approach. Head Neck 2019;41:16–29.
12. Chiu ES, Liu PH, Baratelli R, et al. Circumferential pharyngoesophageal reconstruction with a supraclavicular artery island flap. Plas Reconstr Surg 2010; 125(1):161–6.
13. Yu P, Roblin P, Chevray P. Internal mammary artery perforator (IMAP) flap for tracheostoma reconstruction. Head Neck 2006;28(8):723–9.
14. Yu P. Characteristics of the anterolateral thigh flap in a Western population and its application in head and neck reconstruction. Head Neck 2004;26(9):759–69.

15. Yu P, Robb GL. Pharyngoesophageal reconstruction with the anterolateral thigh flap: a clinical and functional outcomes study. Plas Reconstr Surg 2005;116(7): 1845–55.

16. Yu P, Hanasono MM, Skoracki RJ, et al. Pharyngoesophageal reconstruction with the anterolateral thigh flap after total laryngopharyngectomy. Cancer 2010; 116(7):1718–24.

17. Thomas WW, Calcagno HE, Azzi J, et al. Incidence of inadequate perforators and salvage options for the anterior lateral thigh free flap. Laryngoscope 2020;130: 343–6.

18. Hupkens P, Van Loon B, Lauret GJ, et al. Anteromedial thigh flaps: an anatomical study to localize and classify anteromedial thigh perforators. Microsurg 2010; 30(1):43–9.

19. Hsieh CH, Yang JC, Chen CC, et al. Alternative reconstructive choices for antero-lateral thigh flap dissection in cases in which no sizable skin perforator is available. Head Neck 2009;31(5):571–5.

20. Yu P, Selber J. Perforator patterns of the anteromedial thigh flap. Plas Reconstr Surg 2011;128(3):151e–7e.

21. Sun J, Chew K, Wong C, et al. Vascular anatomy of the anteromedial thigh flap. J Plast Reconstr Aesthet Surg Open 2017;13:113–25.

22. Yu P, Selber J, Liu J. Reciprocal dominance of the anterolateral and anteromedial thigh flap perforator anatomy. Ann Plast Surg 2013;70(6):714–6.

23. Katre C, Shaw R, Batstone M, et al. Rescue of anterolateral thigh flap with absent perforators using anteromedial thigh flap. Br J Oral Maxfac Surg 2008;46(4): 334–5.

24. Anthony JP, Singer MI, Mathes SJ. Pharyngoesophageal reconstruction using the tubed free radial forearm flap. Clin Plast Surg 1994;21:137–47.

25. Lutz BS, Wei FC, Chang SC, et al. Donor site morbidity after suprafascial eleva-tion of the radial forearm flap: a prospective study in 95 consecutive cases. Plas Reconstr Surg 1999;103(1):132–7.

26. Chang SC, Miller G, Halbert CF, et al. Limiting donor site morbidity by suprafas-cial dissection of the radial forearm flap. Microsurg 1996;17(3):136–40.

27. Sieg P, Bierwolf S. Ulnar versus radial forearm flap in head and neck reconstruc-tion: an experimental and clinical study. Head Neck 2001;23(11):967–71.

28. Yu P, Chang EI, Selber JC, et al. Perforator patterns of the ulnar artery perforator flap. Plas Reconstr Surg 2012 Jan;129(1):213–20.

29. Seidenberg B, Rosenak SS, Hurwitt ES, et al. Immediate reconstruction of the cer-vical esophagus by a revascularized isolated jejunal segment. Ann Surg 1959; 149(2):162–71.

30. Hester TR, McConnel FM, Nahal F, et al. Reconstruction of cervical esophagus, hypopharynx and oral cavity using free jejunal transfer. Am J Surg 1980;140(4): 487–91.

31. Reece GP, Bengtson BP, Schusterman MA. Reconstruction of the pharynx and cervical esophagus using free jejunal transfer. Clin Plast Surg 1994;21(1): 125–36.

32. Mays AC, Yu P, Hofstetter W, et al. The supercharged pedicled jejunal flap for to-tal esophageal reconstruction: a retrospective review of 100 cases. Plas Reconstr Surg 2019;144(5):1171–80.

33. Selber JC, Xue A, Liu J, et al. Pharyngoesophageal reconstruction outcomes following 349 cases. J Reconstr Microsurg 2014;30(9):641–54.

34. Sharaf B, Xue A, Solari MG, et al. Optimizing outcomes in pharyngoesophageal reconstruction and neck resurfacing: 10-year experience of 294 cases. Plas Reconstr Surg 2017;139(1):105e–19e.
35. Yu P, Lewin JS, Reece GP, et al. Comparison of clinical and functional outcomes and hospital costs following pharyngoesophageal reconstruction with the anterolateral thigh free flap versus the jejunal flap. Plas Reconstr Surg 2006;117(3): 968–74.

History, Innovation, Pearls, and Pitfalls in Complex Midface Reconstruction

Hilary C. McCrary, MD, MPH[1], Nolan B. Seim, MD,
Matthew O. Old, MD*

KEYWORDS

- Midface • Reconstruction • Free flap • Trauma • Head and neck cancer

HISTORY AND EVOLUTION OF MIDFACE RECONSTRUCTION

The midface is a complex anatomical area with the two maxilla serving as the boney framework with the overlying soft tissue and musculature providing a critical role in facial expression, speech, and mastication.[1] This complex form and function makes the reconstruction of the maxilla one of the more challenging types of reconstructive surgeries that can be performed. Over the course of several decades there has been significant innovation in terms of a head and neck surgeon's ability to effectively reconstruct complex maxilla defects. Prior to the 1990's there were few reconstructive options that existed for patients suffering from neoplasms (a majority being sinonasal or oral cavity squamous cell carcinomas), trauma or osteomyelitis/osteoradionecrosis affecting the midface. Traditionally these defects were commonly managed with the used of an obturator alone.[2] However, with the advent of free flap reconstruction, the options for reconstruction have rapidly increased, which helps overcome many of the functional and cosmetic issues faced with obturator alone. There is still a place for the use of obturators to aid in rehabilitation among patients with small to medium defects with appropriate supportive dentition and structure,[3] but among larger, more complex defects there should be consideration of free flap reconstruction. A recent systematic review evaluated differences between obturators and free flap reconstruction, with free flap reconstruction of the maxilla being associated with decreased pain, with an ability to retain masticatory efficiency, equivalent speech intelligibility, and a decreased level of anxiety when compared to use of an obturator alone.[4]

Patients with complex maxillary defects have a wide variety of options across the reconstructive ladder.[5] The factors that are most important in a surgeon's decision

Department of Otolaryngology–Head and Neck Surgery, The Ohio State University Wexner Medical Center, Columbus, OH, USA
[1] Present address: 1350 East Emerson Avenue, Salt Lake City, UT 84105, USA
* Corresponding author. Department of Otolaryngology, The James Comprehensive Cancer Center and Solove Research Institute, The Ohio State University, 915 Olentangy River Road, Suite 4000, Columbus, OH 43212.
E-mail address: matthew.old@osumc.edu

Otolaryngol Clin N Am 56 (2023) 703–713
https://doi.org/10.1016/j.otc.2023.04.010
0030-6665/23/© 2023 Elsevier Inc. All rights reserved.

for the reconstruction of the midface include the "site, size and soft tissue defect."[6] While prosthetic devices were the first technique utilized for midface/maxilla reconstruction, local flaps were soon utilized in reconstructive efforts, including local flaps from the forehead, cheek, upper lip, or turbinate.[7] While these techniques were effective for small defects, they were of limited utility among larger defect requiring skin, bone, and mucosal coverage. The use of free flaps for maxillary reconstruction has become increasingly popular due to the ability to provide a single-stage reconstruction with excellent aesthetic and functional outcomes. Flaps are also used in situations in which prosthodontic expertise is not available. In 2006, authors Futran and Mendez described an algorithm for how to approach the reconstruction of the midface, with simple palate and infrastructural maxillectomy defects utilizing soft tissue reconstruction and local flaps, whereas, total maxillectomy defects often required vascularized bone flaps for defects without viable dentition for a prothesis or if the orbitozygomatic contour is not intact.[8] These authors advocate for the integration of several different approaches to achieve the best possible outcome for patients. The most commonly used free flaps for maxillary reconstruction include the radial forearm flap, anterolateral thigh flap, fibula flap, latissimus dorsi flap, scapular system flaps, and the rectus abdominis flap.[9,10] Each flap has its own advantages and disadvantages, but the variety of free flap reconstructive options couple with the improving medical modeling technology has allowed for a rapidly changing landscape in midface reconstruction. Nevertheless, complex defects of the maxilla remain a challenging reconstruction for even experienced surgeons.

Within our own institution, we have seen an evolution in the approaches to midface reconstruction. While the advent of virtual surgical planning was starting, we deployed the use of an intraoperative stents to enable the facilitation of free tissue transfer placement.[11] Prior to the initiation of surgery, dental impressions are obtained and upper/lower casts are created using ethyl vinyl acetate mouth guard material. These stents we used intraoperatively to ensure correct position of the maxillary teeth and allowed the reconstructive surgeon to make adjustments during free flap reconstruction, ensuring appropriate alignment for cosmetic and dental restoration. All bone cuts and plating were done free hand which was standard prior to virtual surgical planning and modeling.[12]

Medical modeling has since replaced or augmented most of these techniques and it includes the integration of three-dimensional (3D) modeling, presurgical planning and subsequent plating with preprinted plates or bending hardware to a model. While this approach does require sufficient time for preoperative planning, the value of virtual surgical planning in midface reconstruction cannot be understated given that it enables surgeons to anticipate reconstructive needs intraoperatively and reduce overall operative time. Within our institution, we commonly integrate virtual surgical planning with complex maxillary defects, especially if there is a goal to accomplish dental rehabilitation in addition to closure of the defect.[3]

INTEGRATION OF VIRTUAL SURGICAL PLANNING INTO HEAD AND NECK MICROVASCULAR SURGERY PROGRAM

Integration of virtual surgical planning is not necessary for all midface defects; however, our institution implements it for patients suffering from severe osteoradionecrosis, complex trauma and blast injuries to the midface, complex head and neck cases, or revision surgery. Our system for the integration of virtual surgical planning for our patient's undergoing midface reconstruction includes obtaining high-resolution thin cut maxillofacial computed tomography (CT) and lower extremity CT angiograms to evaluate if the patient is a candidate for a fibula free flap reconstruction. After obtaining proper imaging, a meeting is set up with an engineer (KLS Martin group) to discuss operative plan and beginning the surgical planning process. Often this planning process includes the integration of osseointegrated implants if indicated with our prosthodontists being a critical part of planning for dental rehabilitation (**Fig. 1**). After the initial planning session, the engineer and surgeon will then proceed with creating a 3D model of the patient's anatomy based on their CT imaging, where cutting guides and customized plates can be curated for each specific patient, allowing for the free flap bone segments to have maximal contact with the native bone and aligned osteotomies. The surgeon will then review the plan and make any necessary adjustments. Once the plan is finalized, the engineer will then fabricate the cutting guides and plates, sterilize and integrate the products into the intraoperative toolbox. During the surgery, the cutting guides and plates are used to ensure accuracy and precision in the reconstruction. Fabrication of cutting guides also allows for fibula osteotomies and plating to be performed while the flap is still transfusing in the leg, thus, reducing the overall ischemia time. After the reconstruction is complete, the prosthodontists will then work with the patient to fabricate the necessary prostheses for the patient's rehabilitation. Overall, the integration of virtual surgical planning has allowed us to provide our patients with optimal surgical results that is personalized and tailored to their unique needs.

CLINICAL OUTCOMES AND COST ASSOCIATED WITH VIRTUAL SURGICAL PLANNING

The use of virtual surgical planning within the setting of midface reconstruction has been shown to reduced ischemia and total operative time, and reduced rates of complications, flap failures, and overall time spent in the hospital.[13,14] Studies evaluating anatomical outcomes have also demonstrates superior results. Swenseid and colleagues[15] evaluated a series of midface scapula free flap reconstructions, comparing outcomes among cases that utilized virtual surgical planning versus those that did not, which revealed a significant improvement in the anatomic position of the boney segments, an increase in the number of appositions in which bone segments achieved contact, and a greater average of subunits that were able to be reconstructed. Similar outcomes were appreciated among patients that underwent midface reconstruction using fibula free flaps. Cuéllar and colleagues[16] published a series comparing fibula free flap virtual surgical planning compared to standard surgery showed a significant

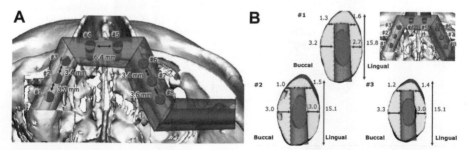

Fig. 1. Virtual surgical planning image with placement of future implants in a complex midface defect allowing for screw hole planning. Image (*A*) demonstrates projected implant placement with planned distance between implants, and Image (*B*) demonstrates the depth of implant placement.

improvement in the anatomical position of the free flap bone, bone apposition, and esthetic outcomes.

While virtual surgical planning has emerged as a promising tool to aid in midface reconstruction, the cost of implementing this technology is a concern across many healthcare systems. A time and cost-analysis was performed by Mazzola and colleagues,[14] which demonstrated a lower mean total cost of surgery, but a higher median total cost of surgery. Other authors have estimated a $5,000-$7,000 higher cost associated with virtual surgical planning, but did state these costs have the potential to be offset by decreased operative time, complications, and overall hospital stay. While a trust cost-benefit analysis still needs to be performed to continue advocating for the use of this planning tool, Mazzola and colleagues[14] felt that virtual surgical planning did not adversely impact the overall cost associated with surgery. Additionally, most head and neck centers have deployed virtual planning as a standard for complex head and neck defects.

COMPLEX MIDFACE RECONSTRUCTION CASE EXAMPLE

The patient is a 17-year-old male that presented to our institution after suffering a gunshot wound to the face, with extensive craniofacial fractures and right lateral frontal lobe injury that prompted a bicoronal craniotomy. The patient was missing a majority of his mandible and maxilla (**Fig. 2**). He had undergone prior surgical debridement, primary closure of defects, fixation of orbital rim fractures, abscess drainages, and placement of external fixation device along the mandible prior to arrival at our institution. A plan was made to first address the large mandible defect prior to the reconstruction of the maxilla to serve as a foundation for ultimate dental rehabilitation. Our prosthodontics colleagues also evaluated the patient in the operating room where impressions for a surgical obturator was completed. Unfortunately, the patient did not tolerate the obturator due to the lack of structures for stability.

Over a month from his initial trauma, the patient proceeded to the operating room for mandible reconstruction using a three-segment fibula from the right leg, which was completed using virtual surgical planning with the plating of the fibula while the free

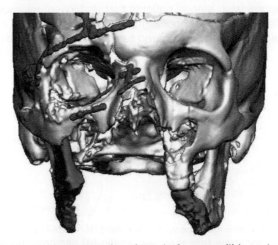

Fig. 2. A 3-D reconstructive pre-operative photo before mandible and maxilla reconstruction image, showing the large midface and mandible defect from the blast injury.

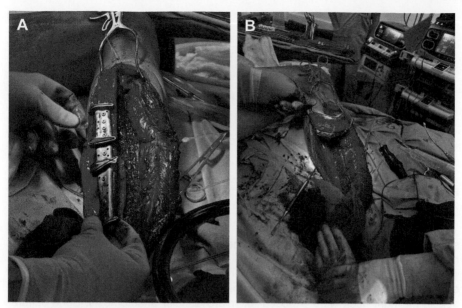

Fig. 3. (*A*) Fibula free flap dissection with placement of the customized cutting guides. (*B*) Fibula free flap still vascularized in the leg with the osteotomies made and the customized reconstruction plate secured to the bone.

flap was still vascularized in the leg (**Fig. 3**). After recovering from the mandible reconstruction, new CT was obtained to allow for virtual surgical planning for his maxillary reconstruction. A plan was made to use the contralateral fibula for the reconstruction of the maxilla/midface using a four-segment fibula (**Fig. 4**). Importantly we ensured the

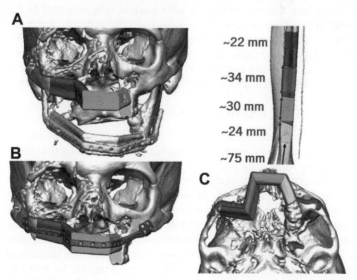

Fig. 4. (*A*) Plans for the midface surgery created from the virtual surgical planning session, showing the four-segment fibula reconstruction with the length of each segment > 2 cm. (*B*) A coronal view of the planned midface reconstruction with the customized plate in place. (*C*) A basal view, showing the complexity of the four-segment fibula reconstruction.

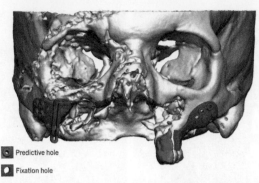

Predictive hole

Fixation hole

Fig. 5. Demonstration of the 3D model with the placement of the cutting guides, to assist with freshening the boney edges to allow for better bone contact during reconstruction.

segments would improve his projection and allow for proper restorative height of the maxilla.

We proceeded to the operating room for his midface reconstruction. The edges of bone at the lateral buttresses were freshened utilizing cutting guides (**Fig. 5**) and vessels in the right neck were exposed for microvascular anastomosis. Bone cultures were taken as well. A left fibula free flap was dissected and prior to harvest, we placed the cutting guides on the fibula and completed our osteotomies, followed by the placement of the midface customized reconstruction plate (**Fig. 6**). Next the free flap was harvested and we placed the fibula and plate in the midface defect, with our screws securing the flap to the zygoma bilaterally (**Fig. 7**). The pedicle was fed into the right neck over the mandible, but given the extensive amount of bone required for the reconstruction of the midface, there was only 8 cm of vascular pedicle. Thus, we harvested a vein graft from the lesser saphenous, which was previously exposed during the fibula free flap dissection. A skin paddle was secured to the oroantral defect, providing excellent closure of the defect. Postoperatively, the patient is found to have excellent projection and restorative height, with appropriate closure of the oroantral fistula (**Fig. 8**). The patient was discharged home on IV antibiotics due to positive bone cultures, which are common in these scenarios. A plan was made to proceed with osseointegrated implants approximately six months after surgery.

PITFALLS AND PEARLS OF MIDFACE RECONSTRUCTION

While there is great potential for success in midface reconstruction even for the most complex of defects, there are many complications and difficulties that can arise in and out of the operating room. The first highlights that there is some complexity in fitting bony segments into the correct portions for reconstruction, particularly if the surgeon is free handing the reconstruction. Among complex defects that require a multi-segment fibular free flap, it is recommended that surgeons limit the amount of muscle harvested with the flap, as any edema of this muscle can cause issues with securing the bone into place. Second, issues with pedicle length in midface reconstruction arise frequently. This can be an issue that is seen commonly with subscapular system flaps.[17] This is what brought into favor the use of the scapular tip free flap based on the angular artery, commonly arising from the thoracodorsal artery, as this flap can have a pedicle length of up to 20 cm in length if the circumflex artery is dissected and sacrificed with flap harvest.[18] However, in patients with a history of radiation or severe trauma where vessel depletion may be a concern, planning for potential vein

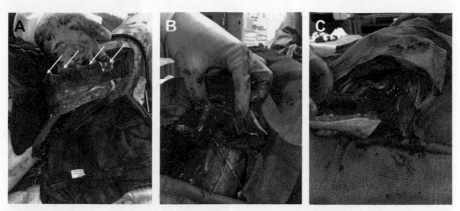

Fig. 6. Intraoperative photos after raising the left fibula free flap, with image (*A*) demonstrating the osteotomies that were created resulting in a four-segment fibula (*white arrows*), (*B*) view of the fibula secured to the plate along the inferior border, and (*C*) view of the skin paddle with the four-segment fibula secured to the customized plate.

grafts and prepping the arm for cephalic vein harvest, or the leg for the saphenous vein harvest should be highly considered. While prior studies have demonstrated that vein grafts are associated with increased risk of free flap complications, including free flap compromise and loss,[19] for complex cases they are frequently a necessity. A multi-institutional review found an 85% success rate with the use of vein graft in complex head and neck reconstruction, with no differences noted between myocutaneous and osteocutaneous free flaps.[20] Another aspect of reconstruction to consider is preventing soft tissue contraction after reconstruction. Soft tissue contraction can be frequently appreciated in patients that have traumatic defects that undergo a delayed reconstruction or prior attempts and local reconstruction.[21] This soft tissue contraction can prompt the need for secondary reconstruction, thus, predicting soft tissue needs in advance can avoid further surgeries down the road.

Osteomyelitis and osteoradionecrosis are commonly seen in patients who have a history of trauma or among those with prior treatment of head and neck cancer, particularly

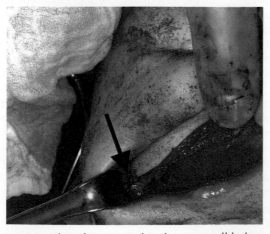

Fig. 7. View of the reconstruction plate secured to the zygoma (*black arrow* indicating a tab hooking onto the zygoma), with the skin paddle visualized, which was used to close the oroantral fistula from the blast injury.

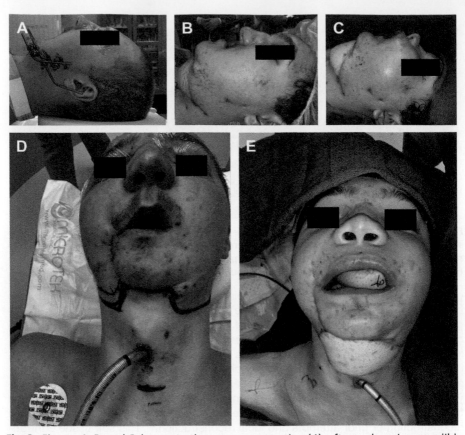

Fig. 8. Figures A, B, and C demonstrating pre-reconstruction (*A*), after undergoing mandible reconstruction (*B*), and his final postoperative profile view after maxilla reconstruction (*C*). Figures D and E demonstrating a pre- (*D*) and postoperative (*E*) frontal view.

among those receiving radiation. While prior rates of osteoradionecrosis were as high as 21% two decades ago, with the advent of more sophisticated radiation treatments, the current prevalence of osteoradionecrosis is estimated to be around 5% or less.[22,23] Given the complexity of operating in what is commonly found to be a chronically infected wound, it is of paramount importance that the bone is cultures so directed therapy can be provided pre- and postoperatively. Importantly, cultures should be obtained from what is considered to be "healthy appearing bone," instead of bone that is going with the specimen. Our institution evaluated patients undergoing microvascular free tissue transfer for radiation or bisphosphonate-related osteonecrosis of the jaw, and found that patients with antibiotic directed therapy obtained from healthy bone were more like to receive proper long-term intravenous antibiotics and had fewer rates of postoperative wound complications.[24] Common pathogens associated with osteomyelitis includes *Candida, Streptococcus,* and *Actinomyces*, with long-term antibiotics being particularly beneficial for the treatment of patients growing *Actinomyces*.

INTERDISCIPLINARY COLLABORATION FOR SUCCESSFUL MIDFACE RECONSTRUCTION

Collaboration is critical to obtain success with midface reconstruction. Our team consists of head and neck microvascular surgery, prosthodontists, radiology, infectious disease, engineers, and medical device representatives. Ultimately, it is the interface of all these specialties that enable these patients to have successful clinical outcomes. We recommend early discussions with a prosthodontist to create an operative plan that allow for bone placement that creates proper restorative height. Furthermore, a protocol with radiology that integrates thin cut high resolution images is a necessity to proceed with virtual surgical planning. This imaging gives surgeons the tools to work with medical engineers and medical device representatives to create customized surgical plans for each unique patient including, the integration of cutting guides and pre-formed reconstruction plates. Finally, for patients with osteomyelitis and osteoradionecrosis, we recommend early integration of infectious disease in their care, with careful discussion about how to proceed with long-term antibiotics if needed after free flap reconstruction.

SUMMARY

While midface reconstruction is challenging, it also is very rewarding, as a successful reconstruction can help restore both form and function. Over the years, there have been great strides in our ability to reconstruct complex defects of the midface, with refinements made in microvascular surgery and free tissue transfer providing arguably the greatest impact in midface reconstruction. While patients with small, simple defects of the maxilla can still be offered an obturator for reconstruction, when evaluating larger, more complex defects of the midface, reconstruction with a free flap should be highly considered. The advent of virtual surgical planning has made the reconstruction of even the most complex maxilla and midface achievable, with growing evidence to support improved anatomical, cosmetic and functional outcomes. While the cost-benefit of this tool is still to be determined most head and neck reconstructive surgeons and centers have integrated it as standard of care for complex defects. We advocate for the use of virtual surgical planning in revision cases, complex cancer cases including osteoradionecrosis or osteomyelitis, or patients with complex trauma and blast injuries to the midface. While pedicle length and the need for vein graft are always potential issues encountered with midface reconstruction, with a proper reconstructive plan these cases can safely and efficiently be performed. Overall, midface reconstruction is an intricate but gratifying procedure that can restore a patient's quality of life.

CLINICSAL CARE POINTS

- Free flap reconstruction has become the standard of care for large defects of the midface, with significant innovation in surgical approaches being achieved over the past decade.

- Given the complexities associated with midface reconstruction, utilization of virtual surgical planning is encouraged among complex ablative cases, blast injuries to the face, and cases that involve osteoradionecrosis or osteomyelitis.

- Common reconstructive delimmas in midface reconstruction include need for a long free flap pedicle for microvascular anastomosis, chronic infection of the bone, anatomical complexity of reconstruction, and long-term issues with soft tissue contracture.

REFERENCES

1. Santamaria E, Cordeiro PG. Reconstruction of maxillectomy and midfacial defects with free tissue transfer. J Surg Oncol 2006;94(6):522–31.

2. Langenbeck B, Krotky H, Olk E. [The air obturator as new type of closure of a large operative defect in the head region]. HNO 1964;12:339–40.

3. Seim NB, Ozer E, Valentin S, et al. Custom presurgical planning for midfacial reconstruction. Facial Plast Surg 2020;36(6):696–702.

4. Cao Y, Yu C, Liu W, et al. Obturators versus flaps after maxillary oncological ablation: a systematic review and best evidence synthesis. Oral Oncol 2018;82:152–61.

5. Eskander A, Kang SY, Teknos TN, et al. Advances in midface reconstruction: beyond the reconstructive ladder. Curr Opin Otolaryngol Head Neck Surg 2017;25(5):422–30.

6. Genden EM. Reconstruction of the mandible and the maxilla: the evolution of surgical technique. Arch Facial Plast Surg 2010;12(2):87–90.

7. Muzaffar AR, Adams WP Jr, Hartog JM, et al. Maxillary reconstruction: functional and aesthetic considerations. Plast Reconstr Surg 1999;104(7):2172–83 [quiz: 2184].

8. Futran ND, Mendez E. Developments in reconstruction of midface and maxilla. Lancet Oncol 2006;7(3):249–58.

9. Hammer D, Vincent AG, Williams F, et al. Considerations in free flap reconstruction of the midface. Facial Plast Surg 2021;37(6):759–70.

10. Nguyen S, Tran KL, Wang E, et al. Maxillectomy defects: virtually comparing fibular and scapular free flap reconstructions. Head Neck 2021;43(9):2623–33.

11. Varma VR, Yiu Y, Van Putten M Jr, et al. Novel approach to maxillary reconstruction using osteocutaneous free tissue transfer with a customized stent. Head Neck 2017;39(9):E96–101.

12. Chan TJ, Long C, Wang E, et al. The state of virtual surgical planning in maxillary reconstruction: a systematic review. Oral Oncol 2022;133:106058.

13. Lawless M, Swendseid B, von Windheim N, et al. Review of cost and surgical time implications using virtual patient specific planning and patient specific implants in midface reconstruction. Plastic and Aesthetic Research 2022;9:26.

14. Mazzola F, Smithers F, Cheng K, et al. Time and cost-analysis of virtual surgical planning for head and neck reconstruction: a matched pair analysis. Oral Oncol 2020;100:104491.

15. Swendseid BP, Roden DF, Vimawala S, et al. Virtual surgical planning in subscapular system free flap reconstruction of midface defects. Oral Oncol 2020;101:104508.

16. Navarro Cuéllar C, Martínez EB, Navarro Cuéllar I, et al. Primary maxillary reconstruction with fibula flap and dental implants: a comparative study between virtual surgical planning and standard surgery in class IIC defects. J Oral Maxillofac Surg 2021;79(1):237–48.

17. Miles BA, Gilbert RW. Maxillary reconstruction with the scapular angle osteomyogenous free flap. Arch Otolaryngol Head Neck Surg 2011;137(11):1130–5.

18. Ferrari S, Ferri A, Bianchi B. Scapular tip free flap in head and neck reconstruction. Curr Opin Otolaryngol Head Neck Surg 2015;23(2):115–20.

19. Maricevich M, Lin LO, Liu J, et al. Interposition vein grafting in head and neck free flap reconstruction. Plast Reconstr Surg 2018;142(4):1025–34.

20. Seim NB, Old M, Petrisor D, et al. Head and neck free flap survival when requiring interposition vein grafting: a multi-instiutional review. Oral Oncol 2020;101:104482.

21. Rodriguez ED, Bluebond-Langner R, Park JE, et al. Preservation of contour in periorbital and midfacial craniofacial microsurgery: reconstruction of the soft-

tissue elements and skeletal buttresses. Plast Reconstr Surg 2008;121(5): 1738–47.

22. Moon DH, Moon SH, Wang K, et al. Incidence of, and risk factors for, mandibular osteoradionecrosis in patients with oral cavity and oropharynx cancers. Oral Oncol 2017;72:98–103.

23. Toneatti DJ, Graf RR, Burkhard JP, et al. Survival of dental implants and occurrence of osteoradionecrosis in irradiated head and neck cancer patients: a systematic review and meta-analysis. Clin Oral Investig 2021;25(10):5579–93.

24. Agarwal R, Freeman TE, Li MM, et al. Outcomes with culture-directed antibiotics following microvascular free tissue reconstruction for osteonecrosis of the jaw. Oral Oncol 2022;130:105878.

Lateral Skull Base and Auricular Reconstruction

Alexandra E. Kejner, MD[a],*, Byung Joo Lee, DMD, MD[b],
Patrik Pipkorn, MD[c]

KEYWORDS

- Lateral skull base • Auricular reconstruction • Optimizing free tissue for prosthetics

KEY POINTS

- Reconstruction of the lateral skull base can be accomplished by means of locoregional tissue reconstruction or free tissue transfer depending on the extent of the original defect, plan for prosthetics, and if there is plan for immediate facial nerve rehabilitation.
- Preservation of the ear canal can be challenging and be a source of infection if not managed appropriately.
- As many of these patients may undergo adjuvant radiotherapy, consideration of flap robustness and bulk are important.

INTRODUCTION

Surgery of the lateral skull base has evolved in scope as the ability to reconstruct has advanced. Neoadjuvant and adjuvant treatments, locoregional and microvascular techniques, as well as prosthetics now allow for more extensive resections and more elegant reconstruction and rehabilitation. Extirpation of tumors in this area can involve removal of cutaneous, cartilaginous, bony, salivary, vascular, and sometimes neurologic structures including dura and cranial nerves and its complexity requires thoughtful consideration of reconstructive options.[1] While this area is not at risk from salivary contamination, potential complications include infection, cerebrospinal fluid leak, meningitis, cranial nerve dysfunction (auditory, vestibular, facial nerve paralysis, dysphagia), in addition to cosmetic concerns.[2]

Prior to more widespread adoption of free tissue transfer, skin grafting, locoregional, and pedicled flaps were more commonly used.[3] Free flaps have become more universally adopted due to the facility of 2 team approaches for simultaneous resection and

[a] Division of Head & Neck Surgery, Medical University of South Carolina, 135 Rutledge Avenue MSC 550, Charleston, SC 29436, USA; [b] Division of Maxillofacial Prosthodontics, MUSC 135 Rutledge Avenue MSC 550, Charleston, SC 29436, USA; [c] Department of Otolaryngology-Head and Neck Surgery, Washington University School of Medicine, 660 South Euclid Avenue, Campus Box 8115, St. Louis, MO 63110, USA
* Corresponding author.
E-mail address: kejner@musc.edu

Otolaryngol Clin N Am 56 (2023) 715–726
https://doi.org/10.1016/j.otc.2023.04.016
0030-6665/23/© 2023 Elsevier Inc. All rights reserved.

harvest with potentially decreased operative time and ease of patient positioning. Microvascular techniques in conjunction with pedicled flaps have expanded the armamentarium of reconstruction as well.[2] Techniques for facial nerve reanimation can also substantially improved the potential quality of life for patients.[4]

Advances in prosthetic rehabilitation have improved cosmetic and functional outcomes for these patients. Since auricular reconstruction is complex and frequently requires multistage procedures to achieve cosmetically acceptable outcomes, prosthetics are frequently the better option. Unfortunately, financial constraints and difficulty in access to an anaplastologist which precludes many patients from proper rehabilitation.

Further refinements in the reconstruction of the lateral skull base and auricle will continue to develop. As biologic agents expand in usage and the number of surviving immunocompromised patients grows, the number of patients at risk for cutaneous malignancies will increase as will the need for advancing this area of reconstruction.[5]

DEFINITIONS

The lateral skull base can be defined as the combination of Regions II and III as described by Irish and colleagues.[6] This area lies directly over the middle cranial fossa, formed by the infratemporal and pterygopalatine fossae. Structures in this area include the internal carotid artery (ICA), the internal jugular vein (IJV), cranial nerves V2, V3, VII, VIII, IX, X, XI, XII.[7]

While these classifications (**Table 1**) can be useful, they do not include consideration for facial nerve deficits and so some reconstructive surgeons advocate for component classification: skin, soft tissue, osseous, cartilaginous, neural (dura and/or cranial nerve) in the context of patient characteristics (including prior radiotherapy, future need for radiotherapy, and prior head and neck surgery).[10,11]

Patel and colleagues designed an algorithm that also took into consideration whether the resection was a primary or a recurrent (secondary) procedure, with anticipated need for free or pedicled flap if postoperative radiotherapy needed or if in a salvage setting, or if a CSF leak with large dural defect was anticipated.[12] Defects at or below the zygomatic arch were also considered and anything above the zygomatic was recommended for free flap due to reach.[12] **Fig. 1** derives from Patel and colleagues's article demonstrates their proposed algorithm.

NONVASCULARIZED FLAPS

The use of dermal fat grafts, free fat grafts, or dermal substitutes can be feasible in small defects or for the ablation of a lateral temporal bone defect. However, fat

Table 1		
Anatomic and structure defect classification		
Homer et al[8] Anatomic Defect Classification		Rosenthal et al[9] Structure Defect Classification
• Advanced skin cancer of external ear including auricle, concha, or periauricular skin	Class I	Parotidectomy + skin loss, preservation of the EAC, ± mastoidectomy.
• Advanced parotid cancer	Class II	LTBR, middle ear obliteration, preservation of auricle.
• Infratemporal fossa and TMJ cancer • Primary EAC • Primary middle ear cancer	Class III	Encompassed LTBR, total auriculectomy, middle ear ablation, ± parotidectomy.

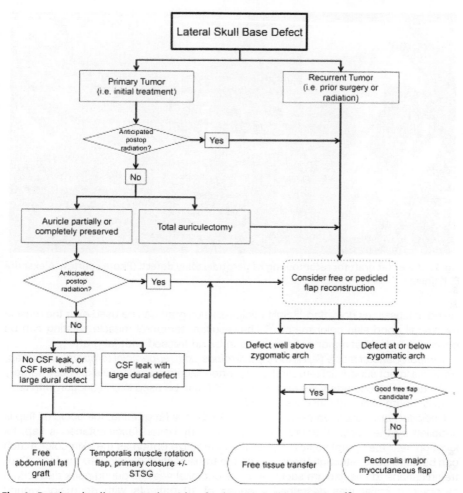

Fig. 1. Patel and colleagues's algorithm for lateral skull base defect.[12]

liquefaction, seroma, and resorption related to radiotherapy can put complications as high as 33%.[13,14] These grafts can be used in conjunction with other rotational flaps to optimize skin color match and increase vascularity.[15]

Ideal for: primary EAC cancer, volume repletion for parotidectomy contour, reinforcing CSF leak repair.

Pitfalls: Risk of liquefaction of fat, resorption of graft for patients undergoing radiation

Example: (**Fig. 2**).

LOCOREGIONAL FLAPS FOR LATERAL SKULL BASE RECONSTRUCTION

Temporalis muscle: Depending on the viability of the deep temporal artery, the temporalis flap is a useful reconstructive tool for defects of the lateral skull base. In a series of 18 patients undergoing temporalis muscle reconstruction, Thompson and colleagues noted a 42.9% complication rate including dehiscence, infection, hematoma, and stitch abscess, although this was not statistically significantly different from submental

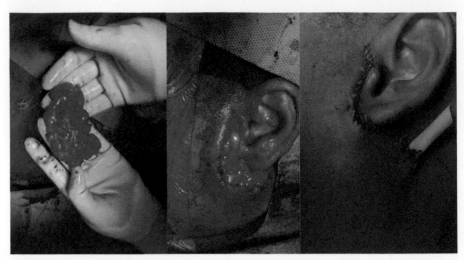

Fig. 2. Use of fat graft for recontouring of parotidectomy defect. (Photo courtesy Alexandra E. Kejner.)

island or latissimus dorsi flap.[16] Split thickness skin graft can be used over the muscle for overall good skin color match.[12] The resultant temporal muscle wasting can be cosmetically frustrating for patients but can be addressed with fat grafting.[14,17]

Temporoparietal fascia flap (TPFF) (plus/minus skin), superficial temporal artery flap: Requires intact superficial temporal artery (often sacrificed in lateral skull base surgery or if external carotid artery sacrificed.) The TPFF can be used in conjunction with temporalis if both skin and muscle are needed.

Occipital flap: Described in conjunction with dermal fat grafting, the occipital flap is supplied by the occipital artery and is an inferiorly based fasciocutaneous flap. Its location near the operative field makes it an attractive option as the skin color match can be quite good although there may be the translocation of hair onto the face. Contraindications to this flap are sacrifice of the occipital vessels during neck dissection. Moore and colleagues described a series of 10 patients with no major wound complications.[15]

Ideal for: Advanced skin cancer of external ear (auricle, concha, periauricular skin), primary EAC, primary middle ear cancer, Class I defects.

Pitfalls: Temporal muscle wasting, unavailability due to intraoperative sacrifice of feeding vessels (superficial temporal artery or occipital)

Example: (**Fig. 3**).

PEDICLED FLAPS

Supraclavicular artery island flap (SCAIF): Based on the transverse cervical vessels, the SCAIF is a versatile flap that has a good skin color match, arc of rotation, and is typically away from radiated fields. The span of the skin typically cannot extend more than 10 × 15 cm and in those situations, alternative donor site may be chosen. Care must be taken during the level IV dissection to avoid injury to the transverse cervical vessels.[11] Emerick and colleagues described 46 reconstructions using the SCAIF flap with minimal wound complications.[18]

Submental artery island flap: Perfused by the submental vessels which branch from the facial artery and vein, the submental flap can be harvested with good skin color

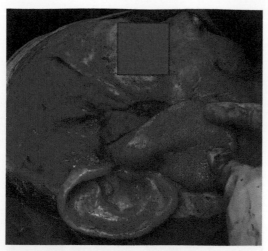

Fig. 3. Use of a hair-bearing tempoparietal fascia flap for reconstruction for a Class I defect (parotidectomy, skin loss, partial temporomandibular joint resection). (Photo courtesy Alexandra E. Kejner.)

match and in conjunction with neck dissection.[19] Ability to use this flap can be limited if there is extensive nodal involvement requiring sacrifice of the feeding vessels and preoperative computed tomography scans can be helpful in assessing its feasibility prior to surgery. See later in discussion for discussion regarding hybrid SMAIF flap.

Pectoralis major muscle flap (PMFF): Widely considered a work-horse flap for head and neck reconstruction, the PMFF has reliable anatomy and can include a skin paddle for reconstruction. Given the location of lateral skull base defects, use of the PMFF can sometimes be limited by vertical extent as well as be a poor skin-color match for this area.[12,20] However, its reliability, ease of harvest, and muscle bulk make it an excellent option for later in discussion zygomatic arch reconstruction.

Trapezius muscle flap: This flap can be either an upper trapezius or lower trapezius flap depending on the extent of defect and arc of rotation needed. First described for lateral skull base by Panje,[21] the flap can be harvested either prone or in the lateral decubitus position. It can cause significant dysfunction of the shoulder as well as pain and this is something that needs to be discussed with the patient prior to surgery. The benefit of the trapezius flap is muscle bulk with reliable vascular supply away from prior radiated areas.[11]

Latissimus dorsi tunneled flap: In head and neck reconstruction this flap is more commonly used as a free flap, however, can also be used as a pedicled flap. The flap can be tunneled through areolar space between the pectoralis minor and major. The flap is then further tunneled through transection and separation of the pectoralis muscles and the clavicle. The flap can then tension-free reach the lateral skull base.[22]

Ideal for: Advanced skin cancer of external ear (auricle, concha, periauricular skin), primary EAC, primary middle ear cancer, Class I, II, and III defects *below the zygoma*.

Pitfalls: Reach above the zygoma (except for hybrid submental artery island flaps), temporal muscle wasting, unavailability due to intraoperative sacrifice of feeding vessels (superficial temporal artery or occipital in advanced parotid cancer), significant shoulder dysfunction possible with trapezius muscle flap, cosmetic deformity from pectoralis flap as well as inability to reach above zygoma.

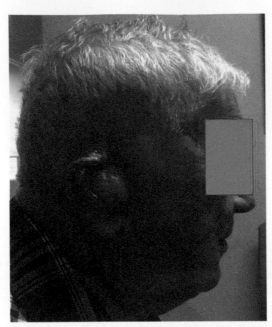

Fig. 4. Use of submental artery island flap for the reconstruction of Class II defect. (Photo courtesy of Kiran Kakarala MD FACS.)

Example: (**Fig. 4**)

FREE FLAPS
Myocutaneous Flaps

Anterolateral thigh (ALT): Based on the descending lateral descending circumflex, the anterolateral thigh is often considered the "work-horse" of free tissue transfer for the lateral skull base and auricle given its potential for chimerism, its ease of harvest in a two-team approach, long pedicle, and its relatively well-hidden donor site with minimal morbidity. An additional advantage of the ALT is that fascia lata can be harvested for static facial reanimation and/or the nerve to vastus lateralis may be harvested either as a cable graft or can be used in a chimeric fashion, utilizing a muscle component on its own perforator for facial nerve reanimation. Hasmat and colleagues described a series of 27 patients in which chimeric vastus lateralis and anterolateral thigh flap were designed for radical parotidectomy with associated skin resection.[23]

Subscapular system: The subscapular system lends itself well to the reconstruction of the lateral skull base again due to its potential for chimerism. Multiple components may be harvested, or a latissimus may be harvested with skin and minimal donor site morbidity. The scapular bone may be used for bony grafting if indicated. The use of the thoracodorsal artery as the main pedicle allows for increased pedicle length, which can be particularly useful for vessel-depleted necks.

Myocutaneous gracilis flap: The gracilis muscle is a long slender muscle in the medial compartment of the thigh. The upper part of the muscle can be harvested as a free flap based on terminal branches of the medial femoral circumflex artery and concomitant veins.[24] Initially described as pedicled flap for groin reconstruction, this flap has found multiple applications in free tissue reconstruction. In head and neck reconstruction it has primary been used in facial re-animation due to its ability to be harvested as an innervated flap through a branch of the obturator nerve. The flap can also be harvested with a skin paddle. Initial experience with the cutaneous component showed frequent distal necrosis, but better understanding through anatomic studies has improved the reliability of the cutaneous component.[25] Thus, if simultaneous dynamic facial reanimation is planned with need for a cutaneous component, this flap should be considered.

Rectus abdominis: The rectus abdominis flap is based on the inferior epigastric artery. This flap can provide a significant amount of muscle bulk and a large area of skin. For a long time, a very popular free flap for skull base reconstruction, this flap has largely been supplanted by the ALT flap due to lower risk of severe complications.[26] This flap is easy to raise, reliable, has a long pedicle and is located far enough from the head and neck area to allow for two team approach. However, the small but significant risk for abdominal hernia has made this decrease in popularity.[27]

Fasciocutaneous Flaps (Forearm, Posterior Tibial, Superficial Inferior Epigastric Artery)

Superficial inferior epigastric artery (SIEA) and muscle-sparing Deep Inferior Epigastric Perforator Flap: The SIEA and DIEP represent a useful donor site as it can provide a large quantity of vascularized fat and can be used for facial recontouring as well as skin replacement. The shorter and smaller pedicle diameter makes this site potentially less desirable than other listed flaps although it has been used extensively for breast reconstruction.[28,29]

Ideal for: Advanced skin cancer of external ear (auricle, concha, periauricular skin), primary EAC, primary middle ear cancer, Class I, II, and III defects.

Pitfalls: Vessel depleted neck, need for two team approach/length of operative time, donor site morbidity (hernia). Example: (**Fig. 5**).

Management of the External Auditory Canal (EAC): Preservation of patency of the external auditory canal in patients whose resection goes up to but does not include the EAC presents a substantial challenge to the reconstructive surgeon, particularly given its propensity to harboring bacteria.[30] If local options available, like the inferior pedicled square screw flap from the preauricular area,[31] these can be helpful in the reconstruction of this area, however, depending on the amount of skin resected, this may not be a viable option. Alternatively, planned obliteration with secondary recanalization can be attempted which can be technically challenging, particularly

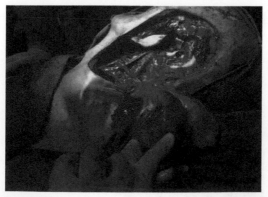

Fig. 5. Use of anterolateral thigh flap for the reconstruction of Class III defect. (Photo courtesy Alexandra E. Kejner.)

given the tendency toward collapse. Various techniques including full-thickness grafting after secondary reconstruction, stenting, and devices to stretch the external auditory canal have also been proposed.[32,33] However, anecdotally, many surgeons over time note transitioning away from EAC preservation given the propensity toward failure.

Example (**Fig. 6**): showing stenting of the neocanal

Facial reanimation: Several options are available at the time of reconstruction and can either be directly from the free flap chosen (gracilis myocutaneous, anterolateral thigh with vastus) as well as nerve grafts adjacent to donor sites (sural, nerve to vastus lateralis, nerve to latissimus, medial antebrachial cutaneous). Other facial reanimation techniques are discussed in later articles.

Lateral skull base bony defects: As noted by Arnaoutakis and colleagues, the indications for bony reconstruction continue to be debated on the bases of defect size, facial deformity, or a policy of always reconstructing any bone defect.[11] Titanium mesh and Polyetheretherketone (PEEK) implants have been utilized to reconstruct lateral temporal bone defects as have PEEK implants. Ceramics including porous hydroxyapatite as a single unit have also debuted as possible replacements for this area.[34] Any implant must be carefully considered as radiation and radiated tissue can have high rates of extrusion.[35]

Prosthetics in Lateral Skull Base Reconstruction

When auricular prosthetic rehabilitation is the end goal, the involvement of maxillofacial prosthodontist and anaplastologist even before resection and reconstruction is highly valuable. Prosthetic rehabilitation team could fabricate preoperative impression, 3D scans, surgical splint, surgical guide for endosseous implants, prototype of future prosthesis, and aid in successful reconstructive planning for optimizing future outcome. Effective prosthetic rehabilitation heavily depends on idealizing the surgical site and free flap design which should include the consideration of the placement of endosseous implants at the time of resection and reconstruction, removal of hair follicles at the future prosthetic site, and minimizing flap thickness to 7 mm or less especially around endosseous implant sites. There is a significantly higher patient acceptance rate for implant-retained prosthesis over adhesive-retained one due to complete elimination of needing medical adhesive and improvement in skin hygiene, retention, support, stability, longevity, and ease of prosthetic placement and maintenance.[36] Therefore, endosseous implant placement should be highly considered when

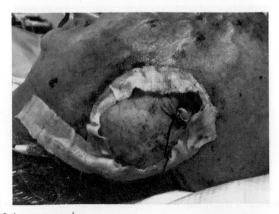

Fig. 6. Stenting of the neocanal.

planning resection and reconstruction. Hair underneath the prosthesis creates hygienic and maintenance issues for patients and thus should be removed. Because tall implant abutments around thick, mobile, free flap may increase skin reaction and implant failure rates, the thickness of the flap around the endosseous implants should be subcutaneously thinned as much as possible.[37] If 7 mm or less thickness of free flap around implants cannot be obtainable initially, patient will require future debulking procedure when uncovering implants. If endosseous implant placement is not feasible, the free flap design must also include few tight surface irregularities that will allow the prosthetic rehabilitation team and the patient to use as a reference to be able to repetitively and correctly position the prosthesis. Patients have the most difficulty correctly positioning and placing the adhesive-retained auricular prosthesis on a smooth free flap as there are minimum reference points other than the differing skin tones from native skin to the flap. With proper multidisciplinary planning and surgical design, optimum auricular prosthetic rehabilitation could be achieved as shown on photos above.

DISCUSSION

Advances in imaging, microvascular technique, prosthetics, and adjuvant therapies have led to improvements in the reconstruction of the lateral skull base. Approaching reconstruction in a thoughtful manner allows for the optimization of patient outcomes and aesthetics. This approach can be evaluated from a structure classification (Class I, II, III as described by Rosenthal and colleagues), or by a "component" approach: cutaneous, osseous, dural, and so forth.[2] Consideration of whether cutaneous, fasciocutaneous, myofasciocutaneous, or osteomyocutaneous is required can help guide choice of donor site as can need for facial nerve reanimation.

Additionally, anatomic considerations must also be considered. Patients with history of prior head and neck surgery or radiation have more limited vascular options regarding recipient vessels or regional, pedicled flaps as these vessels are often sacrificed during standard neck dissection or parotidectomy. Additionally, the use of locoregional flaps in patients with skin cancer or immunocompromised status may ultimately yield equally sun-damaged/at-risk skin for reconstruction as well as be limited if there is a history of multiple skin cancer resections in the past.[38]

Ultimately, the protection of lateral skull base structures including vessels, bone, and brain is of utmost importance. Concerning cosmesis, optimization after reconstruction for prosthetics can improve patient quality of life.

SUMMARY

Reconstruction of the auricular, periauricular structures, and lateral skull base should be approached in a systematic fashion to optimize outcomes. Intraoperative extent of extirpation can change based on tumor spread, thus, approaching this area with knowledge of available options and after having substantial discussion with the patient can optimize outcomes.

CLINICS CARE POINTS

- Choice of reconstruction should include the consideration of components involved, whether facial reanimation is needed, and patient characteristics (prior surgery or radiation that changes viability of certain flaps)[10,11,39]

- If postoperative radiation is likely, a reconstruction with more bulk is preferred to reduce the risk of lateral skull base osteomyelitis and extrusion of hardware.[11,20,35]

- Locoregional flaps including musculocutaneous submental island may reduce overall operative time, hospitalization, and the need for debulking procedures but may be limited in their vertical extent and are reliant on the preservation of the ipsilateral associated facial vessels.[2,11] However, hybrid flaps utilizing a free vessel anastomosis to the ipsilateral external jugular vein have been described for increased span.[40]

- Optimization for prosthetic rehabilitation may take refinements of free flap placement. Consideration for abutment placement at the time of surgery may be feasible in some patients. Irregular surfaces may be more amenable to adhesive-style prosthetics to allow for ease of use by the patient.

DISCLOSURE

The authors have nothing to disclosure

REFERENCES

1. Moncrieff MD, Hamilton SA, Lamberty GH, et al. Reconstructive options after temporal bone resection for squamous cell carcinoma. J Plast Reconstr Aesthet Surg 2007;60(6):607–14.
2. Howard BE, Nagel TH, Barrs DM, et al. Reconstruction of Lateral Skull Base Defects: A Comparison of the Submental Flap to Free and Regional Flaps. Otolaryngol Head Neck Surg 2016;154(6):1014–8.
3. Gal TJ, Kerschner JE, Futran ND, et al. Reconstruction after temporal bone resection. Laryngoscope 1998;108(4 Pt 1):476–81.
4. Thielker J, Wahdan A, Buentzel J, et al. Long-Term Facial Nerve Outcome in Primary Parotid Cancer Surgery: A Population-Based Analysis. Laryngoscope 2021; 131(12):2694–700.
5. Crisafulli S, Bertino L, Fontana A, et al. Incidence of Skin Cancer in Patients With Chronic Inflammatory Cutaneous Diseases on Targeted Therapies: A Systematic Review and Meta-Analysis of Observational Studies. Front Oncol 2021;11:687432.
6. Irish JC, Gullane PJ, Gentili F, et al. Tumors of the skull base: outcome and survival analysis of 77 cases. Head Neck 1994;16(1):3–10.
7. Thurnher D, Novak CB, Neligan PC, et al. Reconstruction of lateral skull base defects after tumor ablation. Skull Base 2007;17(1):79–88.
8. Homer JJ, Lesser T, Moffat D, et al. Management of lateral skull base cancer: United Kingdom National Multidisciplinary Guidelines. J Laryngol Otol 2016; 130(S2):S119–24.
9. Rosenthal EL, King T, McGrew BM, et al. Evolution of a paradigm for free tissue transfer reconstruction of lateral temporal bone defects. Head Neck 2008;30(5): 589–94.
10. Hanasono MM, Silva AK, Yu P, et al. Comprehensive management of temporal bone defects after oncologic resection. Laryngoscope 2012;122(12):2663–9.
11. Arnaoutakis D, Kadakia S, Abraham M, et al. Locoregional and Microvascular Free Tissue Reconstruction of the Lateral Skull Base. Semin Plast Surg 2017; 31(4):197–202.
12. Patel NS, Modest MC, Brobst TD, et al. Surgical management of lateral skull base defects. Laryngoscope 2016;126(8):1911–7.
13. Conger BT, Gourin CG. Free abdominal fat transfer for reconstruction of the total parotidectomy defect. Laryngoscope 2008;118(7):1186–90.

14. Davis RE, Guida RA, Cook TA. Autologous free dermal fat graft. Reconstruction of facial contour defects. Arch Otolaryngol Head Neck Surg 1995;121(1):95–100.
15. Moore MG, Lin DT, Mikulec AA, et al. The occipital flap for reconstruction after lateral temporal bone resection. Arch Otolaryngol Head Neck Surg 2008; 134(6):587–91.
16. Thompson NJ, Roche JP, Schularick NM, et al. Reconstruction Outcomes Following Lateral Skull Base Resection. Otol Neurotol 2017;38(2):264–71.
17. Yin D, Shen G. Aesthetic Effect of Autologous Fat Transplantation on Frontotemporal Depression Filling and Its Influence on SCL-90 and SES of Patients. Emerg Med Int 2022;2022:3374780.
18. Emerick KS, Herr MW, Lin DT, et al. Supraclavicular artery island flap for reconstruction of complex parotidectomy, lateral skull base, and total auriculectomy defects. JAMA Otolaryngol Head Neck Surg 2014;140(9):861–6.
19. Jorgensen MG, Tabatabaeifar S, Toyserkani NM, et al. Submental Island Flap versus Free Flap Reconstruction for Complex Head and Neck Defects. Otolaryngol Head Neck Surg 2019;161(6):946–53.
20. Ch'ng S, Ashford BG, Gao K, et al. Reconstruction of post-radical parotidectomy defects. Plast Reconstr Surg 2012;129(2):275e–87e.
21. Panje WR. Myocutaneous trapezius flap. Head Neck Surg 1980;2(3):206–12.
22. Feng AL, Nasser HB, Rosko AJ, et al. Revisiting pedicled latissimus dorsi flaps in head and neck reconstruction: contrasting shoulder morbidities across mysofascial flaps. Plast Aesthet Res 2021. https://doi.org/10.20517/2347-9264.2021.03.
23. Hasmat S, Low TH, Krishnan A, et al. Chimeric Vastus Lateralis and Anterolateral Thigh Flap for Restoring Facial Defects and Dynamic Function following Radical Parotidectomy. Plast Reconstr Surg 2019;144(5):853e–63e.
24. Mathes SJ, Nahai F. Classification of the vascular anatomy of muscles: experimental and clinical correlation. Plast Reconstr Surg 1981;67(2):177–87.
25. Chidester JR, Leland HA, Navo P, et al. Redefining the Anatomic Boundaries for Safe Dissection of the Skin Paddle in a Gracilis Myofasciocutaneous Free Flap: An Indocyanine Green Cadaveric Injection Study. Plast Reconstr Surg Glob Open 2018;6(12):e1994.
26. Zanoletti E, Mazzoni A, Martini A, et al. Surgery of the lateral skull base: a 50-year endeavour. Acta Otorhinolaryngol Ital 2019;39(SUPPL. 1):S1–146.
27. Chirappapha P, Trikunagonvong N, Prapruttam D, et al. Donor-Site Complications and Remnant of Rectus Abdominis Muscle Status after Transverse Rectus Abdominis Myocutaneous Flap Reconstruction. Plast Reconstr Surg Glob Open 2017;5(6):e1387.
28. Allen RJ, Kaplan J. Reconstruction of a parotidectomy defect using a paraumbilical perforator flap without deep inferior epigastric vessels. J Reconstr Microsurg 2000;16(4):255–7 [discussion: 258-9].
29. Alkureishi LWT, Bhayani MK, Sisco M. Superficial Inferior Epigastric Artery Flap for a Total Parotidectomy Defect. Eplasty 2017;17:e38.
30. Juan KH, Lin SR, Peng CF. [Bacterial flora of the external ear canal. 1. Cancer patients]. Gaoxiong Yi Xue Ke Xue Za Zhi 1990;6(8):418–21.
31. Anazawa U, Omura K, Nishijima Y, et al. External auditory canal reconstruction with inferior pedicled square screw flap from the preauricular area after resection of external auditory canal cancer. Laryngoscope Investig Otolaryngol 2021;6(1): 77–80.
32. Tirelli G, Nicastro L, Gatto A, et al. Stretching stenoses of the external auditory canal: a report of four cases and brief review of the literature. Acta Otorhinolaryngol Ital 2015;35(1):34–8.

33. Minoda R, Haruno T, Miwa T, et al. External auditory canal stenting utilizing a useful rolled, tapered silastic sheet (RTSS) post middle ear surgery. Auris Nasus Larynx 2010;37(6):680–4.
34. Stefini R, Esposito G, Zanotti B, et al. Use of "custom made" porous hydroxyapatite implants for cranioplasty: postoperative analysis of complications in 1549 patients. Surg Neurol Int 2013;4:12.
35. Richmon JD, Yarlagadda BB, Wax MK, et al. Locoregional and free flap reconstruction of the lateral skull base. Head Neck 2015;37(9):1387–91.
36. Chang TLGN, Roumanas E, Beumeur J III. Treatment satisfaction with facial prosthesis. J Prosthet Dent 2005;94:275–80.
37. Westin T, Tjellstrom A, Hammerlid E, et al. Long-term study of quality and safety of osseointegration for the retention of auricular prostheses. Otolaryngol Head Neck Surg 1999;121(1):133–43.
38. Monnier Y, Pasche P, Monnier P, et al. Second primary squamous cell carcinoma arising in cutaneous flap reconstructions of two head and neck cancer patients. Eur Arch Oto-Rhino-Laryngol 2008;265(7):831–5.
39. Vozel D, Pukl P, Groselj A, et al. The importance of flaps in reconstruction of locoregionally advanced lateral skull-base cancer defects: a tertiary otorhinolaryngology referral centre experience. Radiol Oncol 2021;55(3):323–32.
40. Hayden RE, Nagel TH, Donald CB. Hybrid submental flaps for reconstruction in the head and neck: part pedicled, part free. Laryngoscope 2014;124(3):637–41.

Anterior Skull Base Reconstruction

Samuel Racette, MD[a], Sruti Tekumalla, BA[b], Aarti Agarwal, MD[b],
Joseph Curry, MD[b], Donald David Beahm, MD[a],*

KEYWORDS

- Anterior skull base reconstruction • Loca flaps • Free tissue transfer
- Cerebrospinal fluid rhinorrhea

KEY POINTS

- The goals of skull base reconstruction include (1) watertight dural seal, (2) separation of sterile intracranial contents with vascularized tissue, (3) protection of exposed vessels and neural structures, and (4) restoration of facial contour.
- The size and location of the defect influence the decision for reconstruction material and complexity.
- Large defects or defects from open surgery often require vascularized tissue such as regional flaps or free tissue transfer.
- The anatomic spaces violated by ablation play an important role in choice of reconstructive technique.
- Advances in technology, such as virtual surgical planning, can be useful in complex anterior skull base reconstruction.

INTRODUCTION

The goal and challenge in anterior skull base (ASB) reconstruction are the ability to convert a complex three-dimensional defect into a safe and functional wound that is able to form a watertight dural seal, separating intracranial contents from the nonsterile cavities with vascularized tissue, protect exposed vessels and neural structures, restore three-dimensional appearance of bony and soft tissues, and reestablish the orbital and oropharyngeal cavities.[1,2] The ASB is a convex structure formed by the frontal, ethmoid, and sphenoid bones which house the anterior cranial fossa. The sinonasal and orbital intracranial structures are separated by thin osseous bone, and critical neurovascular structures are important to consider during resection and

a Department of Otolaryngology, University of Kansas Medical Center, Kansas City, KS, USA;
b Department of Otolaryngology, Thomas Jefferson University, Philadelphia, PA, USA
* Corresponding author.
E-mail addresses: racettesam@gmail.com (S.R.); sruti.tekumalla@jefferson.edu (S.T.); aarti.agarwal@jefferson.edu (A.A.); joseph.curry@jefferson.edu (J.C.); dbeahm@kumc.edu (D.D.B.)

Otolaryngol Clin N Am 56 (2023) 727–739
https://doi.org/10.1016/j.otc.2023.04.015
0030-6665/23/© 2023 Elsevier Inc. All rights reserved.

reconstruction (**Fig. 1**). Multilayer closure is often necessary to prevent cerebrospinal fluid (CSF) leak and resultant infection.[3]

ANATOMIC CLASSIFICATION AND APPROACH TO RECONSTRUCTION

There are several classification systems used to describe ASB defects, which can be useful in planning for reconstruction. One such system separates defects into four categories with the largest being category 1 and including at least one-half of the ASB with inclusion of orbit or maxilla and smallest category 4 defects are 1.5 cm or smaller.[4] A system focused on complex open defects described by Pusic and colleagues separates defects into middle and anterior cranial fossa. The ASB is further subdivided into central (cribriform and fovea ethmoidalis), lateral (orbital roof), and combined defects.[5] For endoscopic defects, some have used only size to classify defects which impacted the plan for repair, particularly when to use intranasal pedicled flaps.[6]

The approach to ASB reconstruction is often multifactorial, depending on surgeon preference and skill as well as individual patient characteristics, defect surface area and volume, location, presence of dural defect, and native tissue integrity. The disease process may impact this decision with higher rates of postoperative CSF leak being seen in resections of craniopharyngiomas and meningiomas or in cases of tumor resection after radiation therapy.[7,8] The size of the defect may be the most impactful with smaller defects, especially those less than 1 cm, requiring less complex repair. Larger defects and those with high-flow CSF leaks, such as those that connect with the intracranial cisterns and ventricles, have been shown to benefit from multilayered closure and transfer of vascularized tissue via a pedicled flap.[9] More complex defects spanning multiple anatomic sites created through open surgical resection may require free tissue transfer (FTT) for optimal closure.

SURGICAL TECHNIQUE

The approach to the ASB will inevitably be dictated by the pathology being addressed and as such the reconstruction will be dependent on this as well. In the case of CSF

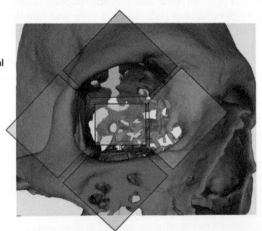

Superior:
- Orbital Roof
- Superior Orbital Fissure
- Frontal Sinus
- Orbital Rim

Lateral:
- Orbital Rim
- Inferior Orbital Fissure
- Middle fossa

Medial:
- Fovea ethmoidalis
- Cribriform plate
- Ethmoid
- Frontal outflow
- Nasal cavity

Orbital apex
- Ophthalmic artery
- Cavernous sinus
- Middle fossa

Inferior:
- Orbital floor
- Inferior orbital rim
- Maxillary sinus

Fig. 1. Anatomic landmarks in anterior skull base reconstruction. Reconstruction considerations include superior (*red*), inferior (*blue*), medial (*brown*), and lateral (*green*) anatomic structures.

leak due to trauma, idiopathic intracranial hypertension, congenital lesion, or arising iatrogenically, it is of paramount importance to identify the location(s) of the defect to adequately address the leak. Beta-2-transferrin is the preferred confirmatory test and initial imaging with high-resolution CT (computerized tomography) scan is recommended. In the instance of a positive beta-2-transferrin and no defect noted on CT or in cases where fluid cannot be collected for beta-2-transferrin, the use of either CT or MR cisternography with intrathecal contrast may be helpful. The use of intrathecal fluorescein intraoperatively can be useful in proper localization of the skull base defect.[10] While in the OR (operating room), a systematic approach and careful inspection of all preoperatively identified areas is recommended to avoid missing the primary lesion or in the instance of multiple defects.

In sinonasal or intracranial tumor resection, whether performed endoscopically or open, the defect is typically apparent and sizeable compared with those as mentioned above. In either instance, the surgeon should prepare the defect through stripping of mucosa and the elimination of any bone septations, which may not allow for an overlay repair to sit flush with the defect. Small bony defects may not be amenable to inlay repair due to size constraints. Careful bipolar cautery of the dural defect and any associated meningocele or encephalocele along with free graft as described below may be sufficient if the site has been properly prepared. This graft can be secured with a variety of commercially available tissue sealants as well as resorbable or non-resorbable packing.

In larger defects, the extracranial site requires preparation in the same way that smaller defects are prepared. A drill may be required to remove bony septations in order for free or vascularized tissue flaps to properly reach and/or heal without a tract allowing for continued leakage of CSF. Intracranial repair will be dictated by the tissue types, which remain, access to the defect, and surgeon preference. Suturing of synthetic dural replacement may be possible in open resections with dural defects, whereas the placement of grafts endoscopically may require larger grafts to be placed intracranially in underlay fashion whether intradural and/or along a remaining bony edges. In most instances of defects involving the dura, it is often preferable to perform a primary dural repair with inlay and/or only grafts followed by extradural repair with free graft or vascularized tissue to create a multilayered repair.[11]

In the remainder of this review, the authors focus on graft options and described techniques which are available to the skull base surgeon and instances in which these may be useful in addressing lesions or defects which may arise in the ASB.

FREE GRAFTS

The use of free grafts is well supported for small defects and low-flow CSF rhinorrhea. Grafts may be obtained from a variety of locations including the nasal floor and lateral nasal wall mucosa, inferior turbinate, middle turbinate, or the nasal septum.[9,12,13] External autografts include fascia lata, fat, and temporalis fascia.[14–17]

Fascia lata offers robust tissue for reconstruction and several harvesting methods have been described.[18,19] Complications after fascia lata are rare and long term relate to cosmetic appearance of the scar. Leg pain and functional limitations should be considered for young and physically active individuals.[20] Temporalis fascia has been shown to be biomechanically similar to dura, whereas fascia lata has been shown to be stiffer and less elastic.[21] Temporalis fascia is frequently used in facial plastic and otologic procedures and is highly reliable, and the morbidity of harvest is low. One algorithm in skull base reconstruction advocates for use of temporalis fascia in low-flow CSF leaks due to small dural tears.[22] Fat grafts are frequently obtained from abdomen although can be obtained from a leg incision if fascia lata is also being harvested. Fat autografting may be used to eliminate dead space after tumor resection and/or as an inlay in repair of CSF leak.[17,23] Postoperative imaging effects should be considered when using fat grafting.

INTRANASAL PEDICLED GRAFTS

The use of vascularized tissue has dramatically improved the ability to surgically close defects of the cranial base.[9] The most common intranasal pedicled flap is the nasoseptal flap, also known as the Hadad-Bassagasteguy flap.[24] Other flap options include the septal flip-flap, inferior turbinate, lateral nasal wall, middle turbinate, and superior turbinate flaps.[25-28]

The nasoseptal flap is based on the posterior septal artery which is a branch from the sphenopalatine artery. Skull base reconstruction with the nasoseptal flap has been shown to decrease incidence of CSF leak in the surgical treatment of a variety of pathologies.[9,29] The flap may be modified in size depending on location and size of the defect (**Fig. 2**). Benefits of the flap include location within the surgical corridor, ease of harvest, long pedicle, degree of possible rotation, and consistent vascularity. Perforations of the flap during harvest have not been shown to impact postoperative CSF leak rates especially when used with multilayered closures as the main benefit of the nasoseptal flap is the transfer of robust and well-vascularized tissue.[30]

The septal flip-flap, originally described in 2016, is a reconstructive option pedicled off the anterior and/or posterior ethmoid artery. It requires that involvement of the tumor or skull base defect does not extend to the contralateral nasal septum. It may be used to reconstruct contralateral cribriform defects yet requires sacrifice of the ipsilateral posterior septal artery.[25]

The inferior turbinate flap and the lateral nasal wall flap may be used in small cribriform, sellar, and clival defects. The flap can be pedicled posteriorly on the inferior turbinate artery or anteriorly on branches of the facial and anterior ethmoid system. A portion of inferior turbinate bone may be included within the harvest. The narrow width of the flap and location of pedicle limit the use of the flap for larger defects.

The middle turbinate flap may contribute to reconstruction of the fovea ethmoidalis, planum sphenoidale, cribriform, and sella and possibly may reach clival defects. It is pedicled posteriorly on the middle turbinate artery which is a branch of the sphenopalatine artery. Anatomic variations of the turbinate and size of defect to repair may

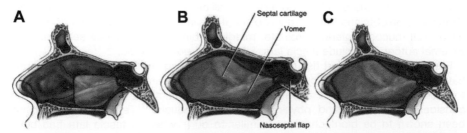

Fig. 2. Nasoseptal flap. Artist rendition of area of harvest with possible modifications including (*A*) primary area of the nasoseptal flap, (*B*) extension anteriorly to include entirety of anterior septum with exclusion of the olfactory strip, and (*C*) extension to nasal floor and lateral nasal wall. (*From* Atlas of Endoscopic Sinus and Skull Base Surgery with permission.[68])

increase difficulty or preclude use of the flap. It is primarily used for small to moderate sized planum, cribriform, or sellar defects.[27]

A superior turbinate flap also referred to as the superior turbinate osteoplastic flap is posteriorly based on several arteries including the posterior lateral nasal artery and posterior ethmoid artery. The flap includes both mucosa and bone of the superior turbinate and is limited by the small size of the turbinate and small rotational arc.[31]

EXTRA-NASAL PEDICLED GRAFTS

Several pedicled flaps from extra-nasal sources have been successfully used and are well described in reconstruction of the ASB.

The temporoparietal fascia flap is supplied by the anterior frontal branch of the superficial temporal artery. The flap can be widened to include the gala aponeurosis over the temporal line. To reach the nasal cavity, the flap must be tunneled. The flap can be lengthened to cover the ASB as well as lateral defects within the nasal cavity.[32]

The pericranial flap is well recognized in the reconstruction of the ASB and is frequently used during open resections. It is supplied by the supra-orbital artery, and branches of the supra-trochlear artery may contribute to the vascular supply. The flap may be elevated from a coronal incision or minimally invasive endoscopic technique.[33] The flap requires bony osteotomies in the anterior table of the frontal sinus to be created and frequently a Draf III (modified endoscopic Lothrop) frontal sinusotomy to prevent mucocele of the frontal sinus due to obstruction from the passage of the flap.[34]

Several alternatives exist including flaps from palatal, pharyngeal, facial artery myomucosal, and buccal fat pad have been described to reconstruct regions of the ASB in situations where more traditional means have been unavailable.[35,36]

FREE TISSUE TRANSFER

FTT allows reliable reconstruction of large defects and can avoid pedicle length restrictions. FTT can include bone which may be used to support native structures, obliterate dead space, and provide a watertight seal.[37] Historically, when compared with regional flaps, FTT has shown improved wound healing and prevention of CNS (central nervous system) complications.[1] Locoregional flaps in some cases are less durable against radiation, whereas FTT is robust enough for rapid initiation of postoperative radiation.[38]

Flap selection is an important consideration. The rectus abdominis flap was the original FTT flap of choice; however, this has largely been supplanted by the anterior lateral thigh (ALT) and radial forearm free flap (RFFF).[37,39,40] The ALT flaps provides a large skin paddle with significant tissue bulk and can be used in a chimeric fashion.[41] It carries minimal donor site morbidity; however, it has a shorter pedicle length than the RFFF. RFFFs are a reliable option when thinner flaps are needed, or the patient's lower extremity precludes use of the ALT. The RFFF is a pliable flap, allowing folding and contour flexibility good for scalp and fascial coverage with a long pedicle (up to 15 cm) and better skin matching than the ALT.[40]

Defects involving the orbital rims, nasal bones, or craniofacial buttresses may be reconstructed with osseous free tissue to improve cosmetic outcomes and functionality. Fibular free flaps (FFFs) are commonly used in these scenarios for their availability of bone stock and option of an accompanying skin paddle harvest. The FFF provides a large, thin skin paddle with a reported size as high as 14 cm by 24 cm and long bony segment up to 25 cm length.[42] The FFF may also be harvested in multiple segments, allowing for precision contouring and possibly greater facial symmetry.[43] The malleable skin paddle of the FFF lends itself well to being de-epithelialized and buried to aid in sealing the skull base while overlaying bone can be used for simultaneous reconstruction of orbitomaxillary defects.[40] A layered approach to osteocutaneous FFF has been described by Shipchandler and colleagues[44] as a favorable choice for long-term outcomes in total maxillectomy patients. Subscapular system free flaps are also uniquely suited for this purpose. Compared with the FFF, the subscapular arterial system is generally protected from atherosclerotic disease, promoting flap longevity.[45] Not only can bone be harvested from the lateral scapular border and scapular tip, but it also allows for chimeric flaps. These can be harvested in various combinations, adding parascapular and scapular skin paddles, latissimus muscle (with or without skin), serratus muscle, and rib. These can also be harvested from separate pedicles, which allow more freedom of movement. The lateral border of the scapula is thicker bone that may be adequate to take dental implants or reconstruct the frontal bar, where the tip is ideal for maxillary reconstruction.[46]

TECHNIQUES

There are several methods which have been described to close defects and repair CSF leak in ASB surgery. These include several methods of multilayered repair, the gasket seal, and button graft. The direct comparison of different techniques is difficult due to high degree of heterogeneity between groups and differences in implementation of repair techniques. Our algorithm for repair is shown in **Fig. 3** with specific techniques and materials dependent on surgeon preference.

There is evidence that the repair of low-flow CSF leak is successful using a variety of techniques and outcomes for these patients are similar to those with no intraoperative CSF leak.[47] Multilayered repair is advocated in repairing more complex defects. Precise dural replacement inlay is imperative to successful repair. Tucking these edges under remaining bone to bolster the repair allows for improved graft stability. This can be further bolstered by onlay of vascularized tissue from one of the grafts as described previously.[16,29,48]

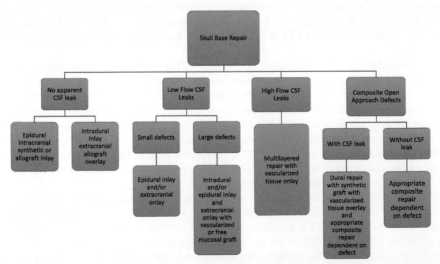

Fig. 3. Skull base repair algorithm. Approach to reconstruction of skull base defects based on the presence of CSF leak, size, and composition of the defect.

The gasket seal technique has been shown to reduce the rate of CSF leak after skull base repair to 4.7%. The technique originally described used fascia lata as the free graft and included placement of intracranial fat to eliminate dead space. The fascial or synthetic free graft onlay of the entire defect is extended well beyond the edges of the bony defect. A rigid reconstruction of a free bone graft or synthetic implant sized to the same size as the defect is then used as a countersink to firmly secure the free graft in place. This technique requires a bony rim.[49]

Button grafts (**Fig. 4**) were originally described in 2010 with two pieces of fascia lata secured together with an inlay component approximately 25% larger than the defect and an onlay component 5% larger. By suturing the grafts together, the grafts stabilize each other and prevent graft migration, which is a major reason for reconstruction failure. The button graft was combined with or without a nasoseptal flap with a CSF leak rate of 10%, representing a significant improvement before the use of the button graft.[50]

COMPLICATIONS
Anterior Skull Base and Sinonasal Cavity

Following reconstruction of the skull base a variety of complications may arise. These include, but are not limited to, graft displacement, flap compromise and breakdown, postoperative CSF leak, pneumocephalus, sinonasal or intracranial infection,

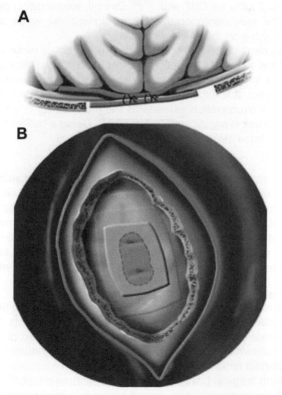

Fig. 4. Button repair technique. Artist illustration of the button repair technique with (*A*) placement of the larger side intradurally and sutured to the smaller portion placed as an overlay. (*B*) Endoscopic view of the button placed within the dural defect. (*Adapted from* Luginbuhl et al., 2010 with permission.[50])

mucoceles, fistula, nasal valve stenosis, and hardware infection.[51] Infection of synthetic implants and cements frequently require revision surgery to remove and reconstruct due to difficulty in clearing the infection with medical treatment alone.

Postoperative CSF leak has been managed with CSF diversion, but many require earlier repair to avoid intracranial infection.[52] Adjuvant treatment of skull base pathology with radiotherapy may lead to breakdown of repairs and subsequent delayed CSF leak. This must be considered and emphasizes the importance of routine vigilant follow-up for this patient cohort. The incidence of complications has been dramatically reduced with the use of vascularized pedicled flaps as the incidence of postoperative CSF leak has been reduced.[53]

Orbit

The challenging nature of volume assessment when resecting multiple orbital walls can put the patient at risk of orbital dystopia, enophthalmos, and diplopia. Careful preoperative planning including VSP can help optimize position of the eye in the final reconstruction. Supporting the orbital contents with a free fascial graft can help with positioning, whereas the bony reconstruction is underway.[54] Reconstructive challenges with exenteration include restoring volume to the orbit, midface, and sinonasal cavities while supporting CNS structures. Exenteration may expose the dura and CSF leak can be an expected intraoperative complication with reported rates of dural exposure of 20.5% and 30.8% for CSF leak.[55,56] Overall, exenteration poses a 0.6% to 16.7% risk for CSF leak postoperatively with highest risk when aggressive skull base requirement or the orbital apex is involved.[57]

If the orbital rims remain intact after exenteration, soft tissue reconstruction is regularly used.[2] Thin flaps are used to maintain orbital concavity and facilitate implants, but when the medial or inferior orbital walls are absent fistula risk increases. When the orbital roof is resected, it is important to ensure adequate tissue volume to prevent CSF leak.[58,59] When exenteration extends to the nasal cavity or paranasal sinuses, naso-orbital fistulas risk is significantly increased.[60] Using a bulkier flap can improve support of the skull base closure.[2]

Dental restoration

The possibility of dental restoration should be kept in mind to optimize postoperative quality of life and functional rehabilitation. There has been a decrease in obturator use over the past two decades with shifts toward osteocutaneous free flap use with immediate placement of dental implants.[61] Scapula and fibula osteocutaneous flaps have been successful at rates as high as 97.6%.[62,63] Advantages of this method include greater access for placement, decreasing the need for periosteum stripping. Implants have been shown to have a longer lifespan when placed before adjuvant radiotherapy.[64]

Use of virtual surgical planning

Virtual surgical planning (VSP) allows visualization of the surgical reconstruction based on multiplanar modalities using 3D imaging computer software (**Fig. 5**). Navigation of patient-specific tumor before reconstruction allows for improved planning. Although VSP has not been shown to decrease surgical complications, studies suggest shorter operative and ischemia times with increased reconstructive accuracy. This is thought to be due to shifting surgical planning to the preoperative phase.[65,66] Although VSP has traditionally been criticized for increased costs, one study showed no significant difference in total cost between VSP and non-VSP midface cases.[67] VSP also has great utility in secondary reconstructions when the anatomy of the defect side has already been altered by using a mirror image of the "normal" side.[66]

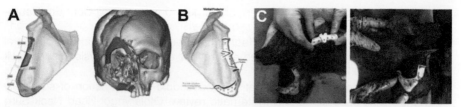

Fig. 5. Virtual surgical planning (VSP) for significant orbito-maxillary defect. (*A*) VSP of three-segment scapula lateral border and tip free flap for orbito-maxillary defect. (*B*) Custom cutting guides placed on VSP scapula model. (*C*) Intraoperative use of cutting guides after harvest of scapular free flap.

SUMMARY

ASB reconstruction requires careful preoperative planning to use the most effective technique for the expected defect. Adherence to the principles of skull base reconstruction is imperative to minimize complications and improve patient outcomes.

CLINICS CARE POINTS

- Multilayered closure should be used when possible for closure of anterior skull base defects.
- The resection of multiple anatomic subsites may require larger repairs including local pedicled tissue transfer or free tissue transfer for adequate closure of the defect and functional reconstruction.
- Multiple techniques have been described for closure of anterior skull base defects, but none demonstrate superiority.

DISCLOSURES

There are no relevant disclosures for any of the authors of this article.

REFERENCES

1. Neligan PC, Mulholland S, Irish J, et al. Flap selection in cranial base reconstruction. Plast Reconstr Surg 1996;98(7):1159–66 [discussion: 1167-1158].
2. Swendseid B, Chaskes M, Philips R, et al. Free tissue transfer for skull base reconstruction - a review. Plastic and Aesthetic Research 2021;8:41.
3. Gullane PJ, Lipa JE, Novak CB, et al. Reconstruction of skull base defects. Clin Plast Surg 2005;32(3):391–9, vii.
4. Nameki H, Kato T, Nameki I, et al. Selective reconstructive options for the anterior skull base. Int J Clin Oncol 2005;10(4):223–8.
5. Pusic AL, Chen CM, Patel S, et al. Microvascular reconstruction of the skull base: a clinical approach to surgical defect classification and flap selection. Skull Base 2007;17(1):5–15.
6. Clavenna MJ, Turner JH, Chandra RK. Pedicled flaps in endoscopic skull base reconstruction: review of current techniques. Curr Opin Otolaryngol Head Neck Surg 2015;23(1):71–7.
7. Munich SA, Fenstermaker RA, Fabiano AJ, et al. Cranial base repair with combined vascularized nasal septal flap and autologous tissue graft following

expanded endonasal endoscopic neurosurgery. J Neurol Surg Cent Eur Neurosurg 2013;74(2):101–8.

8. Yong M, Wu YQ, Su S, et al. The effect of prior radiation on the success of ventral skull base reconstruction: a systematic review and meta-analysis. Head Neck 2021;43(9):2795–806.

9. Soudry E, Turner JH, Nayak JV, et al. Endoscopic reconstruction of surgically created skull base defects: a systematic review. Otolaryngol Head Neck Surg 2014;150(5):730–8.

10. Oakley GM, Alt JA, Schlosser RJ, et al. Diagnosis of cerebrospinal fluid rhinorrhea: an evidence-based review with recommendations. Int Forum Allergy Rhinol 2016;6(1):8–16.

11. Snyderman CH, Wang EW, Zenonos GA, et al. Reconstruction after endoscopic surgery for skull base malignancies. J Neuro Oncol 2020;150(3):463–8.

12. Suh JD, Ramakrishnan VR, DeConde AS. Nasal floor free mucosal graft for skull base reconstruction and cerebrospinal fluid leak repair. Ann Otol Rhinol Laryngol 2012;121(2):91–5.

13. Peris-Celda M, Chaskes M, Lee DD, et al. Optimizing sellar reconstruction after pituitary surgery with free mucosal graft: results from the first 50 consecutive patients. World Neurosurg 2017;101:180–5.

14. El-Banhawy OA, Halaka AN, El-Hafiz Shehab El-Dien A, et al. Subcranial transnasal repair of cerebrospinal fluid rhinorrhea with free autologous grafts by the combined overlay and underlay techniques. Minim Invasive Neurosurg 2004; 47(4):197–202.

15. Kim BK, Kong DS, Nam DH, et al. Comparison of graft materials in multilayer reconstruction with nasoseptal flap for high-flow CSF leak during endoscopic skull base surgery. J Clin Med 2022;11(22):6711.

16. Ringel B, Abergel A, Horowitz G, et al. Skull base reconstruction with multilayered fascia lata: a single-center 17 years experience. J Neurol Surg B Skull Base 2021; 82(Suppl 3):e217–23.

17. Ahn S, Park JS, Kim DH, et al. Surgical experience in prevention of postoperative CSF leaks using abdominal fat grafts in endoscopic endonasal transsphenoidal surgery for pituitary adenomas. J Neurol Surg B Skull Base 2021;82(5):522–7.

18. Skoch J, Avila MJ, Fennell VS, et al. A Minimally invasive endoscopic technique for fascia lata graft acquisition and fascial reapproximation. Oper Neurosurg (Hagerstown) 2020;19(6):735–40.

19. Bhatti AF, Soueid A, Baden JM, et al. Fascia lata harvesting: minimal access for maximum harvest. A new technique. Plast Reconstr Surg 2010;126(5):277e–8e.

20. Giovannetti F, Barbera G, Priore P, et al. Fascia lata harvesting: the donor site closure morbidity. J Craniofac Surg 2019;30(4):e303–6.

21. Puksec M, Semenski D, Jezek D, et al. Biomechanical comparison of the temporalis muscle fascia, the fascia lata, and the dura mater. J Neurol Surg B Skull Base 2019;80(1):23–30.

22. Gil Z, Abergel A, Leider-Trejo L, et al. A comprehensive algorithm for anterior skull base reconstruction after oncological resections. Skull Base 2007;17(1):25–37.

23. Bohoun CA, Goto T, Morisako H, et al. Skull base dural repair using autologous fat as a dural substitute: an efficient technique. World Neurosurg 2019;127: e896–900.

24. Hadad G, Bassagasteguy L, Carrau RL, et al. A novel reconstructive technique after endoscopic expanded endonasal approaches: vascular pedicle nasoseptal flap. Laryngoscope 2006;116(10):1882–6.

25. Battaglia P, Turri-Zanoni M, De Bernardi F, et al. Septal flip flap for anterior skull base reconstruction after endoscopic resection of sinonasal cancers: preliminary outcomes. Acta Otorhinolaryngol Ital 2016;36(3):194–8.

26. Fortes FS, Carrau RL, Snyderman CH, et al. The posterior pedicle inferior turbinate flap: a new vascularized flap for skull base reconstruction. Laryngoscope 2007;117(8):1329–32.

27. Prevedello DM, Barges-Coll J, Fernandez-Miranda JC, et al. Middle turbinate flap for skull base reconstruction: cadaveric feasibility study. Laryngoscope 2009; 119(11):2094–8.

28. Hadad G, Rivera-Serrano CM, Bassagaisteguy LH, et al. Anterior pedicle lateral nasal wall flap: a novel technique for the reconstruction of anterior skull base defects. Laryngoscope 2011;121(8):1606–10.

29. Harvey RJ, Parmar P, Sacks R, et al. Endoscopic skull base reconstruction of large dural defects: a systematic review of published evidence. Laryngoscope 2012;122(2):452–9.

30. Huntley C, Iloreta AM, Nyquist GG, et al. Perforation of a nasoseptal flap does not increase the rate of postoperative cerebrospinal fluid leak. Int Forum Allergy Rhinol 2015;5(4):353–5.

31. Do HF A, Kshettry V, Nyquist GG, et al. Endonasal vascularized flaps for cranial base reconstruction. JHN Journal 2015;10(2):28–31.

32. Fortes FS, Carrau RL, Snyderman CH, et al. Transpterygoid transposition of a temporoparietal fascia flap: a new method for skull base reconstruction after endoscopic expanded endonasal approaches. Laryngoscope 2007;117(6): 970–6.

33. Zanation AM, Snyderman CH, Carrau RL, et al. Minimally invasive endoscopic pericranial flap: a new method for endonasal skull base reconstruction. Laryngoscope 2009;119(1):13–8.

34. Patel MR, Shah RN, Snyderman CH, et al. Pericranial flap for endoscopic anterior skull-base reconstruction: clinical outcomes and radioanatomic analysis of preoperative planning. Neurosurgery 2010;66(3):506–12 [discussion: 512].

35. Kim GG, Hang AX, Mitchell CA, et al. Pedicled extranasal flaps in skull base reconstruction. Adv Oto-Rhino-Laryngol 2013;74:71–80.

36. Pezato R, Dassi C, Stamm AC, et al. New nasopharyngeal flap for posterior skull-base reconstruction: the upper-tongue flap. Int Arch Otorhinolaryngol 2022;26(3): e467–9.

37. Ein L, Sargi Z, Nicolli EA. Update on anterior skull base reconstruction. Curr Opin Otolaryngol Head Neck Surg 2019;27(5):426–30.

38. Moyer JS, Chepeha DB, Teknos TN. Contemporary skull base reconstruction. Curr Opin Otolaryngol Head Neck Surg 2004;12(4):294–9.

39. Teknos TN, Smith JC, Day TA, et al. Microvascular free tissue transfer in reconstructing skull base defects: lessons learned. Laryngoscope 2002;112(10): 1871–6.

40. Bell EB, Cohen ER, Sargi Z, et al. Free tissue reconstruction of the anterior skull base: a review. World J Otorhinolaryngol Head Neck Surg 2020;6(2):132–6.

41. Karonidis A, Ren Chang L. Using the distal part of vastus lateralis muscle as chimeric anterolateral thigh free flap is a more flexible tool for head and neck reconstruction. Eur J Plast Surg 2010;33:1–5.

42. Al Deek NF, Kao HK, Wei FC. The fibula osteoseptocutaneous flap: concise review, goal-oriented surgical technique, and tips and tricks. Plast Reconstr Surg 2018;142(6):913e–23e.

43. Futran ND, Wadsworth JT, Villaret D, et al. Midface reconstruction with the fibula free flap. Arch Otolaryngol Head Neck Surg 2002;128(2):161–6.
44. Shipchandler TZ, Waters HH, Knott PD, et al. Orbitomaxillary reconstruction using the layered fibula osteocutaneous flap. Arch Facial Plast Surg 2012;14(2):110–5.
45. Brown J, Bekiroglu F, Shaw R. Indications for the scapular flap in reconstructions of the head and neck. Br J Oral Maxillofac Surg 2010;48(5):331–7.
46. Tracy JC, Brandon B, Patel SN. Scapular tip free flap in composite head and neck reconstruction. Otolaryngol Head Neck Surg 2019;160(1):57–62.
47. Di Perna G, Penner F, Cofano F, et al. Skull base reconstruction: a question of flow? A critical analysis of 521 endoscopic endonasal surgeries. PLoS One 2021;16(3):e0245119.
48. Cavallo LM, Solari D, Somma T, et al. The 3F (fat, flap, and flash) technique for skull base reconstruction after endoscopic endonasal suprasellar approach. World Neurosurg 2019;126:439–46.
49. Garcia-Navarro V, Anand VK, Schwartz TH. Gasket seal closure for extended endonasal endoscopic skull base surgery: efficacy in a large case series. World Neurosurg 2013;80(5):563–8.
50. Luginbuhl AJ, Campbell PG, Evans J, et al. Endoscopic repair of high-flow cranial base defects using a bilayer button. Laryngoscope 2010;120(5):876–80.
51. Ransom ER, Chiu AG. Prevention and management of complications in intracranial endoscopic skull base surgery. Otolaryngol Clin North Am 2010;43(4):875–95.
52. Tien DA, Stokken JK, Recinos PF, et al. Comprehensive postoperative management after endoscopic skull base surgery. Otolaryngol Clin North Am 2016;49(1):253–63.
53. Zamanipoor Najafabadi AH, Khan DZ, Muskens IS, et al. Trends in cerebrospinal fluid leak rates following the extended endoscopic endonasal approach for anterior skull base meningioma: a meta-analysis over the last 20 years. Acta Neurochir 2021;163(3):711–9.
54. Jelks G, Smith B, McCarthy J. Reconstruction of the eyelids and associated structures. Plastic Surgery 1990;2:1671–784.
55. Limawararut V, Valenzuela AA, Sullivan TJ, et al. Cerebrospinal fluid leaks in orbital and lacrimal surgery. Surv Ophthalmol 2008;53(3):274–84.
56. de Conciliis C, Bonavolontà G. Incidence and treatment of dural exposure and CSF leak during orbital exenteration. Ophthal Plast Reconstr Surg 1987;3(2):61–4.
57. Gill KS, Hsu D, Tassone P, et al. Postoperative cerebrospinal fluid leak after microvascular reconstruction of craniofacial defects with orbital exenteration. Laryngoscope 2017;127(4):835–41.
58. Yuen HK, Cheng AC, Auyeung KC. Late-onset occult cerebrospinal fluid leakage after orbital exenteration. Ophthal Plast Reconstr Surg 2008;24(3):238–40.
59. Tassone P, Gill KS, Hsu D, et al. Naso- or orbitocutaneous fistulas after free flap reconstruction of orbital exenteration defects: retrospective study, systematic review, and meta-analysis. J Neurol Surg B Skull Base 2017;78(4):337–45.
60. Goldberg RA, Kim JW, Shorr N. Orbital exenteration: results of an individualized approach. Ophthal Plast Reconstr Surg 2003;19(3):229–36.
61. Alani A, Owens J, Dewan K, et al. A national survey of oral and maxillofacial surgeons' attitudes towards the treatment and dental rehabilitation of oral cancer patients. Braz Dent J 2009;207(11):E21 [discussion: 540-541].
62. Burgess M, Leung M, Chellapah A, et al. Osseointegrated implants into a variety of composite free flaps: a comparative analysis. Head Neck 2017;39(3):443–7.

63. Lanzer M, Gander T, Grätz K, et al. Scapular free vascularised bone flaps for mandibular reconstruction: are dental implants possible? J Oral Maxillofac Res 2015;6(3):e4.

64. Ch'ng S, Skoracki RJ, Selber JC, et al. Osseointegrated implant-based dental rehabilitation in head and neck reconstruction patients. Head Neck 2016; 38(Suppl 1):E321–7.

65. Eskander A, Kang SY, Teknos TN, et al. Advances in midface reconstruction: beyond the reconstructive ladder. Curr Opin Otolaryngol Head Neck Surg 2017;25(5):422–30.

66. Swendseid BP, Roden DF, Vimawala S, et al. Virtual surgical planning in subscapular system free flap reconstruction of midface defects. Oral Oncol 2020;101: 104508.

67. Alnemri A, Philips R, Sussman S, et al. Analysis of cost and outcomes in bony versus soft tissue midface free flap reconstruction. Head Neck 2022;44(8): 1896–908.

68. Sansoni ER, Harvey RJ. Large skull base defect reconstruction with and without pedicled flaps. In: Chiu AG, Palmer JN, Adappa ND, editors. *Atlas of endoscopic Sinus and Skull base Surgery.* 2nd edition. Philadelphia, PA: Elsevier; 2019. p. 285–97.

Scalp and Calvarium Reconstruction

Ciaran Lane, MD, MSc[a],*, Alice Lin, MD[b,1], Neerav Goyal, MD, MPH[a,1]

KEYWORDS

- Scalp reconstruction • Calvarium reconstruction • Microvascular reconstruction
- Plastic surgery • Cranioplasty

KEY POINTS

- The primary goal of scalp and calvarium reconstruction is to provide a protective barrier for the brain.
- Use the simplest reconstruction method while meeting patient goals.
- Stage reconstruction in infected wounds or with unclear tumor margins.
- Consider vascularized tissue in patients with prior radiation or poor wound healing.
- Biocompatible materials provide good strength and cosmesis for large calvarium defects.

BACKGROUND

The scalp is an unprotected area of the body leaving it prone to trauma and skin cancer. Those at risk for skin cancer tend to have more than one skin cancer in a lifetime, and the number increases with advanced age. Thus, scalp reconstruction becomes more complex over a patient's lifetime as age and medical comorbidities accumulate. Mohs surgery is the most common treatment of skin cancer often performed in the outpatient setting. Patients may require adjuvant treatment with radiation therapy, thereby limiting reconstructive options. The thickness of the scalp also decreases in the elderly resulting in increased laxity, providing less protection of the calvarium, and increasing the risk of operative complications. In those patients with thin scalps or thin reconstructions, there can be a tendency of the reconstruction to breakdown, expose bone, and prolong healing. Choosing the best reconstruction for the scalp and calvarium needs to be individualized to the patient with attention to the history and

[a] Department of Otolaryngology–Head and Neck Surgery, The Pennsylvania State University, College of Medicine, 500 University Drive MC H091, Hershey, PA 17033, USA; [b] Department of Clinical Sciences, Kaiser Permanente School of Medicine, 4900 Sunset Boulevard 6th Floor, Los Angeles, CA 90027, USA
[1] Co-Senior authors.
* Corresponding author.
E-mail address: lanec345@myumanitoba.ca

Otolaryngol Clin N Am 56 (2023) 741–755
https://doi.org/10.1016/j.otc.2023.04.003
0030-6665/23/© 2023 Elsevier Inc. All rights reserved.

postoperative plan in coordination with the longitudinal multidisciplinary care of the patient to maximize success.

ANATOMY
Borders of the Scalp

- Anterior–Superior orbital rim
- Posterior–Superior nuchal line
- Lateral–External auditory meatus

Layers of the Scalp

- S–**S**kin
- C–sub**C**utaneous tissue
- A–galea **A**poneurosis
- L–**L**oose areolar tissue
- P–**P**eriosteum

The forehead constitutes the non–hair-bearing portion of the scalp. There are 5 layers to the scalp. Local reconstruction relies on the rich vascular network just superficial to the galeal layer. In addition, the loose areolar layer allows an easy plane of dissection for wide undermining. The periosteal layer is tightly adherent to the bone via Sharpey fibers and can provide a clear margin for deeply infiltrative tumors.

BLOOD SUPPLY
Blood Supply to Skin and Galea

- Anterior–supraorbital and supratrochlear a. (branches of internal carotid a.) (**Fig. 1**)
- Lateral–superficial temporal a. and postauricular a. (branches of external carotid a.)
- Posterior–occipital a. (branch of external carotid a.)

Blood supply to the pericranium and calvarial bone comes from the middle meningeal artery. The pericranium is independent of the vascular network associated with

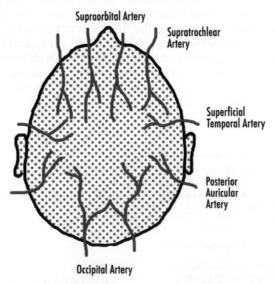

Fig. 1. Arterial blood supply of the scalp.

the galea except anteriorly where there are deep branches from the supraorbital and supratrochlear arteries in the galea-frontalis layer course deeply to supply the pericranium at or just superior to the orbital rim creating the blood supply of the anteriorly based pericranial flap.[1,2]

Calvaria

The calvaria is the superior portion of the frontal, parietal, and occipital cranial bones and is underlying the scalp. There are 3 layers of bone: the outer and inner layers are made of compact bone and the middle layer is a layer of cancellous bone called the diploic space. The diploic space contains bone marrow and a network of draining veins, the diploic veins, and hence is a much more vascular layer than the inner and outer table. The outer table tends to be thicker than the inner table as the inner table is thinned by underlying major blood vessels and arachnoid granulations of the brain.

PATIENT EVALUATION

The initial reconstruction evaluation of a scalp or calvarium defect should involve a thorough history and examination of the patient. Reconstruction can be performed primarily or in a delayed fashion. Delayed reconstruction may be preferred when the wound is grossly infected or while awaiting the final margins of a tumor resection.[3] This decision may involve a discussion between the reconstructive and ablative surgeon.

History

The initial history should include a detailed record of earlier head and neck surgery to gain insight into previous healing issues, earlier reconstructions, and the availability of donor vessels. Medical comorbidities such as vascular disease, immunosuppression due to disease, transplant status, and so forth, diabetes, and colonization with virulent bacteria are important to elicit. Lifestyle factors such as smoking or alcohol dependence will contribute to perioperative risk. Even a temporary abstention from smoking surrounding the surgery and reconstruction can improve reconstructive outcomes.

Examination

The examination should include an estimate of defect size, depth, location, and involvement of hair-bearing scalp. An evaluation of local tissue scalp laxity and vascularity can be helpful in considering local flaps. The location of the defect is important when considering regional options to ensure appropriate tension-free closure. In addition to evaluating the defect, the evaluation should include potential donor sites for skin grafts or free flaps as well as potential local donor vessels for microvascular anastomosis. If one is considering a free flap, it is also important to evaluate the need for a vein graft or vascular loop.[4,5]

Imaging

Photo documentation is helpful in surgical planning and in surveillance visits. To evaluate skin cancer, patients should have computed tomography imaging or MRI to evaluate for bony or dura involvement, respectively. Angiography can be considered to evaluate for free flap donor vessels in a patient with multiple prior surgeries or vascular comorbidities.

Reconstructive Goals

The primary goal of reconstructing the scalp and calvarium is restoring the protective barrier for the brain and calvarium with a secondary goal of esthetics such as color, shape, contour, and hair-bearing ability. The barrier system involves both the integrity of the calvarium and overlying coverage to prevent desiccation and infection.[6] When discussing reconstructive options, framing reconstructive outcomes based on these goals can help set patients' expectations. It is important to be prepared with multiple reconstructive options if intraoperative conditions preclude success with one technique.

SCALP RECONSTRUCTION
Secondary Intention

Healing by secondary intention is a relatively low-risk method and can produce favorable results.[7] This technique involves wound and dressing management and social support for weeks to months depending on the size of the wound. This may not be a good option for patients who require adjuvant therapy such as radiation. Wound contracture occurs with healing by secondary intention, and it is important to consider this effect on adjacent functional or esthetic structures such as the eyebrow or hairline.[8]

Wound Vacuum-Assisted Closure

Wound vacuum-assisted closure promotes blood flow and the formation of granulation tissue. Vacuum-assisted closure can be used in combination with skin grafting or as a temporizing measure for patients who are not candidates for immediate free tissue transfer.[9] This technique can be successful even when used directly on dura mater. Patients will need regular changes of the vac dressing.[10]

Skin Grafting

Skin grafts are a reliable and straightforward method of reconstruction. It is ideal for high-risk pathologic condition as in the case of melanoma, very high-risk nonmelanoma skin cancer, and skin sarcomas because it provides the best ability to monitor for recurrence. Clear wound margins also allow for more precise adjuvant radiation. In a patient with alopecia, the esthetic result of skin grafts can be favorable.

Graft success is predicated on adequate wound bed preparation, it should be vascular and without active infection. A cerclage suture can contract the wound bed and decrease the total skin graft needed while also stabilizing the wound bed against the shear forces of surrounding muscles or accidental pulling forces during sleep. Skin grafts do not integrate onto bare calvarium and in cases where there is no overlying vascularized tissue, the outer cortex of the cranium can be burred down to the diploic layer to supply the skin graft in a single-stage reconstruction (Fig. 2).[11]

Dermal Regeneration Matrix

Dermal regeneration matrices are composed of an outer layer of silicone with an inner layer consisting of bovine collagen and glycosaminoglycan derived from shark cartilage[12] and can be used directly on the bare calvarial bone.[13–15] In combination with skin grafting, these matrices create a thicker reconstructive bed, which may be more tolerant to trauma or adjuvant radiation and esthetically may better match the thickness of the native scalp.[16] Skin grafting in a delayed fashion after vascularization of the matrix results in an increased graft take compared with when grafting primarily. Meticulous wound care, with clean dressings or the application of a wound vacuum-assisted device, can prevent infection, the major cause of graft failure. Dermal regeneration matrix has mixed results in a previously radiated field[17] (Fig. 3).

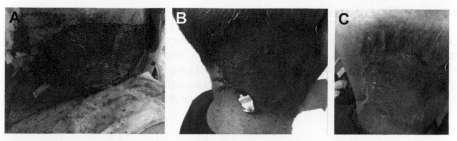

Fig. 2. Grafting on scalp defect over latissimus muscle. (*A*) Meshed split thickness skin graft on latissimus muscle. (*B*) Early postoperative result. (*C*) Late postoperative result.

PRIMARY CLOSURE

Primary closure is simple and useful in defects 3 cm or less in width (**Fig. 5**A). It can provide a good esthetic result in the hair-bearing scalp, with a tension-free closure required to prevent alopecia. The scalp has both tight and loose regions with variable mechanical

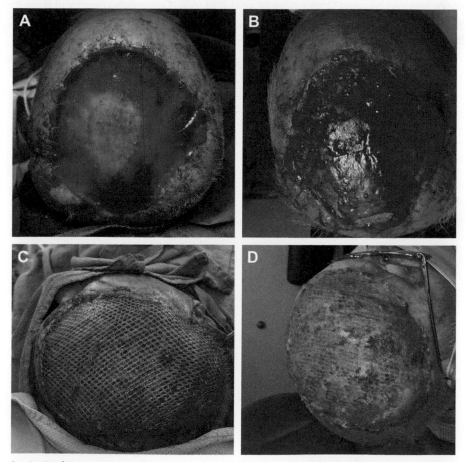

Fig. 3. Grafting on bone scalp defects. (*A*) Integra dermal matrix grafted on burred vascularized calvaria bone. (*B*) Granulation tissue formation weeks after integra grafting. (*C*) Meshed split thickness skin graft on bed of vascularized granulation tissue. (*D*) Early postoperative result of split thickness skin graft.

properties.[18] This limits the mechanical creep and even a small defect may require significant undermining to achieve closure. Blunt dissection in the loose areolar tissue plane allows for wide undermining with minimal disruption of the vasculature. Subsequent galeotomies, relaxing incisions in the galea, can be performed to allow further movement of the scalp skin. Galeotomies should be performed sharply and precisely with care to not disrupt the vascular network just superficial to the galea. Advanced suturing techniques such as the pully stitch may assist in a tight closure.[19]

LOCAL FLAPS

For small to medium size defects in non-radiated patients, local flaps provide the best color and tissue match to the native tissue. Local flaps have the advantage of preserving areas of hair-bearing scalp and may even improve alopecia in select patients. These flaps are supplied by a rich vascular network and can provide robust coverage of bare bone or implants. Local flaps do not require a general anesthetic, which is useful in elderly or patients with comorbidities. If the donor site of the flap cannot be closed primarily without significant tension, skin grafting of the pericranium of the donor site can be used to close the wound (**Fig. 5**D). Commonly used local flaps in the scalp include the O-Z, double hatchet, pinwheel, orticochea, rotational, and snail flaps (**Figs. 4**A-F, and **5**B,C).[20,21]

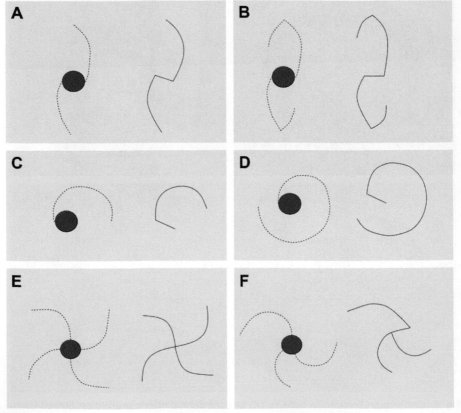

Fig. 4. Local scalp flap design and closure patterns. (*A*) O-Z, (*B*) double hatchet, (*C*) rotation, (*D*) snail, (*E*) pinwheel, and (*F*) orticochea.

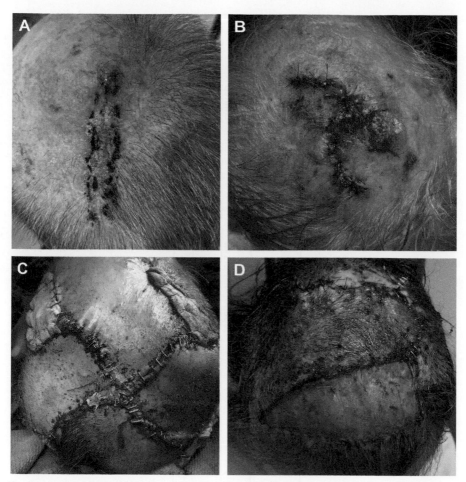

Fig. 5. Local reconstruction of scalp defect. (*A*) Primary closure. (*B*) Double hatchet flap. (*C*) Pinwheel flap. (*D*) Rotational flap with skin grafting of donor site.

Regional Flaps

Medium-to-large posterior scalp defects may be candidates for regional pedicled flap reconstruction. Pedicled flaps have cost savings, reduce operating time, and require fewer revision surgeries in comparison to free flaps when used in head and neck reconstruction.[22] One of the main drawbacks of the pedicled flap is the distance from the donor site. The pedicled trapezius and latissimus flaps arch of rotation limit them to posterior scalp defects. The Juri flap has excellent reach but its thin nature limits its use to small defect sizes (**Table 1**).

FREE FLAPS
Flap Selection

Free flap selection should consider the defect size, donor site morbidity, pedicle length, and esthetic considerations. The radial forearm free flap may be appropriate for a medium-sized defect and has advantages in pedicle length. Large-size scalp

Table 1
Regional pedicled flaps in scalp reconstruction

Flap	Pedicle	Maximal Dimensions	Reach	Advantages	Disadvantages
Trapezius	Dorsal scapular artery Transverse cervical artery	30 × 10 cm	Occipital prominence Superior helical rim	Muscular flap	Non-hair-bearing Limited reach
Latissimus dorsi	Thoracodorsal artery	20 × 40 cm	Scalp vertex	Esthetic result Large thin muscle	Non-hair-bearing Donor site morbidity
Temporo-parieto-occipital (Juri)	Superficial temporal artery	4 × 25 cm	Entire scalp	Hair-bearing scalp	Limited width

defects or defects over bioprosthetic implants may require a thicker free flap, such as the latissimus dorsi or anterolateral thigh flap, with underlying muscle to prevent implant exposure. Donor site morbidity needs to be balanced against maintaining activities of daily living. Flap thickness and volume are additional considerations to match the esthetics of local tissue (**Figs. 6–8, Table 2**). In general, the latissimus dorsi and anterolateral thigh flaps are favored for scalp reconstruction due to the range of flap volume harvestable and pedicle length available with minimal donor site morbidity.

Donor Vessels

One key consideration in assessing the candidacy for free flap reconstruction is the distance from potential donor vessels. The superficial temporal artery is an accessible donor vessel; however, in patients with previous radiation or neurosurgical procedures, the integrity may be compromised. In the elderly, this artery can also be calcified or noncompliant. For venous anastomosis, the superficial temporal vein is often of variable caliber. The retromandibular vein, posterior auricular vein, and facial vein are alternative options. Vein grafting can be used to extend pedicle length toward the higher caliber neck vessels; however, the technique may be associated with increased flap failure rates.[4] In the vessel-depleted patients, arteriovenous loops may be used to provide length to the neck vessels.[5]

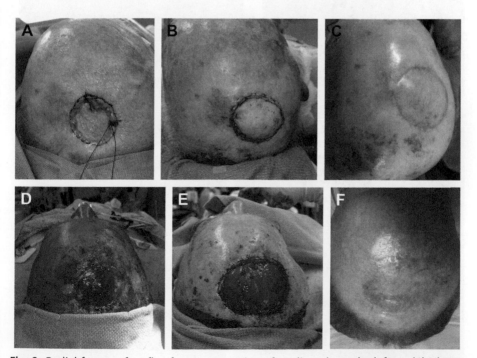

Fig. 6. Radial forearm free flap for reconstruction of medium-size scalp defects. (*A*) Ulcerative wound of the scalp vertex with planned excision margins and orientation stitches. (*B*) Inset of radial forearm flap with subcutaneous tunnel to the superficial temporal vessels. (*C*) Postoperative result of radial forearm. (*D*) Tumor of the scalp vertex. (*E*) Inset of radial forearm free flap with split thickness skin graft harvested from flap. (*F*) Postoperative result of radial forearm flap.

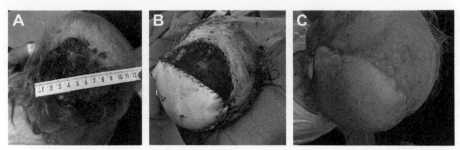

Fig. 7. Anterolateral thigh free flap for reconstruction of large posterior scalp defect. (*A*) Tumor of posterior scalp. (*B*) Musculocutaneous anterolateral thigh inset. Note: Vastus lateralis muscle juxtaposed to cutaneous skin paddle to extend flap width. (*C*) Postoperative result of anterolateral thigh flap.

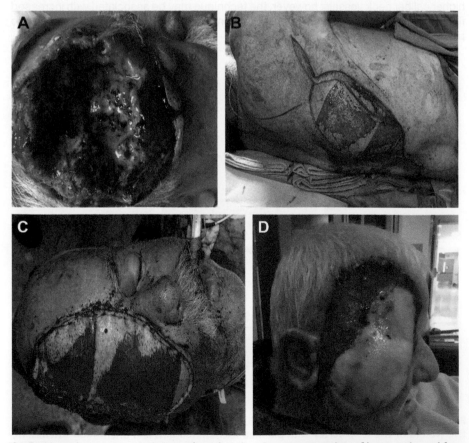

Fig. 8. Musculocutaneous latissimus dorsi free flap for reconstruction of large scalp and face defect. (*A*) Tumor eroding right temple. (*B*) Musculocutaneous latissimus dorsi harvest. Note: Skin graft taken from flap to minimize donor site morbidity. (*C*) Inset of latissimus dorsi flap in temple and orbit. (*D*) Postoperative result of latissimus dorsi free flap.

Table 2
Free flaps in scalp reconstruction

Flap	Flap Types	Maximal Dimensions	Pedicle Length	Donor Site	Advantages	Disadvantages
Latissimus dorsi	Musculocutaneous Muscle only	20 × 40 cm	6–16 cm	Closed primarily	Large thin muscle Esthetic result Chimeric flap	Limitations in positioning Functional arm morbidity
Anterolateral thigh	Adipofascial Fasciocutaneous Musculocutaneous Muscle only	8 × 22 cm	12–22 cm	Closed primarily	Limited donor site morbidity Fascia use in dura reconstruction	Tissue bulk dependent on body habitus Limited width
Parascapular	Fasciocutaneous	15 × 25 cm	3–7 cm	Closed primarily	Chimeric flap Limited donor site morbidity	Limitations in positioning Short pedicle
Radial forearm	Fasciocutaneous	8 × 18 cm	4–14 cm	Grafting required	Thin and pliable flap Long pedicle length	Limited dimensions Hand weakness and paresthesia
Rectus abdominus	Musculocutaneous Muscle only	30 × 10 cm	5–7 cm	Closed primarily	Fascia use in dura reconstruction Large surface area	Short pedicle Ventral hernia Flap volume

CALVARIUM RECONSTRUCTION (CRANIOPLASTY)

Calvarium reconstruction may be performed primarily or in a delayed fashion for infected wounds. Key considerations for calvaria reconstruction are the size and location of the defect and the integrity of the underlying structures.

Free Bones Grafts

Autologous split calvaria free bone grafts can be harvested from the parietal bone due to the relative thickness of this donor bone,[23] and integrate well for small bony defect.[24] Alternative sites for free bone grafts include the sternum, rib, and iliac crest. The advantages of using bone grafts include their strength and biocompatibility, although grafts can have issues with resorption over time and have increased rates of failure as compared with bioprosthetic implants.[24,25]

Biosynthetic Grafts

Large full-thickness defects can be reconstructed with biocompatible materials such as titanium mesh and polyetheretherketone (PEEK). These 2 materials have become popular due to their simple nature, strength, and low infection rates. Titanium has some concerns related to the risk of implant exposure and heat conductance, and causing of artifact on imaging. Although PEEK does not have these risks, both materials carry the risk of infection and often require removal if infected.[26,27] The use of three-dimensional (3D) modeling and customization of the implants has improved cosmesis.[24]

Vascularized Bone Flap

The use of autologous vascularized bone free flaps in compromised defects can help overcome infection concerns. The subscapular system has the advantage of being harvested in combination with serratus muscle and rib on a single vascular pedicle.[28] This complex reconstruction technique may have a role in select cases.

Virtual Surgical Planning

Virtual surgical planning (VSP) in combination with 3D modeling and fabrication allows for the use of patient customized cranial reconstruction. As a result, VSP offers the advantages of decreased operating time, improved precision, and improved functional and cosmetic outcomes for complex reconstruction of the calvarium and orbit.[29,30] Preoperative VSP can be combined with intraoperative image navigation to increase the precision of implant placement while avoiding critical structures (**Fig. 9**).

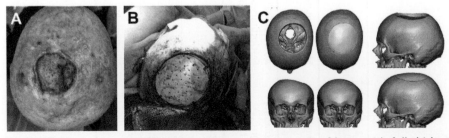

Fig. 9. Calvarium bone reconstruction. (*A*) Osteoradionecrosis of bone with full thickness defect. (*B*) Inset of PEEK customized biosynthetic implant. (*C*) Virtual surgical plan for customized PEEK implant. Image courtesy of DePuy Synthes.

SUMMARY

Scalp and calvarium reconstruction encompass the full spectrum of the reconstructive ladder. This region is anatomically challenging to reconstruct due to its thin nature, mechanical properties, and distance from large vessels. The reconstructive populations are commonly elderly, previously radiated, and have poor healing potential. A thorough patient evaluation is necessary to understand a patient's reconstruction goals. The reconstructive surgeon should consider a variety of reconstructive options and select the simplest reconstructive approach, which meets the patient's goals.

CLINICS CARE POINTS

- Meticulous wound care is needed to avoid infection for skin graft.
- Galeotomies can be used to improve laxity in regions of tight scalp.
- Local flaps provide excellent color and tissue match for small to medium sizes defects.
- Large defects may require free flap reconstruction which has advantages for radiated patients.
- Biosynthetic grafts provide strength and protection of the underlying structure in calvarium reconstruction.

DISCLOSURE

The authors have no conflicts of interest to declare.

REFERENCES

1. Potparíc Z, Fukuta K, Colen LB, et al. Galeo-pericranial flaps in the forehead: a study of blood supply and volumes. Br J Plast Surg 1996;49(8):519–28.
2. Yoshioka N, Rhoton AL. Vascular Anatomy of the Anteriorly Based Pericranial Flap. Oper Neurosurg 2005;57(suppl_1):11–6.
3. Denewer A, Khater A, Farouk O, et al. Can we put a simplified algorithm for reconstruction of large scalp defects following tumor resection? World J Surg Oncol 2011;9(1):129.
4. Furr MC, Cannady S, Wax MK. Interposition vein grafts in microvascular head and neck reconstruction. Laryngoscope 2011;121(4):707–11.
5. Moubayed SP, Giot JP, Odobescu A, et al. Arteriovenous fistulas for microvascular head and neck reconstruction. Plast Surg (Oakv) 2015;23(3):167–70.
6. Dedhia R, Luu Q. Scalp reconstruction. Curr Opin Otolaryngol Head Neck Surg 2015;23(5):407–14.
7. Snow SN, Stiff MA, Bullen R, et al. Second-intention healing of exposed facial-scalp bone after Mohs surgery for skin cancer: Review of ninety-one cases. J Am Acad Dermatol 1994;31(3):450–4.
8. Smart RJ, Yeoh MS, Kim DD. Paramedian Forehead Flap. Oral Maxillofac Surg Clin N Am 2014;26(3):401–10.
9. Andrews BT, Smith RB, Goldstein DP, et al. Management of complicated head and neck wounds with vacuum-assisted closure system. Head Neck 2006; 28(11):974–81.

10. Powers AK, Neal MT, Argenta LC, et al. Vacuum-assisted closure for complex cranial wounds involving the loss of dura mater: Report of 5 cases. J Neurosurg 2013; 118(2):302–8.

11. Molnar JA, DeFranzo AJ, Marks MW. Single-stage approach to skin grafting the exposed skull. Plast Reconstr Surg 2000;105(1):174–7.

12. Burke JF, Jung WK. Successful Use of a Physiologically Acceptable Artificial Skin in the Treatment of Extensive Burn Injury. Ann Surg 1981;194(4):413–28.

13. Corradino B, Di Lorenzo S, Leto Barone AA, et al. Reconstruction of full thickness scalp defects after tumour excision in elderly patients: Our experience with Integra® dermal regeneration template. J Plast Reconstr Aesthet Surg 2010;63(3): e245–7.

14. Kosutic D, Beasung E, Dempsey M, et al. Single-layer Integra for one-stage reconstruction of scalp defects with exposed bone following full-thickness burn injury: A novel technique. Burns 2012;38(1):143–5.

15. McClain L, Barber H, Donnellan K, et al. Integra Application for Reconstruction of Large Scalp Defects. Laryngoscope 2011;121(S5):S353.

16. Hahn HM, Jeong YS, Lee IJ, et al. Efficacy of split-thickness skin graft combined with novel sheet-type reprocessed micronized acellular dermal matrix. BMC Surg 2022;22(1):358.

17. Aronson S, Ellis MF. Hostile Scalp Wound Reconstruction Using Acellular Dermal Matrix for Soft Tissue Augmentation. J Craniofac Surg 2020;31(3):e309–12.

18. Falland-Cheung L, Scholze M, Lozano PF, et al. Mechanical properties of the human scalp in tension. J Mech Behav Biomed Mater 2018;84:188–97.

19. Kannan S, Mehta D, Ozog D. Scalp Closures With Pulley Sutures Reduce Time and Cost Compared to Traditional Layered Technique—A Prospective, Randomized, Observer-Blinded Study. Dermatol Surg 2016;42(11):1248–55.

20. Varela-Veiga A, Suárez-Magdalena O, Suárez-Amor Ó, Monteagudo B. Double Hatchet Flap For The Reconstruction Of Scalp Defects. Actas Dermo-Sifiliográficas Engl Ed 2017;108(9):878–80.

21. Badhey A, Kadakia S, Abraham MT, et al. Multiflap closure of scalp defects: Revisiting the orticochea flap for scalp reconstruction. Am J Otolaryngol 2016;37(5): 466–9.

22. Gabrysz-Forget F, Tabet P, Rahal A, et al. Free versus pedicled flaps for reconstruction of head and neck cancer defects: a systematic review. J Otolaryngol - Head Neck Surg 2019;48(1):13.

23. Weber RS, Kearns DB, Smith RJH. Split Calvarium Cranioplasty. Arch Otolaryngol Head Neck Surg 1987;113(1):84–9.

24. Liu L, Lu ST, Liu AH, et al. Comparison of complications in cranioplasty with various materials: a systematic review and meta-analysis. Br J Neurosurg 2020; 34(4):388–96.

25. van de Vijfeijken SECM, Münker TJAG, Spijker R, et al. Autologous Bone Is Inferior to Alloplastic Cranioplasties: Safety of Autograft and Allograft Materials for Cranioplasties, a Systematic Review. World Neurosurg 2018;117: 443–52.e8.

26. Thien A, King NKK, Ang BT, et al. Comparison of Polyetheretherketone and Titanium Cranioplasty after Decompressive Craniectomy. World Neurosurg 2015; 83(2):176–80.

27. Sanus GZ, Tanriverdi T, Ulu MO, et al. Use of CortossTM as an Alternative Material in Calvarial Defects: The First Clinical Results in Cranioplasty. J Craniofac Surg 2008;19(1):8.

28. Kim PD, Blackwell KE. Latissimus-Serratus-Rib Free Flap for Oromandibular and Maxillary Reconstruction. Arch Otolaryngol Neck Surg 2007;133(8):791.
29. Chim H, Wetjen N, Mardini S. Virtual Surgical Planning in Craniofacial Surgery. Semin Plast Surg 2014;28(03):150–8.
30. Yashin KS, Ermolaev AYu, Ostapyuk MV, et al. Case Report: Simultaneous Resection of Bone Tumor and CAD/CAM Titanium Cranioplasty in Fronto-Orbital Region. Front Surg 2021;8:718725.

Facial Nerve Reconstruction

Guanning Nina Lu, MD[a],*, John Flynn, MD[b]

KEYWORDS

- Facial paralysis • Facial nerve dysfunction • Facial reanimation • Synkinesis

KEY POINTS

- Primary, tension-free facial nerve repair is preferred when possible for best outcomes.
- For flaccid facial paralysis of less than 2 years duration where primary nerve repair or grafting is impossible, nerve substitution procedures are preferred to restore facial tone and motion.
- For flaccid facial paralysis of more than 2 years duration, patients typically require free muscle or tendon transfer. Static options may also be considered depending on patient scenario.

INTRODUCTION AND BACKGROUND

Facial paralysis has a multitude of causes including traumatic, neoplastic, infectious, rheumatologic, and most commonly, idiopathic (Bell's Palsy). The facial nerve is responsible for innervation of the muscles of facial expression, posterior belly of digastric, stylohyoid, and stapedius as well as parasympathetic and gustatory innervation. Loss of facial function results in facial asymmetry, oral incompetence, poor speech articulation, nasal airway obstruction, and ocular exposure injuries. In addition to these physical symptoms, facial paralysis negatively affects psychological well-being and quality of life.[1] An increase in depression and anxiety occurs in 30% to 60% of patients.[2]

Given the diverse causes of facial paralysis, a thorough diagnostic workup is paramount when the cause is not readily apparent. Assessment of the patient using history and physical examination is critical in identifying the cause of facial paralysis. In cases of acute onset unilateral paralysis without other neurologic changes, one should suspect Bell's Palsy. In situations where patients do not follow the typical course of recovery after Bell's Palsy, it is imperative to rule out neoplastic processes. Management is frequently tailored to the cause and duration of facial paralysis.

In this review, we provide a contemporary description of facial nerve reconstruction for immediate and delayed presentations of flaccid facial palsy.

[a] University of Washington, 325 9th Avenue 4 West, Seattle, WA 98104, USA; [b] University of Kansas Medical Center, 4000 Cambridge Street, Kansas City, KS 66103, USA
* Corresponding author.
E-mail address: ninalu@uw.edu

Otolaryngol Clin N Am 56 (2023) 757–767
https://doi.org/10.1016/j.otc.2023.04.004
0030-6665/23/Published by Elsevier Inc.

IMMEDIATE RECONSTRUCTION

Oncologic ablative procedures and traumatic lacerations are the most common causes of flaccid facial paralysis requiring immediate reconstruction. Traumatic transections of the facial nerve are best repaired within 72 hours of injury because distal nerve branches may be stimulated before Wallerian degeneration occurs. When feasible, concurrent facial nerve reconstruction following ablative surgery is preferred. When performed concurrently with oncologic resection, there is the potential for shorter duration of facial paralysis and the possibility of improved functional outcomes.[3] Despite this fact, there is evidence to suggest that a limited number of patients undergo concurrent facial nerve reconstruction at the time of ablation.[4] Reconstructive management varies by location of facial nerve insult.

IMMEDIATE RECONSTRUCTION FOLLOWING INTRATEMPORAL INJURY

During intratemporal surgery, there is potential for loss of continuity between the facial nerve nucleus and the peripheral facial nerve. An intratemporal facial nerve insult can occur due to excision of tumors within the internal acoustic canal or secondary to temporal bone trauma, cholesteatoma, and iatrogenic injuries.

If discontinuity of the intratemporal facial nerve occurs, the optimal repair includes restoring continuity of the peripheral facial nerve. When feasible, primary, tension-free, end-to-end epineural coaptation of the proximal and distal ends of the facial nerve give the patient the best possible outcome.[5] When tension-free coaptation cannot occur, an interposition nerve graft allows for restoration of the peripheral facial nerve. The choice of donor interposition nerve graft depends on the length required but typically the great auricular nerve (GAN) or sural nerve provides adequate length and caliber.[6] A limitation to nerve grafts includes their need for revascularization. When performed over a long segment of temporal bone, there is possibility of central necrosis and endoneurial fibrosis.[7] Following interposition nerve grafting, most authors report the ability to achieve House-Brackman Grade III outcome in at least 50% of their patients.[6] In instances where continuity between the proximal and distal facial nerve are unable to be restored, nerve transfer procedures could be considered but this rarely occurs in the intratemporal region and can be completed in a delayed fashion.

IMMEDIATE RECONSTRUCTION FOLLOWING EXTRATEMPORAL INJURY

Similar to intratemporal facial nerve injuries, extratemporal facial nerve injuries are ideally reconstructed immediately. Immediate repair not only minimizes the time duration of facial muscle denervation but allows repair to be guided by stimulable facial nerve branches. This allows a better understanding of the muscle groups each facial nerve branch innervates. Extratemporal facial nerve injury most frequently occurs following ablative resection of parotid or cutaneous malignancies. Other causes include traumatic or iatrogenic insults.

In many instances, facial nerve reconstruction is delayed following ablative malignant resection.[4] This may be due to the need for facial nerve margin analysis and/or subsequent radiation. However, studies have demonstrated that positive nerve margins and adjuvant radiation do not adversely affect facial nerve reconstructive outcomes.[8,9] Frozen section facial nerve margin analysis can assist the surgeon in reconstructive technique selection during immediate repair.

NERVE GRAFTING

When possible, primary tension-free epineural coaptation between distal and proximal ends of disrupted facial nerve using microscopic repair with 9-0 or 10-0 nylon suture is optimal. This scenario may develop in instances of penetrating trauma to the facial nerve. Ablative oncologic resection typically requires facial nerve segmental excision, which renders tension-free primary repair unachievable. Interposition or cable nerve grafting is indicated in this situation.

Nerve grafts can be harvested from either sensory or motor nerves. Early studies suggested that motor nerves may allow for better regeneration but this has been contested by more recent studies.[10,11] Some authors have opted for reversal of nerve graft polarity (antidromic orientation) but experimentally this has not shown significant benefit. In a rabbit model comparative study, there was no significant difference in compound motor action potential, nerve conduction velocity or total number of axons between the orthodromic and antidromic nerve grafts.[12]

There are many options for donor nerve grafting. Due to donor site proximity, the GAN can be easily harvested for nerve grafting. There is an excellent size match between the facial nerve and GAN diameter. Graft length can reach between 7 and 10 cm, and the branching pattern may be exploited for repair of multiple distal branches. When a longer nerve graft is necessary, the sural nerve provides length of up to 40 cm and can be used for repair of multiple nerve branches.[13] Harvest of the sural nerve requires a separate incision but has minimal donor site morbidity. Often, the nerve can be harvested through a small single incision using a fascia stripper or endoscope.[14]

Other commonly used donor nerves include motor nerve to vastus lateralis, lateral antebrachial cutaneous nerve, and the anterior division of the medial antebrachial cutaneous nerve.[15,16]

NERVE TRANSFERS

In some situations, the proximal facial nerve is not accessible or available for reconstructive purposes. When this occurs, nerve transfer procedures should be considered if the distal facial nerve and muscle are intact. The nerve to masseter (NTM) and hypoglossal nerve are donor sources for extratemporal nerve repair (**Fig. 1**). Cross facial nerve grafting (CFNG) is not typically used at the time of facial nerve reconstruction in the immediate setting but may be used in a delayed fashion for increased spontaneity.

The NTM is reliably found in the subzygomatic triangle bounded by the zygomatic arch, frontal branch of the facial nerve, and the temporomandibular joint.[17] A convenient starting point for dissection was found at 3 cm anterior to the tragus at a level of 1 cm inferior to the zygomatic arch. The NTM averages greater than 2700 myelinated fibers providing robust axonal volume.[18,19] Because of this axonal load, the NTM offers excellent bite-driven dynamic oral commissure excursion. There is limited ability of resting tone restoration as well as spontaneity of movement. Because of these limitations, concurrent nerve grafting and NTM transfer have been proposed to improve outcomes following radical parotidectomy.[20] During NTM harvest, care should be taken to maintain the anterior branch to preserve masseteric bulk and function.[21]

Hypoglossal nerve transfer to the main trunk of the facial nerve may be considered if a proximal stump of the facial nerve is not available for grafting. The technique for hypoglossal nerve transfer has evolved from the classic description of complete transection of the hypoglossal nerve and coaptation to the main trunk of the facial nerve. Modern techniques have favored partial transection of the hypoglossal nerve with

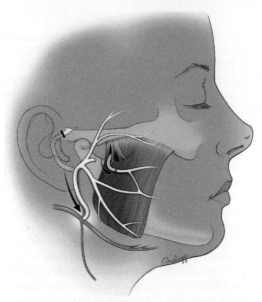

Fig. 1. Simultaneous masseter and hypoglossal nerve transfer. (Illustration ©Chris Gralapp.)

end-to-side anastomosis with the facial nerve.[22] Direct facial coaptation requires adequate length of the facial nerve main trunk for inferior mobilization to the hypoglossal nerve and requires mastoidectomy to utilize the mastoid segment of the facial nerve. Inadequate length may necessitate interposition grafting. The hypoglossal nerve provides superior resting tone compared with NTM.

STATIC SUSPENSION

Static procedures can significantly complement dynamic procedures. Due to the time duration of neural regeneration, which may take up to 6 months, static procedures offer immediate relief. In addition to facial symmetry, oral competence, nasal obstruction, and speech articulation are improved. There are various means to provide static support to the face but fascia lata grafts are preferred to allografts due to lower infection and extrusion rates.[23]

Multivector facia lata static suspension allows for functional restoration of perioral positioning and nasal valve incompetence while also aesthetically improving philtrum positioning and recreating a nasolabial fold (**Fig. 2**). Fascia lata harvest is performed through a minimally invasive technique.[24] It can then be divided into separate bands measuring 1×14 cm in length. Fascia lata bands are secured medially at the oral commissure, nasolabial fold, and nasal valve. Laterally, these are secured to the temporalis fascia. Another band is secured medially at the philtrum and laterally along the perichondrium of the intertragal notch. Each separate fascia lata band must be secured at the proper vector and tension for optimal restoration of the paralyzed face. Immediate return of resting symmetry can be obtained with this technique while awaiting neural regeneration from nerve graft or nerve transfer procedures.

PERIOCULAR RECONSTRUCTION

Paralytic lagophthalmos following facial nerve injury can lead to inadequate corneal protection. Over the long-term, this puts patients at risk of exposure keratopathy,

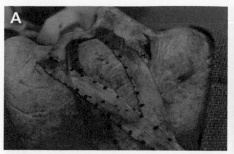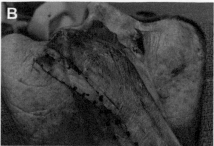

Fig. 2. Fascia lata static facial suspension. (*A*) Fascia lata bands for the philtrum stabilization, nasal valve suspension, and oral commissure. (*B*) Addition of wide band of fascia lata for recreation of the nasolabial fold.

especially those with poor Bell phenomenon and trigeminal anesthesia. Periocular care begins with proper lubrication and moisturization such as preservative free artificial tears and ophthalmic ointment. When surgical intervention has not been performed, eyelid taping or patching is recommended at night.

Surgical intervention traditionally begins with upper eyelid weighting (**Fig. 3**). Upper eyelid weights can be gold or platinum. Platinum eyelid weights have several advantages including lower allergy rate and greater density.[25] Because of the greater density, platinum eyelid weights can achieve the same weight while maintaining a lower profile. Platinum chains are also described, and these allow for better contouring and possibly allows for lesser corneal astigmatism.[26] Palpebral spring placement has the added benefit of not requiring gravity for eyelid closure but their associated complications have made this a less commonly used technique.[27] Traditional placement of the upper eyelid weight is in the pretarsal space but supratarsal placement has proven advantageous to reduce external visibility and reduce risk of astigmatism.[28]

Paralysis of the lower eyelid protractors causes unopposed lower eyelid retractor activation. There are various techniques for surgical correction of this retraction. Traditionally, lateral canthoplasty, lateral tarsal strip, and tarsoconjunctival flaps have been performed.[29] Lower eyelid sling suspension has also proven beneficial in both primary and revision correction of paralytic lagophthalmos.[30] Tarsorrhaphy can be considered in cases of refractory ocular surface disease, although many would consider this esthetically unsatisfactory. Alternatively, a scleral lens can achieve excellent results without compromising esthetics.[31]

DELAYED RECONSTRUCTION

Immediate nerve reconstruction should be used at the time of known facial nerve disruption as in the case of traumatic transection and parotid tumor extirpation. However, many other circumstances causing facial paralysis involve delayed treatment paradigms and management varies based on timing of presentation, probability of spontaneous recovery, anatomic continuity of facial nerve, and viability of facial musculature. The length of time of flaccid paralysis is of utmost importance in surgical decision-making because the reinnervation potential of the facial musculature is a key differentiator of management (**Fig. 4**).

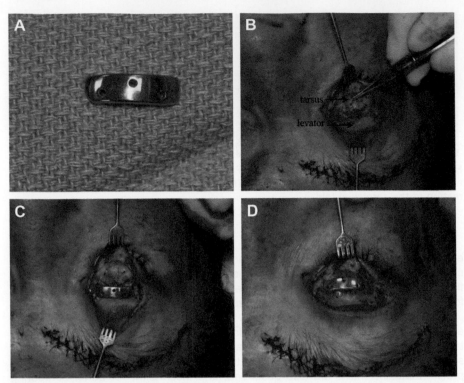

Fig. 3. Upper eyelid weighting. (*A*) Upper eyelid gold weight. (*B*) Exposure of the tarsal plate. (*C*) Gold weight resting in place over the tarsal plate. (*D*) Gold weight sutured in place. (Massry GG. Surgical management of the eye. In: Slattery B, editor. The facial nerve. New York: Thieme Publishers; 2013. p. 171.)

Timing of Intervention

Patients with intact facial nerve and muscle but prolonged facial paralysis present a management dilemma for facial nerve reconstruction. Traditionally, patients are observed for spontaneous facial recovery for 12 months before facial nerve intervention. However, a prolonged facial palsy risks increased facial musculature degeneration, possible decreased success of subsequent facial reanimation surgery, as well as lengthens the physical and psychosocial harms of facial palsy experienced by the patient.

Attempts have been made to identify early predictors of long-term facial paralysis outcomes, particularly following vestibular schwannoma surgery. A retrospective chart review of 281 patients by Rivas and colleagues[32] evaluated spontaneous facial nerve recovery in patients with an intact facial nerve but postoperative facial palsy following vestibular schwannoma resection. The authors found that the rate of recovery was predictive of facial nerve outcomes beyond 1 year. The authors found that a failure of a HB Grade 6 to improve by 6 months is associated with a greater-than 80% chance of poor outcome long-term greater than a year. Patients with HB Grade 6 paralysis failing to improve by 6 months had a greater-than 80% chance of a poor long-term outcome beyond a year. Their model overall predicted poor outcome in patients with initial HB Grades 5 and 6 with 97% sensitivity and 97% specificity. This study was followed by a prospective study of 62 patients with uninterrupted facial nerves after

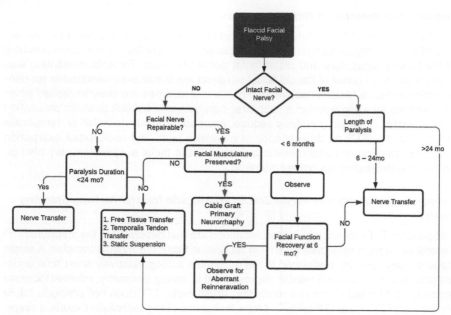

Fig. 4. Management algorithm for flaccid facial palsy.

cerebellopontine angle (CPA) tumor resection and postoperative facial paralysis.[33] Patients who showed no signs of recovery by 6 months but declined facial reanimation surgery demonstrated at best HB grade 5 after 18 months of observation. Those patients who did undergo a nerve transfer achieved HB 2-4 results with a mean score of HB 3. The authors did not find a clinical difference in nerve outcome when performed early (<12 months of paralysis) versus late (>12 months of paralysis) but noted that patients experienced a shortened duration of paralysis. They found that masseteric to facial nerve transfers showed earlier signs of reinnervation (5.6 months mean) compared with hypoglossal to facial nerve transfers (10.8 months mean). A retrospective study of 60 patients reviewed hypoglossal nerve transfers performed after cerebellopontine angle tumor extirpation.[3] The authors compared 34 patients with nerve transection and hypoglossal to facial nerve anastomosis within 14 days with 26 patients with anatomically intact facial nerve but poor postoperative function who underwent hypoglossal to facial anastomosis after 14 days of injury. They found a 4.97-fold greater odds of achieving HB 3 or less in the early surgery group (95% CI 1.5–16.9; $P = .01$). A study of 7 patients comparing masseter nerve transfer before or after 6 months of paralysis found a significantly increase oral commissure excursion in the early group.[34] Although definitive conclusions cannot be drawn from these studies alone, there has been a paradigm shift to earlier intervention in persistent flaccid facial palsy at 6 months rather than waiting until 12 months. This shift is, in part, influenced by the popularization of masseter to facial nerve transfer. When performed to a redundant buccal branch of the facial nerve, a masseter nerve transfer does not preclude further spontaneous facial nerve regeneration and does not meaningfully weaken the smile even in the case of spontaneous facial nerve regeneration. This concept is extrapolated from historical experience in CFNG wherein a redundant buccal branch from a normally functioning facial nerve is transected to provide donor axons and does not meaningfully weaken the smile.

Reinnervation Potential of Facial Musculature

Key determinants of management for flaccid facial paralysis are the duration and degree of facial paralysis. Longer duration of paralysis affects the reinnervation potential of the facial musculature and distal facial nerve branches. Patients presenting less than 2 years from onset of flaccid facial paralysis are considered candidates for reinnervation of native facial musculature. However, outcomes are likely improved when interventions take place within a year after paralysis onset. Adult patients presenting after 2 years of flaccid paralysis require functional muscle transfer or temporalis tendon transfer (TTT) as do scenarios of extensive head and neck tumor extirpation involving resection of facial mimetic muscles. Static facial suspension may also be considered depending on patient scenario.

Temporalis Tendon Transfer Versus Gracilis Free Muscle Transfer for Long-Standing Paralysis

Orthodromic TTT techniques and modifications are well described in the literature.[35–38] Several key advantages distinguish this technique from free muscle transfer: A single stage surgery routinely performed in the outpatient setting, relatively short time under anesthesia, immediate and reliable improvement in resting symmetry, minimal incisions required, and limited donor site morbidity. Additionally, TTT does not preclude future placement of free muscle if desired. Major limitations of this technique include a single, fixed vector for oral commissure insertion, lack of true spontaneity, adequate length may require fascia lata extension, and variability in commissure excursion.

Although numerous donors for free muscle transfer have been described in the literature, the gracilis free muscle transfer (GFMT) has become the preferred technique in most institutions (**Fig. 5**). Donor nerve selection has also varied and includes sources such as cross facial nerve graft, masseteric, hypoglossal, deep temporal, spinal accessory, and phrenic. Ipsilateral facial nerve is used when feasible but not available in most scenarios. Beyond an ipsilateral facial nerve source, CFNG is the only source of truly spontaneous movement. Single innervation with CFNG requires a 2-stage approach to first place the nerve graft from the contralateral face at least 4 months before muscle transplantation. Given the use of 2 neurorrhaphy sites and axonal loss across a long graft, single innervation with CFNG is less reliable. Masseteric nerve innervation allows for a large source of axons and increases reliability of GFM but does not allow for true spontaneity. Dual innervation with both CFNG and masseteric nerve

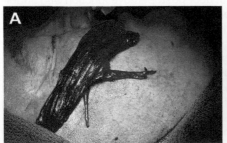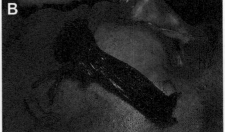

Fig. 5. GFMT. (*A*) Muscle oriented for nerve to master coaptation with nerve to gracilis. (*B*) Muscle oriented for cross face nerve graft coaptation with nerve to gracilis. (*Reproduced from* Jowett N, Hadlock TA. Free Gracilis Transfer and Static Facial Suspension for Midfacial Reanimation in Long-Standing Flaccid Facial Palsy. Otolaryngol Clin North Am. 2018 Dec;51(6):1129-1139. https://doi.org/10.1016/j.otc.2018.07.009.)

is a safe, reliable, and consistent technique with most patients achieving spontaneity.[39] Key advantages to GFMT over TTT include the ability to achieve true spontaneity, unencumbered placement of muscle vectors for individualization based on patient characteristics, and meaningful commissure excursion. Disadvantages include the need for microvascular equipment and expertise, a staged procedure and numbness of the lower leg with CFNG innervation, lengthy time under anesthesia, risk of midfacial bulk and asymmetry, and delay in patient benefit from surgery.

Aberrant Facial Nerve Reinnervation

Depending on the degree of facial nerve injury, spontaneous recovery may be accompanied by abnormal reinnervation resulting in postparalytic facial nerve syndrome. This includes synkinesis, hyperkinesis, hypertonicity, spasm, contracture, facial pain, and gustatory epiphora. Development of secondary dysfunction starts as early as 3 to 4 months postparalysis and continues for up to 2 years. Treatment includes facial neuromuscular retraining, selective weakening of maladaptive muscle movement with botulinum toxin or surgery, and augmenting facial movement with free muscle transfer.

SUMMARY

Facial palsy causes profound facial disfigurement, functional compromise, and psychosocial distress. Surgeons operating in the head and neck will inevitably care for patients with facial palsy. Many options exist for facial paralysis rehabilitation regardless of the timing of presentation. Treatment of facial paralysis improves patients' quality of life, reduces functional impairments, and prevents devastating ophthalmologic consequences. Facial paralysis patients should be evaluated systematically by a multidisciplinary team for best outcomes.

CLINICS CARE POINTS

- Facial paralysis has significant negative effects on psychological well-being and quality of life.

- Facial nerve transection is ideally repaired within 72 hours, prior to the onsent of wallerian degeneration.

- In patients with complete flaccid facial paralysis with an intact facial nerve after acoustic neuroma surgery, facial nerve recovery at 6 months is predictive of ultimate outcome.

- Recovery after facial nerve injury may result in postparalytic facial nerve syndrome and development of secondary dysfunction can develop for up to 2 years.

DISCLOSURE

None.

REFERENCES

1. Lyford-Pike S, Nellis JC. Perceptions of patients with facial paralysis: predicting social implications and setting goals. Facial Plast Surg Clin North Am 2021; 29(3):369–74.
2. Walker D, Hallam M, Ni M, et al. The psychosocial impact of facial palsy: our experience in one hundred and twenty six patients. Clin Otolaryngol 2012; 37(6):474–7.

3. Yawn RJ, Wright HV, Francis DO, et al. Facial nerve repair after operative injury: impact of timing on hypoglossal-facial nerve graft outcomes. Am J Otolaryngol 2016;37(6):493–6.
4. Lu GN, Villwock MR, Humphrey CD, et al. Analysis of facial reanimation procedures performed concurrently with total parotidectomy and facial nerve sacrifice. JAMA Facial Plast Surg 2019;21(1):50–5.
5. Christopher LH, Slattery WH, Smith EJ, et al. Facial nerve management in patients with malignant skull base tumors. J Neuro Oncol 2020;150(3):493–500.
6. Prasad SC, Balasubramanian K, Piccirillo E, et al. Surgical technique and results of cable graft interposition of the facial nerve in lateral skull base surgeries: experience with 213 consecutive cases. J Neurosurg 2018;128(2):631–8.
7. Best TJ, Mackinnon SE, Evans PJ, et al. Peripheral nerve revascularization: histomorphometric study of small- and large-caliber grafts. J Reconstr Microsurg 1999;15(3):183–90.
8. Hontanilla B, Qiu SS, Marré D. Effect of postoperative brachytherapy and external beam radiotherapy on functional outcomes of immediate facial nerve repair after radical parotidectomy. Head Neck 2014;36(1):113–9.
9. Wax MK, Kaylie DM. Does a positive neural margin affect outcome in facial nerve grafting? Head Neck 2007;29(6):546–9.
10. Nichols CM, Brenner MJ, Fox IK, et al. Effects of motor versus sensory nerve grafts on peripheral nerve regeneration. Exp Neurol 2004;190(2):347–55.
11. Ali SA, Rosko AJ, Hanks JE, et al. Effect of motor versus sensory nerve autografts on regeneration and functional outcomes of rat facial nerve reconstruction. Sci Rep 2019;9(1):8353.
12. Kim J, Choi YE, Kim JH, et al. Nerve repair and orthodromic and antidromic nerve grafts: an experimental comparative study in rabbit. BioMed Res Int 2020;5046832.
13. Humphrey CH, Kriet JD. Nerve repair and cable grafting for facial paralysis. Facial Plast Surg 2008;24(2):170–6.
14. Hadlock T, Cheney ML. Single-incision endoscopic sural nerve harvest for cross face nerve grafting. J Reconstr Microsurg 2008;24(7):519–23.
15. David AP, Seth R, Knott PD. Facial reanimation and reconstruction of the radical parotidectomy. Facial Plast Surg Clin North Am 2021;29:405–14.
16. Revenaugh PC, Knott D, McBride JM, et al. Motor nerve to the vastus lateralis. Arch Facial Plast Surg 2012;14(5):365–8.
17. Collar RM, Byrne PJ, Boahene KD. The subzygomatic triangle; rapid, minimally invasive identification of the masseteric nerve for facial reanimation. Plast Reconstr Surg 2013;132(1):183–8.
18. Borschel GH, Kawamura DH, Kasukurthi R, et al. The motor nerve to the masseter muscle: an anatomic and histomorphometric study to facilitate its use in facial reanimation. J Plast Reconstr Aesthet Surg 2012;65(3):363–6.
19. Snyder-Warwick AK, Fattah AY, Zive L, et al. The degree of facial movement following microvascular muscle transfer in pediatric facial reanimation depends on donor motor nerve axonal density. Plast Reconstr Surg 2015;135(2):370e–81e.
20. Owusu JA, Troung L, Kim JC. Facial nerve reconstruction with concurrent masseteric nerve transfer and cable grafting. JAMA Facial Plastic Surgery 2016;5(18):335–9.
21. Klebuc M. The evolving role of the masseter-to-facial (V-VII) nerve transfer for rehabilitation of the paralyzed face. Ann Chir Plast Esthet 2015;60(5):436–41.
22. Jandali D, Revenaugh PC. Facial reanimation: an update on nerve transfers in facial paralysis. Curr Opin Otolaryngol Head Neck Surg 2019;27(4):231–6.

23. Langille M, Singh P. Static facial slings: approaches to rehabilitation of the paralyzed face. Facial Plast Surg Clin North Am 2016;24(1):29–35.
24. Amir A, Gur E, Gatot A, et al. Fascia lata sheaths harvest revisited. Operat Tech Otolaryngol Head Neck Surg 2000;11(4):304–6.
25. Siah WF, Nagendran S, Tan P, et al. Late outcomes of gold weights and platinum chains for upper eyelid loading. Br J Ophthalmol 2018;102(2):164–8.
26. Bladen JC, Norris JH, Malhotra R. Cosmetic comparison of gold weight and platinum chain insertion in primary upper eyelid loading for lagophthalmos. Ophthal Plast Reconstr Surg 2012;28(3):171–5.
27. Demirci H, Frueh BR. Palpebral spring in the management of lagophthalmos and exposure keratopathy secondary to facial nerve palsy. Ophthal Plast Reconstr Surg 2009;25(4):270–5.
28. Rozen S, Lehrman C. Upper eyelid postseptal weight placement for treatment of paralytic lagophthalmos. Plast Reconstr Sug 2013;131(6):1253–65.
29. Dedhia R, Shipchandler T, Tollefson T. Eyelid coupling using a modified tarsoconjunctvical flap in facial paralysis. Facial Plast Surg Clin North Am 2021;29(3): 447–51.
30. Bartholomew R, Ein L, Jowett N. Lower eyelid sling for primary and revision correction of paralytic lagophthalmos. Facial Plast Surg Aesthet Med 2022. https://doi.org/10.1089/fpsam.2022.0096.
31. Allen R. Controversies in periocular reconstruction for facial nerve palsy. Curr Opin Opthalmol 2018;29(5):423–7.
32. Rivas A, Boahene KD, Bravo HC, et al. A model for early prediction of facial nerve recovery after vestibular schwannoma surgery. Otol Neurotol 2011;32(5):826–33.
33. Albathi M, Oyer S, Ishii LE, et al. Early nerve grafting for facial paralysis after cerebellopontine angle tumor resection with preserved facial nerve continuity. JAMA facial Plastic Surgery 2016;18(1):54–60.
34. Zhang S, Hembd A, Ching CW, et al. Early masseter to facial nerve transfer may improve smile excursion in facial paralysis. Plast Reconstr Surg Glob Open 2018; 6(11):e2023.
35. Boahene KD, Farrag TY, Ishii L, et al. Minimally invasive temporalis tendon transposition. Arch Facial Plast Surg 2011;13(1):8–13.
36. Labbé D, Huault M. Lengthening temporalis myoplasty and lip reanimation. Plast Reconstr Surg 2000;105(4):1289–97 [discussion: 1298].
37. McLaughlin CR. Surgical support in permanent facial paralysis. Plast Reconstr Surg 1953;11(4):302–14.
38. Byrne PJ, Kim M, Boahene K, et al. Temporalis tendon transfer as part of a comprehensive approach to facial reanimation. Arch Facial Plast Surg 2007; 9(4):234–41.
39. Boonipat T, Robertson CE, Meaike JD, et al. Dual innervation of free gracilis muscle for facial reanimation: What we know so far. J Plast Reconstr Aesthetic Surg 2020;73(12):2196–209.

Laryngotracheal Reconstruction for Subglottic and Tracheal Stenosis

Mollie C. Perryman, MD, Shannon M. Kraft, MD,
Hannah L. Kavookjian, MD*

KEYWORDS

- Tracheal stenosis • Subglottic stenosis • Laryngotracheal reconstruction

KEY POINTS

- Laryngotracheal stenosis is the clinical endpoint of symptomatic airway narrowing, most commonly iatrogenic due to intubation or tracheostomy.
- LTS is most commonly treated using endoscopic surgical interventions.
- Open surgeries most often include resection of the stenotic segment with reanastomosis. Augmentation of the stenotic segment can be accomplished using grafting or free flaps.
- Emerging techniques in laryngotracheal reconstruction are tracheal transplantation and tissue engineering.

INTRODUCTION

Laryngotracheal stenosis (LTS) is the common endpoint for processes which create narrowing of the larynx, subglottis, and/or trachea (**Table 1**). The most common etiology of LTS is iatrogenic, specifically stenosis related to endotracheal intubation or tracheostomy (54.7%). Idiopathic subglottic stenosis (18.5%), autoimmune disorders (18.5%), and polytrauma (8%) account for most of the remaining causes of adult LTS.[1] Surgery is the mainstay of treatment, and the optimal technique (**Fig. 1**) is dictated by the location, length, and grade[2,3] (**Table 2**) of the stenosis.

LARYNGOTRACHEAL RESECTION
Endoscopic Resection

Endoscopic management of LTS has a high success rate and minimal risks.[4–6] Durability can be variable with many patients requiring multiple interventions throughout their lifetime. Endoscopic interventions consist of suspension microlaryngoscopy,

Department of Otolaryngology–Head & Neck Surgery, University of Kansas, The University of Kansas Medical Center, 3901 Rainbow Boulevard, MS 3010, Kansas City, KS 66160, USA
* Corresponding author.
E-mail address: hkavookjian@kumc.edu

Otolaryngol Clin N Am 56 (2023) 769–778
https://doi.org/10.1016/j.otc.2023.04.018
0030-6665/23/© 2023 Elsevier Inc. All rights reserved.

Table 1	
Etiology of adult laryngotracheal stenosis	
Autoimmune	Amyloidosis
	Granulomatosis with polyangiitis
	Immunoglobulin G4 (IgG-4) disease
	Relapsing polychondritis
	Rheumatoid arthritis
	Sarcoidosis
	Systemic lupus erythematosus
Iatrogenic	Intubation
	Tracheotomy
	Radiation therapy
Idiopathic neoplasm/tumor	
Trauma	Caustic or thermal injury blunt or penetrating trauma

bronchoscopy, excision of stenosis, and dilation. This technique encompasses several minor variations[4,6–11] and adjunctive therapies, such as topical mitomycin C[12] or steroid injection.[13] More recently, serial intralesional steroid injections[14,15] or medical management[16] have been used postoperatively in an attempt to prolong the dilation interval.

Endoscopic laryngotracheoplasty (the Maddern procedure) is a durable, scarless treatment for recurrent or refractory idiopathic subglottic stenosis. This technique includes complete endoscopic resection of the subglottic mucosa and scar while maintaining the cartilaginous framework of the larynx and trachea. A graft and the silicone stent are placed within the lumen to facilitate healing and prevent scar recurrence.[17,18]

Tracheal Resection

For stenosis not amenable to endoscopic management, surgical resection with primary anastomosis is the preferred method to reestablish a patent, functional airway. In tracheal resection, the diseased segment is exposed through a cervical incision. A sternotomy may be required for lesions that extend into the thoracic cavity. The stenosis is skeletonized circumferentially and resected (**Fig. 2**). Limiting posterior mobilization of the membranous wall to less than 1 cm beyond the length of stenosis reduces the risk of tracheal devascularization.[19,20] The anastomosis is created first along the membranous wall and then the anterior wall.

A tension-free anastomosis is paramount for successful surgery. Approximately 2 cm of trachea can be primarily resected, but up to 50% of the trachea (approximately 5 cm) can be resected with the addition of lengthening maneuvers.[21] Flexing the neck

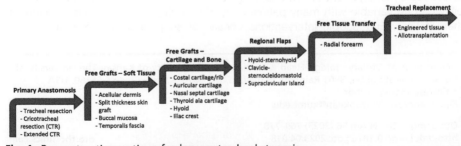

Fig. 1. Reconstruction options for laryngotracheal stenosis.

Table 2 Commonly used endoscopic grading systems for laryngotracheal stenosis	
Cotton-Myer System	
Grade	**Lumen Obstruction**
I	0–50%
II	50–70%
III	71–99%
IV	100%
McCaffrey System	
Stage	**Locations**
I	Subglottic OR tracheal, <1 cm
II	Subglottic >1 cm
III	Subglottic extending into trachea
	Subglottic/tracheal with extension into glottis with
IV	fixation of one/both vocal cords

15 to 30° provides 2 to 4 cm of downward displacement of the trachea, making up most of this length.[22] If a longer segment must be removed, release maneuvers can be used.[23,24] For cervical tracheal resection, release of the suprahyoid muscles will drop the laryngeal framework and release 1 to 2 cm of length.[25,26] This maneuver can result in postoperative dysphagia.[20,21,23] For intrathoracic stenosis, releasing the inferior pulmonary ligament, intrapericardial hilum, and intracartilaginous tracheal ligament can recapture another 2 to 4 cm of tracheal length.[20,21,25,27] Heavy sutures can be placed externally between the skin overlying the mandible and sternum to prevent excessive neck extension in the postoperative period.[21,22]

Cricotracheal Resection

Cricotracheal resection (CTR) is indicated when the stenosis involves both the trachea and cricoid. Surgery involves a partial or complete resection of the diseased cricoid with or without an additional segment of trachea (see **Fig. 2**). When partial cricoidectomy is performed, the inner lamina can be thinned using a high-speed cutting bur to remove underlying scar and fibrosis from the lumen, leaving the outer table of cartilage intact.[20] CTR carries an increased risk of injury to the recurrent laryngeal nerves as they enter near the cricothyroid joint. This risk can be mitigated with identification of the nerves and by maintaining dissection medial to the cricothyroid muscles. The role of intraoperative nerve monitoring is unclear.[28] After resection of the diseased segment, the trachea is advanced cranially, and anastomosis to the residual cricoid or thyroid cartilage is performed.[19,20] CTR often requires perioperative tracheostomy due to transient postoperative glottic edema.

Extended Cricotracheal Resection

When the stenosis extends superiorly into the subglottis/glottis, an extended CTR (ExtCTR) combines the tracheal resection/CTR techniques with expansion grafting to reconstruct the airway. The posterior cricoid is approached via a laryngofissure and divided, allowing placement of a posterior graft to expand the subglottis. The stenotic trachea is resected, and healthy trachea is anastomosed to the cricoid remnant and thyroid cartilage. A stent or endotracheal tube is placed for structural support of the expanded airway.[20]

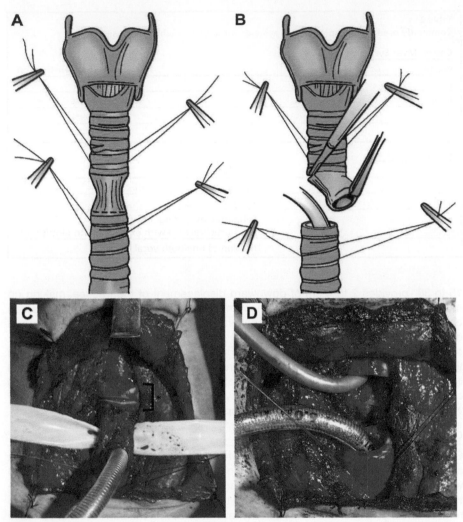

Fig. 2. Schematic of tracheal and cricotracheal resection. Figure adapted from Surgical Management of Upper Airway Stenosis, Cummings Otolaryngology Head and Neck Surgery, 7th Edition. Tracheal stenosis is identified and isolated (A) then excised along inferior (dashed line) and superior borders (B). Cricotracheal stenosis (C) with partial resection of the cricoid (*) and inferior tracheal stenosis. Distal and proximal ends are reapproximated (D) for primary anastomosis. (*From* Robert A. Saadi, Surgical management of upper airway stenosis, Paul W. Flint et, Cumming otolaryngology: Hean and Neck, 7th edition, Elsevier, Inc.)

LARYNGOTRACHEOPLASTY

Expansion grafting can be used alone or in combination with resection (such as in ExtCTR) to augment the airway. Ideal reconstruction materials should provide (1) rigidity to maintain airway patency, (2) flexibility to allow for movement of the neck, and (3) an epithelialized lining for the lumen. Laryngotracheoplasty with autologous tissue including free grafts, composite grafts, pedicled grafts, and free flaps has been described using a variety of methods. Autologous grafts have the benefits of no rejection risk, variable harvest sites (potentially from the same operative field), and potential for both rigid and soft tissue reconstruction.

Single- Versus Double-Staged Reconstruction

Single-stage reconstruction refers to avoiding tracheostomy tube placement at the time of surgery. This may require intubation for several days until glottic edema has resolved. Double-stage reconstruction involves placement of a tracheostomy ± indwelling stent at the time of reconstruction. Stents used in the treatment of LTS include Montgomery laryngeal stents, "t-tubes," endotracheal tubes, or laryngeal keels. These can then be modified to fit a patient's unique anatomy.[29] The stent is kept in place for weeks to months to support airway healing and is removed during a second procedure. Indications for a double-stage procedure include multi-level stenosis, significant comorbid neurological, or respiratory conditions, craniofacial malformations, or salvage procedures.[20] CTR and ExtCTR are often performed as double-staged reconstructions.

Free Mucosal Grafts

Soft tissue grafts can be used to reconstruct the lining of the airway, cover areas of exposed cartilage, and facilitate wound healing. Split thickness skin grafting of the larynx has been used for decades to cover exposed cartilage and prevent formation of granulation tissue or recurrent scar.[30] After harvesting a graft of approximately 0.08 to 0.12 inch thickness, the graft is wrapped around a stent with the dermal side out. Placing the stent within the airway then holds the dermal surface against the exposed cartilage, facilitating wound healing, and mucosal coverage. The stent is then removed transorally after adequate time for skin graft "take" to the surrounding tissue.

Cartilage, Bone, and Composite Grafts

The structural rigidity and native curvature of the autologous cartilage grafts are ideal for maintaining airway patency. Costal and auricular cartilage is well suited for tracheal reconstruction due to straightforward harvest and the amount of tissue available for reconstruction (**Fig. 3**). Animal models have shown durable cartilage viability with relining of respiratory epithelium 4 months postoperatively.[31] Over time, cartilage can resorb, prompting exploration of prosthetic materials for structural support.[32,33]

Composite grafts have the benefit of providing both rigidity and a mucosal lining. These can be free grafts or pedicled flaps, such as hyoid-sternohyoid flap. The hyoid was first used as a grafting material for laryngotracheal reconstruction in 1938[34] and was resurrected in the 1970s to provide durable results in a series of 20 patients.[35–38] The hyoid provides a rigid, vascularized graft when taken as a composite with the infrahyoid muscles,[39] making it more robust. The graft can be trimmed to fit the defect,[40] but care must be taken to preserve the periosteum to reduce the risk of bone necrosis.[40,41] The procedure can be combined with a posterior cricoid split to augment the subglottic airway.[38] The hyoid–sternothyroid flap is limited by the length of the sternohyoid pedicle and the length of bone that can be harvested (~3 cm).[42] The main contraindications include prior Sistrunk procedure, thyroid surgery, or radiotherapy.[40]

Free Flaps

For tracheal defects longer than 5 to 6 cm, primary resection with tension-free anastomosis is often unable to be performed. In these cases, reconstruction options are limited and include autologous tissue transfer, engineered tissue/synthetic prostheses,

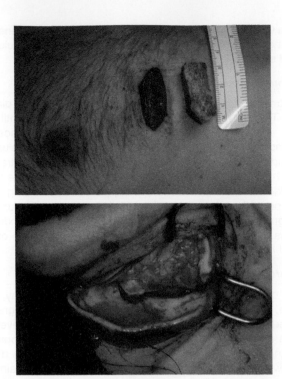

Fig. 3. Costal and auricular cartilage harvest. These autologous grafts can provide additional cartilage for laryngotracheal reconstruction.

and allogenic transplantation. Microvascular flaps provide a source of vascularized tissue for reconstruction of long-segment stenosis. A skin paddle can be incorporated to recreate the airway lining.[43,44] The flap can be augmented with additional tissue to provide rigid support of the airway lumen.[32,33,44–47] In multistage surgeries, cartilage is harvested, fashioned into the appropriate structure, and implanted in the subcutaneous layer of the flap. After 4 to 8 weeks, the composite graft can be harvested and used for reconstruction.[44,47,48] Single-staged procedures implant cartilage grafts into the subdermal layer of the flap at the time of reconstruction.[46] Defects ranging from 7 to 12 cm have been repaired using a tubed fasciocutaneous forearm flap with embedded costal cartilage to create a neo-trachea.[49]

There are limitations to free flap reconstruction. Intraluminal stenting is usually required, which can cause granulation tissue and accumulation of secretions.[45,50] The keratinized squamous cell epithelium of a skin graft lacks mucociliary clearance and can produce keratin debris in the airway. De-epithelializing the skin paddle can improve this.[50]

TRACHEAL REPLACEMENT
Tissue Engineering

Tissue engineered tracheal grafts (TETGs) are alternatives to the tracheal replacement methods discussed previously. Tissue engineering requires a scaffold, which incorporates seeded or native cells to generate a functional graft.[51,52] Silicone,[53] tubed polypropylene,[54] and cryopreserved aortic allograft[55] have all been used in attempts to create a tracheal scaffold. Although short-term outcomes were promising, TETGs have had limited durable success to date due to poor incorporation of artificial materials into the airway, resorption of engineered cartilage,[56] delayed/incomplete graft reepithelialization,[57] and restenosis.[58]

Tracheal Transplantation

Early forays into tracheal transplantation began in the 1970s, but the first successful surgery was not performed until 2008.[59] Transplantation can be performed in single or multistage procedures depending on the intended blood supply. In single-stage reconstruction, the blood supply (superior thyroid arteries and veins, thyrocervical trunk, internal jugular veins, and carotid arteries), esophagus, thyroid gland, and overlying strap muscles are harvested with the donor airway.[60] The lumen of the esophagus is resected, leaving only the esophageal muscularis and the vascular anastomoses between the esophageal muscle and trachea. After the microvascular anastomoses are completed, the donor airway is inset. Multistaged procedures begin with harvest of the fresh cadaveric trachea.[60–62] The graft is implanted into an alternative recipient site, such as the forearm, where a fascial free flap is used to vascularize the donor airway. Additional procedures, such as mucosal or skin grafts, may be necessary to create a mucosal lining for the trachea. Immunosuppression strategies vary, and patients require long-term monitoring for organ rejection and airway patency.

SUMMARY

LTS is the common endpoint for any process that results in the narrowing of the airway at the level of the glottis, subglottis, or trachea. Although endoscopic procedures are effective in opening the airway lumen, open resection and reconstruction can be necessary to reconstitute a functional airway. When resection and anastomosis are insufficient due to extensive length or location of the stenosis, autologous grafts can be used to expand the airway. Future directions in airway reconstruction include tissue engineering and allotransplantation.

CLINICS CARE POINTS

- Airway stenosis can be managed endoscopically in many patients with low morbidity.
- Tracheal resection and cricotracheal resection are the primary methods to treat laryngotracheal stenosis less than 5 to 6 cm long.
- Autologous grafts for airway expansion must provide a rigid support and provide an epithelial lining for the reconstructed airway.
- Tracheal transplantation and tissue engineering may provide alternatives for the reconstruction of longer segment stenoses in the future.

DISCLOSURES

The authors have no financial or commercial disclosures relevant to this article.

REFERENCES

1. Gelbard A, Francis DO, Sandulache VC, et al. Causes and consequences of adult laryngotracheal stenosis. Laryngoscope 2015;125(5):1137–43.

2. Myer CM, Oconnor DM, Cotton RT. Proposed grading system for subglottic stenosis based on endotracheal-tube sizes. Ann Otol Rhinol Laryngol 1994;103(4): 319–23.
3. McCaffrey TV. Classification of laryngotracheal stenosis. Laryngoscope 1992; 102(12 Pt 1):1335–40.
4. Gelbard A, Donovan DT, Ongkasuwan J, et al. Disease homogeneity and treatment heterogeneity in idiopathic subglottic stenosis. Laryngoscope 2016;126(6):1390–6.
5. Herrington HC, Weber SM, Andersen PE. Modern management of laryngotracheal stenosis. Laryngoscope 2006;116(9):1553–7.
6. Dwyer CD, Qiabi M, Fortin D, et al. Idiopathic subglottic stenosis: an institutional review of outcomes with a multimodality surgical approach. Otolaryng Head Neck 2021;164(5):1068–76.
7. Gelbard A, Shyr Y, Berry L, et al. Treatment options in idiopathic subglottic stenosis: protocol for a prospective international multicentre pragmatic trial. BMJ Open 2018;8(4):e022243.
8. Nouraei SA, Sandhu GS. Outcome of a multimodality approach to the management of idiopathic subglottic stenosis. Laryngoscope 2013;123(10):2474–84.
9. Ekbom DC, Bayan SL, Goates AJ, et al. Endoscopic wedge excisions with CO2 laser for subglottic stenosis. Laryngoscope 2021;131(4):E1062–6.
10. Sandhu G. Endoscopic tracheoplasty for treating tracheotomy-related airway stenosis. Operative Techniques in Otolaryngology - Head and Neck Surgery 2011; 22(2):128–30.
11. Nouraei SA, Sandhu GS. Outcome of endoscopic resection tracheoplasty for treating lambdoid tracheal stomal stenosis. Laryngoscope 2013;123(7):1735–41.
12. Ubell ML, Ettema SL, Toohill RJ, et al. Mitomycin-c application in airway stenosis surgery: analysis of safety and costs. Otolaryngol Head Neck Surg 2006;134(3): 403–6.
13. Wierzbicka M, Tokarski M, Puszczewicz M, et al. The efficacy of submucosal corticosteroid injection and dilatation in subglottic stenosis of different aetiology. J Laryngol Otol 2016;130(7):674–9.
14. Bertelsen C, Shoffel-Havakuk H, O'Dell K, et al. serial in-office intralesional steroid injections in airway stenosis. JAMA Otolaryngol Head Neck Surg 2018;144(3): 203–10.
15. Luke AS, Varelas EA, Kaplan S, et al. Efficacy of office-based intralesional steroid injections in the management of subglottic stenosis: a systematic review. Ear Nose Throat J 2021;26. https://doi.org/10.1177/01455613211005119. 145561321 1005119.
16. Bowen AJ, Xie KZ, O'Byrne TJ, et al. Recurrence following endoscopic laser wedge excision and triple medical therapy for idiopathic subglottic stenosis. Otolaryngol Head Neck Surg 2022;167(3):524–30.
17. Davis RJ, Lina I, Motz K, et al. Endoscopic resection and mucosal reconstitution with epidermal grafting: a pilot study in idiopathic subglottic stenosis. Otolaryngol Head Neck Surg 2022;166(5):917–26.
18. Kavookjian H., Endoscopic laryngotracheoplasty (Maddern procedure) for idiopathic subglottic stenosis. Operative Techniques, In: Otolaryngology - Head and Neck Surgery, In Press.
19. Grillo H. Surgery of the Trachea and Bronchi. BC Decker; 2004.
20. Sandhu GS, Nouraei SAR. Laryngeal and Tracheobronchial Stenosis. Plural Publishing, Incorporated; 2015.
21. Mathisen DJ. Surgery of the Trachea. Current Problems in Surgery 1998;35(6): 455–542.

22. Mulliken J. The limits of tracheal resection with primary anastomosis: further anatomical studies in man. J Thorac Cardiovasc Surg 1968;55(3):418–21.
23. Ch'ng S, Wong GL, Clark JR. Reconstruction of the trachea. J Reconstr Microsurg 2014;30(3):153–62.
24. Madariaga MLL, Soni ML, Mathisen DJ, et al. Evaluation of release maneuvers after airway reconstruction. Ann Thorac Surg 2022;113(2):406–12.
25. Broussard B, Mathisen DJ. Tracheal release maneuvers. Ann Cardiothorac Surg 2018;7(2):293–8.
26. Rosen FS, Pou AM, Buford WL. Tracheal resection with primary anastomosis in cadavers: the effects of releasing maneuvers and length of tracheal resection on tension. Ann Otol Rhinol Laryngol 2003;112(10):869–76.
27. Miller RH, Lipkin A, Nouvertne MJ. Tracheal resection. Opening a patient's airway. AORN J 1987;45(4):907–9, 912-909.
28. Cavanaugh K, Park AH. Recurrent laryngeal nerve monitoring during cricotracheal resection. Ann Otol Rhinol Laryngol 2000;109(7):654–7.
29. Folch E, Keyes C. Airway stents. Ann Cardiothorac Surg 2018;7(2):273–83.
30. Olson NR. Skin grafting of the larynx. Otolaryngol Head Neck Surg 1991;104(4): 503–8.
31. Zalzal GH, Cotton RT, McAdams AJ. The survival of costal cartilage graft in laryngotracheal reconstruction. Otolaryngol Head Neck Surg 1986;94(2):204–11.
32. Yu P, Clayman GL, Walsh GL. Human tracheal reconstruction with a composite radial forearm free flap and prosthesis. Ann Thorac Surg 2006;81(2):714–6.
33. Maciejewski A, Szymczyk C, Poltorak S, et al. Tracheal reconstruction with the use of radial forearm free flap combined with biodegradative mesh suspension. Ann Thorac Surg 2009;87(2):608–10.
34. Looper EA. Use of the hyoid bone as a graft in laryngeal stenosis. Arch Otolaryngol Head Neck Surg 1938;28(1):106–11.
35. Ward PH, Canalis R, Fee W, et al. Composite hyoid sternohyoid muscle grafts in humans. Its use in reconstruction of subglottic stenosis and the anterior tracheal wall. Arch Otolaryngol 1977;103(9):531–4.
36. Burstein FD, Canalis R, Ward PH. Composite hyoid-sternohyoid interposition graft revisited: UCLA experience 1974-1984. Laryngoscope 1986;96(5):516–20.
37. Freeland AP. Composite hyoid-sternohyoid graft in the correction of established subglottic stenosis. J R Soc Med 1981;74(10):729–35.
38. Freeland AP. The long-term results of hyoid-sternohyoid grafts in the correction of subglottic stenosis. J Laryngol Otol 1986;100(6):665–74.
39. Wong ML, Finnegan DA, Kashima HK, et al. Vascularized hyoid interposition for subglottic and upper tracheal stenosis. Ann Otol Rhinol Laryngol 1978;87(4 Pt 1): 491–7.
40. Keghian J, Lawson G, Orban D, et al. Composite hyoid-sternohyoid interposition graft in the surgical treatment of laryngotracheal stenosis. Eur Arch Oto-Rhino-Laryngol 2000;257(10):542–7.
41. Cansiz H, Yener HM, Sekercioglu N, et al. Laryngotracheal reconstruction with a muscle-pedicle hyoid bone flap: a series of 23 patients. Ear Nose Throat J 2004; 83(6):424–7.
42. Ouyang D, Liu TR, Liu XW, et al. Combined hyoid bone flap in laryngeal reconstruction after extensive partial laryngectomy for laryngeal cancer. Eur Arch Oto-Rhino-Laryngol 2013;270(4):1455–62.
43. Yamada A, Harii K, Itoh Y, et al. Reconstruction of the cervical trachea with a free forearm flap. Br J Plast Surg 1993;46(1):32–5.

44. Teng MS, Malkin BD, Urken ML. Prefabricated composite free flaps for tracheal reconstruction: a new technique. Ann Otol Rhinol Laryngol 2005;114(11):822–6.

45. Yu P, Clayman GL, Walsh GL. Long-term outcomes of microsurgical reconstruction for large tracheal defects. Cancer 2011;117(4):802–8.

46. Fukunaga Y, Sakuraba M, Miyamoto S, et al. One-stage reconstruction of a tracheal defect with a free radial forearm flap and free costal cartilage grafts. J Plast Reconstr Aesthet Surg 2014;67(6):857–9.

47. Fujiwara T, Nishino K, Numajiri T. Tracheal reconstruction with a prefabricated and double-folded radial forearm free flap. J Plast Reconstr Aesthet Surg 2009;62(6): 790–4.

48. Olias J, Millan G, da Costa D. Circumferential tracheal reconstruction for the functional treatment of airway compromise. Laryngoscope 2005;115(1):159–61.

49. Fabre D, Kolb F, Fadel E, et al. Successful tracheal replacement in humans using autologous tissues: an 8-year experience. Ann Thorac Surg 2013;96(4):1146–55.

50. Beldholm BR, Wilson MK, Gallagher RM, et al. Reconstruction of the trachea with a tubed radial forearm free flap. J Thorac Cardiovasc Surg 2003;126(2):545–50.

51. Bianco P, Robey PG. Stem cells in tissue engineering. Nature 2001;414(6859): 118–21.

52. Zdrahala RJ, Zdrahala IJ. In vivo tissue engineering: Part I. Concept genesis and guidelines for its realization. J Biomater Appl 1999;14(2):192–209.

53. Neville WE, Bolanowski JP, Kotia GG. Clinical experience with the silicone tracheal prosthesis. J Thorac Cardiovasc Surg 1990;99(4):604–12 [discussion: 612-3].

54. Kanemaru S, Hirano S, Umeda H, et al. A tissue-engineering approach for stenosis of the trachea and/or cricoid. Acta Otolaryngol Suppl 2010;(563):79–83. https://doi.org/10.3109/00016489.2010.496462.

55. Martinod E, Paquet J, Dutau H, et al. In vivo tissue engineering of human airways. Ann Thorac Surg 2017;103(5):1631–40.

56. Omori K, Tada Y, Suzuki T, et al. Clinical application of in situ tissue engineering using a scaffolding technique for reconstruction of the larynx and trachea. Ann Otol Rhinol Laryngol 2008;117(9):673–8.

57. Schwartz CM, Dorn BA, Habtemariam S, et al. The wound healing capacity of undifferentiated and differentiated airway epithelial cells in vitro. Int J Pediatr Otorhinolaryngol 2018;112:163–8.

58. Gonfiotti A, Jaus MO, Barale D, et al. The first tissue-engineered airway transplantation: 5-year follow-up results. Lancet 2014;383(9913):238–44.

59. Delaere P, Vranckx J, Verleden G, et al, Leuven Tracheal Transplant G. Tracheal allotransplantation after withdrawal of immunosuppressive therapy. N Engl J Med 2010;362(2):138–45.

60. Genden EM, Miles BA, Harkin TJ, et al. Single-stage long-segment tracheal transplantation. Am J Transplant 2021;21(10):3421–7.

61. Delaere P, Lerut T, Van Raemdonck D. Tracheal Transplantation: State of the Art and Key Role of Blood Supply in Its Success. Thorac Surg Clin 2018;28(3): 337–45.

62. Vranckx JJ, Delaere P. The current status and outlook of trachea transplantation. Curr Opin Organ Transplant 2020;25(6):601–8.

Reconstruction After Skin Cancer Resection of the Head and Neck

David I. Zimmer, MD, DVM[a],*, Aaron M. Wieland, MD[b],
Jamie A. Ku, MD[a]

KEYWORDS

- Reconstruction • Skin cancer • Head and neck • Forehead • Cheek • Lip • Nose
- Eyelid

KEY POINTS

- Reconstruction of skin cancer defects of the face focuses on both functional and aesthetic outcomes.
- Reconstructive techniques can vary greatly from the simplest primary closure to the most complex free flap reconstruction based on defect location, size, shape, thickness, and anatomic functional subunits involved.
- Each reconstructive surgeon must have a thorough understanding of the unique challenges as well as the range of optimal reconstruction options for each type of defect and ultimately develop their own algorithm to achieve the most desirable results in a reliable, consistent, and reproducible fashion.

INTRODUCTION

Skin cancer is the most common overall malignancy in the United States, and this is also true when it comes to the head and neck region.[1] Surgical techniques for resection of skin cancers have made great advances over the last 100 years, with the advent of Mohs micrographic surgery playing a particularly important role.[2] Although it has been shown that patients can be cured from these cancers, they are still left with obvious and notable defects involving the head, face, and neck.

Defects of the head and neck play an exceptionally important role in the form, function, and psychological well-being of patients. Therefore, reconstructive surgeons must have a thorough understanding of the reconstructive ladder and unique challenges that

[a] Head and Neck Institute, Cleveland Clinic, 9500 Euclid Avenue A71, Cleveland, OH 44106, USA; [b] Division of Otolaryngology Head and Neck Surgery, Section of Head and Neck Surgical Oncology, University of Wisconsin, 600 Highland Avenue, BX7375 Clinical Science Center-K4, Madison, WI 53792-3284, USA
* Corresponding author.
E-mail address: zimmerd4@ccf.org

Otolaryngol Clin N Am 56 (2023) 779–790
https://doi.org/10.1016/j.otc.2023.04.006
0030-6665/23/© 2023 Elsevier Inc. All rights reserved.

accompany reconstruction of defects within these regions. The size, shape, thickness, and location of defects all play a role in the decision for reconstruction along with various patient factors.

Anatomically and aesthetically, the head and neck can be divided into central and peripheral subunits that are constituted according to their location, skin quality, thickness, color, texture, and contour.[3] The anatomy of each subunit carries unique challenges, and the decision on how to proceed with reconstruction should be individualized based on patient factors and surgeon comfort.

This review does not seek to depict all available reconstructive options available but instead provides surgeons with a manner to approach common areas of reconstruction based on the regions of defects encountered.

DISCUSSION
Forehead

The forehead is a single subunit that can be divided into 4 different regions: central, paramedian, temporal, and glabellar.[3,4] The primary goals of reconstruction involving the forehead include preservation of sensory and motor innervation, hiding incisions and scars within natural borders and creases, and avoiding distortion of the eyebrows or hairline.

Areas of the forehead can be good candidates to heal via secondary intention, especially concave areas, such as the temporal region. Wound contracture is to be expected in these instances, so care should be taken to avoid this method near the brow or hairline. Primary closure is an excellent option when smaller defects (<3 cm) are present.[5] Wide undermining is possible given the robust blood supply to the forehead. Subcutaneous dissection is possible for smaller defects and provides better laxity of skin, but subfascial dissection should be used for larger defects.[6] Care should be taken while undermining near the temporal region of the forehead, as the frontal branch of the facial nerve courses just beneath frontalis in this region. Vertically designed incisions are also preferred for primary closure defects to avoid distortion of the eyebrows.[3]

Skin grafting can be used in patients who have a granulating tissue bed under their defect but is rarely used owing to poor results in skin color and texture match. Horizontal advancement flaps are commonly used in reconstruction of forehead defects, as their horizontal movement avoids distortion of the hairline or eyebrows while also providing the benefit of camouflaging incisions in naturally occurring rhytids. A-to-T and O-to-T rotation/advancement flaps are options for closure of larger defects near the hairline or brow as the cross-limbs of the T can be placed within the frontal hairline or rhytids over the brow. The incision can extend within these areas across the entire forehead to assist with advancement of tissue.[7]

Tissue expanders can be used to assist with closure of forehead defects; however, utilization requires a staged approach and often a significant amount of time for tissue expansion to adequately occur. For very large defects, free flaps are also a valuable option.

Cheek

The cheek is a subunit that is large and well-vascularized and that often becomes more lax as people age, giving surgeons the advantage of concealing scars in deepened relaxed skin tension lines. The cheek is also similar to other anatomic subunits in that it has visible bilateral symmetry, which must be kept in mind during reconstruction of defects.

The cheek is bounded laterally by the preauricular crease, superiorly by the orbit and zygomatic arch, inferiorly by the mandible, and medially by the lips and nasolabial fold.[8] The cheek as a subunit can generally be subdivided into 3 zones based on texture, mobility, and skin laxity. Zone 1 is considered the infraorbital and perioral cheek area; zone 2 is the preauricular area, and zone 3 is the buccomandibular area.[9]

Defects in all 3 zones can be considered for primary closure. In a retrospective review of more than 400 cases of post–Mohs cheek reconstruction performed by a single surgeon over a 10-year period, more than 50% of cases were repaired via primary closure.[8] Gentle undermining as needed should be performed, and planned vertical defects are generally preferred, as they push excess tissue superiorly and help avoid any excess tension on the inferior lid. Tacking sutures should be performed during initial planning to evaluate for tension on the lid. If any tension exists, further undermining should performed, or another technique should be evaluated.

Geometric flap closures, such as rhomboid or bilobed flaps, have historically been discussed in literature and have been used with great success, especially when orientation of the flap is designed based on aesthetic subunits and relaxed skin tension lines.[8,10,11]

When possible, however, a longer linear scar from primary closure is often better tolerated, as geometric flap closures can result in unavoidable scars with limbs oriented perpendicular to relaxed skin tension lines and with geometric shapes that are not generally found on the native face (**Fig. 1**).

For defects larger than 3 to 4 cm, facial advancement or cervicofacial advancement flaps provide an excellent option for reconstruction. This locoregional advancement-rotation flap allows skin from the cheek, neck, and even chest to be rotated to fill large defects of the cheek. This skin is excellent in color and texture match, and posteriorly based flaps can often successfully be hidden in natural creases and subunit borders. Extreme care has to be taken, however, to avoid downward pull on the area of the lower eyelid. Every effort should be made to avoid tension in this area and can often be achieved by designing the incision above the lateral canthus or suspending the flap to the lateral orbital periosteum[3] (**Fig. 2**).

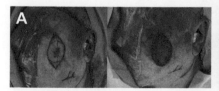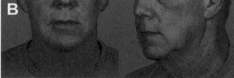

Fig. 1. Primary closure using relaxed skin tension lines. (*A*) Planned defect and surgical defect following excision of skin cancer. (*B*) Final healed surgical scar within relaxed skin tension line.

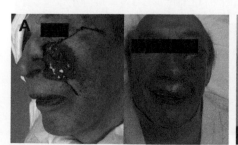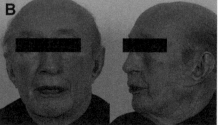

Fig. 2. Facial advancement flap. (*A*) Facial defect with planned advancement flap followed by flap closure. (*B*) Final healed scar.

Lip

The lip is a complex anatomic structure bordered superiorly by the nasal base, inferiorly by the labiomental crease, and laterally by the nasolabial sulcus. It is made up of 4 subunits, including the 2 lateral elements of the upper lip, the central upper lip philtrum, and the lower lip.[3] The lip as a central structure plays an important role in cosmesis but is also incredibly important functionally. On cross-section, the lip comprises skin, subcutaneous tissue, muscle, and oral mucosa. Defects are therefore often

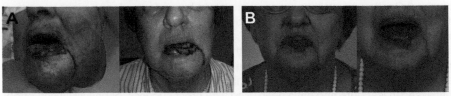

Fig. 3. Rotational flap from the chin. (*A*) Lower lip defect followed by immediate closure. (*B*) Final healed scar.

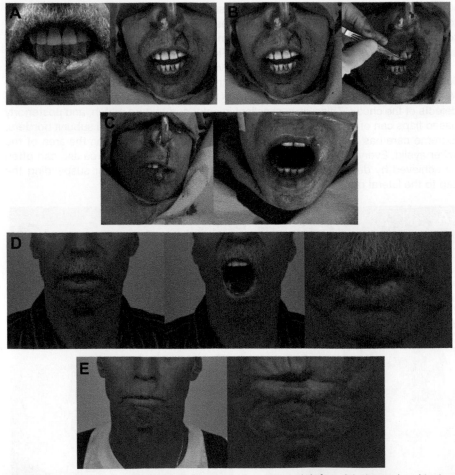

Fig. 4. Abbe flap. (*A*) Lower lip cancer followed by excisional defect. (*B*) Planned and incised upper lip flap. (*C*) Flap following inset and later division. (*D*) Functional use of lip at rest, opening mouth, and puckering lips. (*E*) Final healed scar at rest and during puckering of lips.

grouped based on their location and depth: cutaneous only, vermillion-mucosa only, or full thickness; as well as the size of the defect: less than one-half, one-half to two-thirds, total, or near total.[12]

Cutaneous-only defects can be closed primarily or by using A-to-T and O-to-T-advancement flaps if they are near the vermilion. Larger defects of the upper lip can be reconstructed using melolabial advancement flaps, and larger defects of the lower lip can use rotational flaps from the chin or cheek (**Fig. 3**). For vermillion-mucosa–only defects, closure can be achieved via primary closure for small defects or via mucosal advancement flaps with dissection to the gingivolabial sulcus as needed. Mucosal advancement flaps work well but do run the risk of distorting the vermillion via wound contracture depending on the size of the defect. Interpolated cross-lip mucosal flaps and ventral/lateral tongue flaps have also been described, but they require a second surgery and food restriction, which relegate their use to combined mucosa-muscle defects where bulkiness is required.[3,13]

Full-thickness defects of the lip follow a well-established algorithm, which is approached based on the percentage of the lip missing and its location along the lip. Full-thickness defects less than a third of the total lip length not involving commissure can generally be closed primarily.[14] Defects larger than one-third of the lip length cannot be reconstructed using solely advancement of tissue, so tissue borrowing becomes necessary. The Abbe flap is useful for defects larger than one-third but less than two-thirds of the total lip length that do not involve the commissure (**Fig. 4**).

The Estlander flap is preferred for defects, including the oral commissure, and can be performed as a single-stage procedure, although a second commissuroplasty is often needed if distortion is present owing to the innate inclusion of the modiolus (**Fig. 5**). A Gillies "fan" flap is a modification of the Estlander flap, which is formed

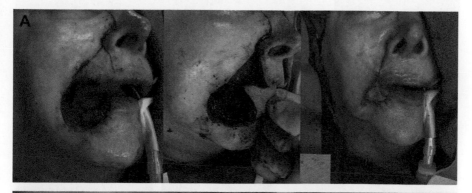

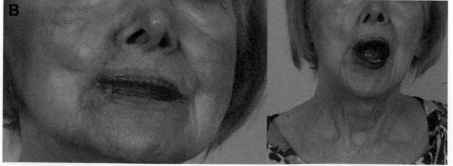

Fig. 5. Estlander flap. (*A*) Oral commissure defect with planned rotational flap, flap division, and immediate inset. (*B*) Final healed scar at rest and during mouth opening.

by recruitment of ipsilateral lip elements with more tissue from the nasolabial area than the opposing lip.[3]

A Karapandzic flap is also a good option for defects comprising between one-third and two-thirds of the total lip length and not involving the commissure. Curved circumoral incisions are made parallel to the nasolabial sulcus allowing remaining and opposing lip tissue to be mobilized to reestablish the lip with care taken to preserve the superior and inferior labial blood supply and buccal nerve branches. The disadvantage of the Karapandzic flap is its ability to cause microstomia.

Defects that encompass greater than 80% of the lip are challenging to repair owing to insufficient remaining lip tissue and difficulty maintaining functional oral competence. The Bernard–von Burrow–Webster flap is a regional flap often used for near total or total lip reconstruction in which remaining lip tissue and cheek tissue are advanced with the utilization of multiple Burrow triangles to mobilize extra cheek tissue. Free flaps are also used for significantly large defects not amenable to the above options.

Ear

The ear provides complex but unique challenges when it comes to reconstruction. The ear is made up of 5 distinct zones, including the helical rim, superior, middle, and lower third of the auricle, and the lobule. Cartilage is present within the upper two-thirds of the ear, and fibrofatty soft tissue and skin constitute the lower third. As in other areas of the head and neck, the location of the defect and its depth of involvement guide reconstructive strategies.[15]

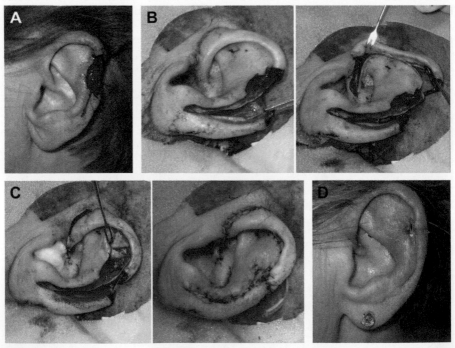

Fig. 6. Helical advancement flaps. (*A*) Surgical defect from skin cancer resection. (*B*) Incisions for planned helical advancement flaps. (*C*) Deep and final closure of helical advancement flaps. (*D*) Final healed surgical scar. (Krieger, Laraine (20050518173349058) 2005060911251 4992.)

Defects involving only the skin and that are less than 3 cm in diameter (with intact perichondrium underneath) are candidates to heal via secondary intention or as recipient sites for skin grafts.[6] This is best used on concave surfaces like the concha bowl, where the underlying cartilage can oppose wound contracture. It is not well used on areas such as the external auditory canal or helical rim, as wound contracture is likely to cause stenosis for the former or contour deformities for the latter.[16] Defects that overlie the antihelix can be allowed to form a granulation bed before being skin grafted.

Helical defects can be managed with wedge excisions or helical advancement flaps (**Fig. 6**). Wedge resections are appropriate for defects that are less than 15% of the auricular height.[16] Although these wedge resections may make the reconstructed ear noticeably smaller than the contralateral ear, it is not commonly recognized owing to the infrequency with which both ears are able to be fully visualized and compared at the same time. For larger defects that are greater than 2 cm, a staged reconstruction can be performed using a postauricular flap with or without cartilage grafts, including composite grafts from the contralateral ear.

For defects of the lobule, primary closure and wedge excisions are readily used. For total or subtotal defects, principles of congenital auricular reconstruction are used. Good success has been described using costal cartilage as a cartilage framework, a temporoparietal fascia (TPF) flap to cover the graft, and finally, a skin graft placed over the TPF in a 2-stage procedure or a single-stage operation.[17]

Nose

The nose has immense importance, as it is a central aesthetic feature of the face as well as serves a critical role in the upper airway respiration and humidification. When it comes to reconstruction, form and function must be balanced. It is helpful to think of nasal reconstruction by assessing the internal lining, structural support, and external nasal subunit defect.[4] All 3 layers of cover, lining, and support must be reestablished for a functionally and aesthetically sound reconstruction. In addition, patient factors, such as comorbid conditions and cooperation, play an important role in the decision for which manner of reconstruction may be undertaken, especially when it comes to performing single-stage versus complex multistaged procedures.

Defects that involve the internal nasal lining can be reconstructed in several ways. Small defects near the alar rim can be closed by recruitment of bipedicled mucosal flaps from the nasal vault depending on the size of the defect. Larger defects can be closed via a septal mucoperichondrial flap, which has often served as the workhorse of restoring internal nasal lining. The only downside of this flap, however, is that it requires a second stage to take down the pedicle and finish inset.[18] Staged turn in flaps, such as the 3-staged folded forehead flap, can help re-create internal lining using extra external skin. A combination of flaps, such as a nasolabial fold flap with a paramedian forehead flap, allows for utilization of each flap to create an internal and external lining for larger defects as well.[18]

In defects that cause structural deformity, structural support must also be replaced. If native cartilage of the nose is involved during ablation, anatomic grafting should be performed. If the alar rim is involved during ablation, then it is also often necessary to perform nonanatomic grafting as well. The most common site to obtain donor cartilage is from the ear. Large amounts of cartilage can be obtained from the conchal cartilage of the ear. Native nasal septal cartilage can also be harvested and used, especially if a septal mucoperichondrial flap is already being used. For larger structural defects or anterior septal defects, rib cartilage can also be harvested and used for reconstruction.

If internal lining and structural support are appropriately addressed, then the external lining and soft tissue defects can then be managed. As a starting point, it is useful to think of the 9 nasal subunits and to use the subunit principle popularized by Burget and Menick.[19,20]

This principle advocates for replacement of an entire subunit if greater than 50% of that subunit is missing.[19] Although this is widely used, the primary purpose of this technique is to disguise incisions along the borders of subunits; considerations of size, structures missing, and location should also always be taken into account.

For external skin defects, skin grafts can be used, often taken from preauricular skin for color thickness match. These are most successful when used for defects high on the lateral nasal sidewall where underlying bone and periosteum combat retraction. Skin grafting to the remainder of the nose, especially the lower third, has been controversial given its propensity for contraction. Local rotational flaps, such as the bilobed flap or banner flap, have been well described in literature and can have decent outcomes for smaller dorsal nasal defects. However, they can also be prone to pin-cushioning, concavity of the donor site, and a measure of unpredictability when it comes to overall results[18] (**Fig. 7**). For small defects, less than 1.5 cm, banner flaps can be acceptable when these defects are located on the tip or supratip, but meticulous undermining and direct closure also yield very successful results for small defects.

For full-thickness defects of the nasal dorsum, which are above the tip defining elements of the nose and less than 2 cm, the dorsal nasal flap has become the procedure of choice for many surgeons.[21] These flaps are developed in the deep submuscular plane above the periosteum with wide undermining of the nasal dorsum in order to provide sufficient laxity for closure of the defect. This allows for the flap to function most effectively at the smooth planes of the nasal dorsum and sidewalls[18] (**Fig. 8**).

For alar defects, nasolabial fold flaps provide an excellent reconstructive option, especially in older patients who already have a defined nasolabial fold. The flap should always be superiorly designed with the border planned at the deepest point of the nasolabial fold. These flaps are especially helpful if you are also reconstructing with cartilage, as it provides a vascularized external cover. These flaps should be thinned carefully to just under the dermal layer so as to not provide excess bulk, but also with care taken to preserve the subdermal plexus. Composite grafts from the root of the helix can also be obtained and used to reconstruct alar rim defects.

In younger patients who lack a nasolabial fold as well as for larger or distal nasal tip defects, the paramedian forehead flap remains the gold standard for reconstruction. The excellent color and texture match, the robust blood supply, the reach of the flap, and the amount of skin that can be used mark the most significant benefits of

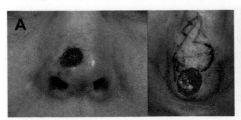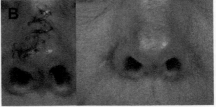

Fig. 7. Bilobed flap. (*A*) Surgical defect and planned bilobed flap. (*B*) Immediate closure and final healed surgical scar.

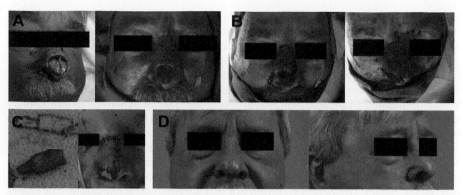

Fig. 8. Dorsal nasal flap with composite graft from left ear for ala. (*A*) Surgical defect on nasal dorsum. (*B*) Dorsal nasal flap following incision and advancement. (*C*) Composite graft taken from ear and inset into alar defect along with closure of composite graft and dorsal nasal flap. (*D*) Final healed surgical scar.

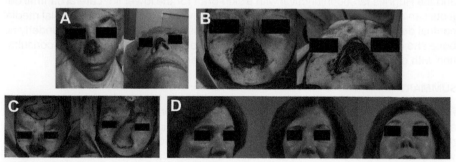

Fig. 9. Nasal reconstruction with cartilage grafting for structural support and a paramedian forehead flap for external reconstruction. (*A*) Surgical defect following skin cancer reconstruction involving skin and underlying cartilage. (*B*) Reconstruction of underlying structural constructs with cartilage grafts. (*C*) Planned and inset paramedian forehead flap. (*D*) Final healed surgical defect after inset and division of forehead flap.

this highly used flap. Its drawbacks primarily stem from the necessity for a 2- or 3-stage procedure along with its cosmesis for patients before division and inset[4,18] (**Fig. 9**).

Eyelid

The eyelid plays an important functional role in protecting and supporting the globe in addition to its prominent aesthetic importance. When reconstructing eyelid defects, it is again important to take into account the structures involved as well as the total size of the defect. It is helpful to think of the eyelid in terms of an anterior lamella (skin, subcutaneous tissue, and the underlying orbicularis) and the posterior lamella (tarsal plate and conjunctiva).[22]

For partial-thickness defects involving the anterior lamella, full-thickness skin grafts from the contralateral eyelid can be harvested via a blepharoplasty incision and used for reconstruction with good color match and low morbidity. For partial-thickness posterior lamellar defects, lateral advancement flaps can be used from the remaining tarsus or conjunctiva as well as free tarsoconjunctival grafts from the contralateral eye. It is important to note that 2 free grafts should not be used in conjunction to reconstruct the anterior and posterior lamellar defects, but instead a combination of an advancement flap and a graft should be used.[4,22]

For full-thickness defects of the upper and lower eyelid, there are different options depending on the size of the defect. For smaller defects, such as those less than 20% in younger individuals and less than 30% in older individuals or those with lax lids, primary closure provides the best aesthetic and functional results. If there is concern for excess tension, a lateral canthotomy or cantholysis can be used to help provide extra length.

For larger but not complete defects of the upper and lower lid, such as those 30% to 50% horizontal width, Tenzel lateral advancement flaps can be used.[4] These flaps require raising skin and soft tissue lateral to the lateral canthus and recruits it to help fill the defect. Dissection is carried out in a suborbicularis plane until just before the orbital rim and then transitioned to a subcutaneous plane to avoid injury to the zygomatic branch of the facial nerve.[3]

For larger defects comprising 50% to 100% of the horizontal width of the upper and lower lid, lid-sharing procedures are often best used: the Cutler-Beard for the upper lid and the Hughes tarsoconjunctival with a skin graft for the lower lid. Lateral canthal defects can often be addressed with rotational or advancement flaps. Superficial medial canthal defects are well suited for skin grafts as discussed above given the underlying bone and concave nature. For deeper defects involving the lacrimal system, consultation with oculoplastic colleagues is often necessary.

SUMMARY

Reconstructive surgeons are tasked with preserving or restoring form, function, and aesthetics following skin cancer ablation. Reconstruction of skin cancer defects can range from primary closure to complex free flaps and everything in between. The vast quantity of reconstructive techniques available can seem daunting to master. However, by approaching each defect in a logistical, systematic manner, surgeons can develop a set of reliable techniques to address any defects they may face.

CLINICS CARE POINTS

- Although many geometric flap closures exhist and have historically been used with great success in certain areas of the a head and neck, a longer linear scar from primary closure is often better tolerated, as geometric flap closures can result in unavoidable scars with limbs oriented perpendicular to relaxed skin tension lines and with geometric shapes that are not generally found on the native face.

- When utilizing local tissue rearrangement for reconstruction of defects, it is important to balance the amount of tension being applied in the area of reconstruction as well as the donor site. It is tempting to believe that tension in a certain area will "settle out," but contracture of scars during healing rarely allow for settling of tissue. Therefore, the amount of tension placed on donor tissue and native tissue surrounding the defect must constantly be considered during planning and reconstruction.

- Patient factors should continue to play a central role when it comes to decision making regarding reconstruction. Each patient's anatomy, defect, and goals of reconstruction are different. Therefore, although there are well used techniques based on anatomical subsites, a surgeon must approach each patient and defect with a critical mind in order to obtain the best outcomes.

DISCLOSURE

The authors have no commercial or financial conflicts of interest or special funding to disclose.

ACKNOWLEDGMENT

The authors would like to especially thank Dr Michael Fritz for his excellence in head and neck reconstruction and education over the years. All of the reconstructions depicted throughout the article were provided by Dr Fritz and are a testament to his dedication to his craft.

REFERENCES

1. Ouyang YH. Skin cancer of the head and neck. Semin Plast Surg 2010;24(2): 117–26.
2. Golda N, Hruza G. Mohs Micrographic Surgery. Dermatol Clin 2023;41(1): 39–47.
3. Eskiizmir G, Baker S, Cingi C. Nonmelanoma skin cancer of the head and neck: reconstruction. Facial Plast Surg Clin North Am 2012;20(4):493–513.
4. Meaike JD, Dickey RM, Killion E, et al. Facial Skin Cancer Reconstruction. Semin Plast Surg 2016;30(3):108–21.
5. TerKonda RP, Sykes JM. Concepts in scalp and forehead reconstruction. Otolaryngol Clin North Am 1997;30(4):519–39.
6. Rogers-Vizena CR, Lalonde DH, Menick FJ, et al. Surgical treatment and reconstruction of nonmelanoma facial skin cancers. Plast Reconstr Surg 2015;135(5): 895e–908e.
7. Angelos PC, Downs BW. Options for the management of forehead and scalp defects. Facial Plast Surg Clin North Am 2009;17(3):379–93.
8. Rapstine ED, Knaus WJ 2nd, Thornton JF. Simplifying cheek reconstruction: a review of over 400 cases. Plast Reconstr Surg 2012;129(6):1291–9.
9. Roth DA, Longaker MT, Zide BM. Cheek surface reconstruction: best choices according to zones. Operat Tech Plast Reconstr Surg 1998;5(1):26–36.
10. Chu EA, Byrne PJ. Local flaps I: bilobed, rhombic, and cervicofacial. Facial Plast Surg Clin North Am 2009;17(3):349–60.
11. Heller L, Cole P, Kaufman Y. Cheek reconstruction: current concepts in managing facial soft tissue loss. Semin Plast Surg 2008;22(4):294–305.
12. Coppit GL, Lin DT, Burkey BB. Current concepts in lip reconstruction. Curr Opin Otolaryngol Head Neck Surg 2004;12(4):281–7.
13. Baker SR. Flap classification and design. Local flaps in facial reconstruction. Philadelphia: Mosby Elsevier; 2007. p. 71–105.
14. Cupp CL, Larrabee WF Jr. Reconstruction of the lips. Operat Tech Otolaryngol Head Neck Surg 1993;4(1):46–53.
15. Lee EI, Xue AS, Hollier LH Jr, et al. Ear and nose reconstruction in children. Oral Maxillofac Surg Clin North Am 2012;24(3):397–416.
16. Shonka DC Jr, Park SS. Ear defects. Facial Plast Surg Clin North Am 2009;17(3): 429–43.
17. Ali SN, Khan MA, Farid M, et al. Reconstruction of segmental acquired auricular defects. J Craniofac Surg 2010;21(2):561–4.
18. Thornton JF, Griffin JR, Constantine FC. Nasal reconstruction: an overview and nuances. Semin Plast Surg 2008;22(4):257–68.

19. Burget GC, Menick FJ. The subunit principle in nasal reconstruction. Plast Reconstr Surg 1985;76(2):239–47.
20. Losco L, Bolletta A, Pierazzi DM, et al. Reconstruction of the Nose: Management of Nasal Cutaneous Defects According to Aesthetic Subunit and Defect Size. A Review. Medicina (Kaunas) 2020;56(12). https://doi.org/10.3390/medicina56120639.
21. Rohrich RJ, Griffin JR, Ansari M, et al. Nasal reconstruction—beyond aesthetic subunits: a 15-year review of 1334 cases. Plast Reconstr Surg 2004;114(6): 1405–16.
22. Gündüz K, Demirel S, Günalp I, et al. Surgical approaches used in the reconstruction of the eyelids after excision of malignant tumors. Ann Ophthalmol 2006;38:207–12.

Current Trends in Head and Neck Trauma

Gregory I. Kelts, MD, Travis R. Newberry, MD*

KEYWORDS

- Facial trauma • Orbital fracture • Mandible fracture • Laryngotracheal trauma

KEY POINTS

- Operative intervention in head and neck trauma should aim to restore premorbid form and function.
- Head and neck trauma encompasses a broad range of tissue types with significant functional implications.
- Knowledge of current trends in management is essential for optimal patient care and long-term outcomes.
- Advances in materials, computer-aided surgery, and bioengineering combined with improved surgical techniques allow for continued changes in practice patterns that improve patient outcomes.

INTRODUCTION

Head and neck trauma is an important part of Otolaryngology training, and most of the junior Otolaryngologists report a desire to incorporate trauma as a part of their practice.[1] The primary goal in management of head and neck trauma is to return form and function, with cosmesis being an important consideration. To accomplish this goal, many patients require multiple procedures and benefit from a multidisciplinary team approach to rehabilitation. In this article, the authors present a collection of up-to-date and evidence-based practice trends surrounding management of head and neck trauma.

DISCUSSION
Soft Tissue Trauma

Soft tissue injuries in the head and neck are common and range from simple lacerations to complex injuries involving a broad range of tissue types. Initial management

Department of Otolaryngology-Head and Neck Surgery, San Antonio Uniformed Services Health Education Consortium, 3551 Roger Brooke Drive, JBSA-Fort Sam Houston, TX 78234, USA
* Corresponding author.
E-mail address: tnewb33@gmail.com

Otolaryngol Clin N Am 56 (2023) 791–800
https://doi.org/10.1016/j.otc.2023.04.011
0030-6665/23/© 2023 Elsevier Inc. All rights reserved.

focuses on control of hemorrhage, extensive wound cleansing, and conservative debridement. The wound should be meticulously cleaned of all foreign materials, but only clearly nonviable native tissue should be removed.[2] Primary closure of wounds is often possible even in large and complex lacerations. If primary closure is not possible, wounds can heal via secondary intention with delayed reconstruction, if needed.

Lacerations involving nose, periorbita, eyelid, lips, and ears are particularly challenging, and a detailed discussion regarding management is beyond the scope of this review. In general, primary repair with meticulous technique yields the best outcome but surgeons should have a clear understanding of relevant anatomy and function when addressing these injuries. The periorbita and eyelid are particularly complex and require careful attention to avoid secondary injuries to the lacrimal system or long-term complications such as entropion or ectropion. In these cases, multidisciplinary care is often in the patient's best interest.

Avulsion injuries in the head and neck, although uncommon, are particularly challenging. If the avulsed tissue is available and vessels are identified, microvascular repair and reimplantation in a timely fashion is often recommended. If a vein is unavailable for anastomosis, leach therapy may be effective to ease venous congestion of the flap.[3] If the avulsed tissue is not available or not viable, regional flaps or microvascular free tissue transfer is necessary. Current trends in reconstructive surgery are to accomplish definitive repair within 2 weeks to avoid significant contracture and infection.[4]

Injuries in the region of the parotid gland deserve special attention due to the location of the facial nerve and Stenson duct. Injuries to the gland parenchyma can be managed conservatively with a closed suction drain, antisialagogues, anticholinergics, Botox, and/or pressure dressings. Exploration of the parotid duct is warranted for penetrating injuries of the cheek, particularly those posterior to the anterior border of the masseter.[5] Transoral canulation of the duct or irrigation allows the surgeon to easily identify injuries. Primary repair within the first 24 hours with closure over a catheter (silastic tubing, angiocatheter, feeding tube, and so forth) is the preferred method of repair for injuries distal to the parotid gland parenchyma.[6,7] The catheter is secured to the oral mucosa and left in place for 2 to 3 weeks. If primary repair is not possible, the proximal duct is ligated and supportive management initiated while parotid atrophy occurs.[8] If injuries are not diagnosed at the time of trauma, or repair is not possible, the literature suggests that nonoperative management is successful although complication rates are higher, and healing occurs over a prolonged period.[9]

Known or suspected injuries to the facial nerve should be explored within 72 hours to allow for stimulation of the distal branches before Wallerian degeneration. However, if early repair is not feasible, attempts at repair weeks after injury can still yield positive results.[10,11] End-to-end primary anastomosis is the treatment of choice for clean transections but the anastomosis must be tension-free through full range of motion.[12] If tension-free primary anastomosis is not possible or if there is a damaged section of the nerve, autograft transposition using sensory nerves is common practice.[13] Bioengineered or decellularized autografts have the advantage of providing an interposition option without donor nerve morbidity, and the use of stem cells or neurotrophic factors in conduits shows promise.[14] Additional studies using bioengineered products for facial nerve injury are needed, but the potential for future success is exciting.[15]

Craniomaxillofacial Trauma

Management of maxillomandibular fractures aims to restore masticatory function, maintain proper occlusion, and achieve cosmetically pleasing results. The initial step in management often involves reduction of the fracture with maxillomandibular fixation (MMF). Erich arch bars have been the gold standard for MMF for decades and remains a valuable option for intermaxillary fixation. However, bone-supported arch bars have shown equal efficacy with reduced operative time.[16] A potential pitfall to bone-supported arch bars is causing damage to teeth and tooth roots. Care should be taken when using alternate MMF techniques to avoid this complication (**Fig. 1**).

Mandibular fractures

Fixation of the mandible with plates and screws reduces or eliminates the time needed in MMF. Plate osteosynthesis of the mandible dates to the late nineteenth century with significant advancements in materials and techniques in the past 50 years.[17] Mandibular angle fractures remain an area of interest due to the higher rates of complications compared with other fracture sites. Two techniques have emerged as standard treatment of angle fractures. In 1978, Champy described a technique using miniplate fixation of the mandibular angle following Champy lines of osteosynthesis.[18] Placement of monocortical miniplates along the superior oblique ridge or superior lateral border of the mandible provides stability of the fracture and allows for secondary bone healing. Care should be taken to ensure the fracture is stabilized or a second miniplate used for additional support. Three-dimensional miniplate fixation has shown better results than using paired miniplates at the mandibular angle.[19] These "box" or "strut" plates provide stability in 3 dimensions, leading to a semirigid fixation. Alternatively, rigid fixation can be achieved using a 2.4 reconstruction plate or the combination of a 2.0 miniplate superiorly and a 2.0 locking plate along the inferior border; this remains the treatment of choice for complicated fractures or in patients with concerns for compliance (**Fig. 2**).

Optimal management of condylar fractures remains controversial although current practice trends tend to be moving toward open repair. There are a variety of classification systems for condylar fractures ranging from simple to complex. Most of the classification systems recognize 3 segments of the condyle–condylar head, condylar

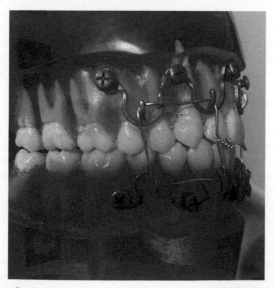

Fig. 1. An example of a bone anchored maxillomandibular fixation device.

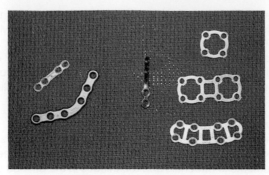

Fig. 2. Options for repair of mandibular angle fractures include rigid plating (*left*), Champy plates (*middle*), and 3D plates (*right*).

neck, and condylar base or subcondyle. Further classification regarding degree of displacement and or dislocation is recognized in more modern systems.[20] Management controversy largely revolves around closed versus open reduction. Absolute indications for open reduction include displacement of mandibular fracture intracranially, presence of a foreign body, inability to obtain proper occlusion, and lateral capsular displacement of the condyle.[21] Other relative indications for open reduction exist depending on the cited source. Improvements in surgical technique and plating materials have led to increased interest in open reduction of fractures. Current literature suggests open treatment may improve malocclusion, protrusion, and laterotrusion but shows no advantage over closed reduction for maximum mouth opening or pain.[22] Evidence suggests that 2 plate fixation, or use of lambda/delta plates, is preferred over single plate fixation.[23]

Orbital fractures

Orbital trauma accounts for a large percentage of craniomaxillofacial trauma, and significant recent advancements in preoperative and intraoperative technique aim to improve patient outcomes.[24] The complex 3-dimensional anatomy, thin bone, and soft-tissue volume create difficulties for the surgical repair. Perhaps more than any other craniomaxillofacial fracture, orbital trauma requires multidisciplinary care to ensure optimal patient outcomes. Urgent repair is indicated for inferior rectus entrapment and concern for symptomatic oculocardiac reflex. Otherwise, timing of repair is controversial, and observation beyond 2 weeks may be reasonable.[25]

Restoration of the premorbid orbital volume is often difficult and incorrect approximation could lead to under or overcorrection. Advancements in imaging techniques and virtual surgical planning have allowed better understanding of fracture patterns and repair strategies. Three-dimensional reconstructions allow better conceptualization of the fracture but do not provide information on premorbid orbital volume in relation to the fractured fragments. Mirror image overlay techniques in which radiographic images of the nontraumatized side are overlayed on the affected orbit allow surgeons better understanding of volume changes.[26] Understanding the volume change is important, but determining the best way to restore the orbital volume remains a difficult task (**Fig. 3**).

Virtual surgical planning (VSP) is the process of creating a 3-dimensional, computer-generated model in a software system that allows manipulation of the virtual patient. Current VSP capabilities allow surgeons to import commercially available implants into the virtual environment in order to test various implants for correct volume

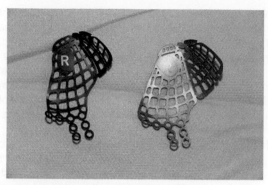

Fig. 3. An example of preformed orbital plates designed to reduce operative time and restore standard orbital volumes.

restoration[27]; this allows the surgeon to identify the most anatomically correct implant as well as identify the optimal placement of the implant before surgery. More recently, researchers are exploring patient-specific implants to see if better outcomes are achieved with printed implants rather than those commercially available.[28,29] Finally, models of the fracture, soft tissue overlays, and implant can be used to perform simulated surgery before the actual procedure.

Intraoperatively, the use of endoscopes, either transorbital or transnasal, can help to ensure plate positioning. In addition, advances in image guidance systems allow for patient-specific implants to be positioned using image guidance to ensure correct placement.[30] Alternatively, the use of image guidance using mirror overlayed image allows "tracing" of commercially available implants to verify correct position and shape.[31] Once in place, intraoperative computed tomography (CT) can verify correct placement and compare the expected simulated position with the final implant position. Indeed, intraoperative CT has already proved advantageous in orbital surgery with or without virtual surgical planning preoperatively.[32]

Frontal sinus fractures

Frontal sinus fractures are relatively rare due to the overall strength of the anterior table. Isolated fractures of the anterior table that do not include the frontal sinus outflow tract are primarily of cosmetic concern. Delayed treatment of these fractures is generally supported, as many cosmetic concerns resolve with time.[33] If the frontal sinus outflow tract is involved, serial imaging should ensure pneumatization of the frontal sinus without mucocele formation.[34] Posterior table fractures pose greater risk for mucocele formation and cerebrospinal fluid (CSF) leak. Current trends favor observation of minimally displaced fractures—even in the presences of CSF leak.[35] Although traditional open approaches remain the standard for operative repair, endonasal approaches are gaining favor. Indeed, even in fractures involving the posterior table with CSF leak, advanced endoscopic techniques allow successful treatment via a transnasal approach.[36]

Laryngotracheal Trauma

Laryngotracheal injuries are relatively uncommon and typically related to blunt trauma.[37] Initial evaluation must focus on airway stability with a low threshold for advanced airway access. Tracheostomy is the safest option for definitive airway management in known or suspected laryngotracheal trauma. If intubation is considered, it should be performed under endoscopic guidance to ensure correct placement past the site of injury while minimizing the risk of additional endolaryngeal damage.

Laryngotracheal injuries often involve multiple structures and frequently have associated injuries. A thorough trauma evaluation and secondary survey are necessary to avoid overlooking critical problems. CT evaluation of the head and neck with or without angiography will identify associated fractures of the hyoid, thyroid, and cricoid cartilages and could identify vascular injuries. Evaluation of the esophagus via esophagoscopy and barium swallow is also critical due to the frequently associated injury of the esophagus.

A thorough evaluation of the airway is necessary to identify the site and extent of laryngotracheal injuries. The Schaefer Classification for Laryngeal injuries first published in 1992 is still widely used today.[38] Other classification systems exist based on extent of trauma, mechanism of injury, and location of injury. Identification and early treatment of airway trauma is important to minimize long-term complications related to breathing, swallowing, and phonation. Early treatment with conservative measures includes head of bed elevation, voice rest, proton pump inhibitors, humidified air, and inhaled corticosteroids.

Laryngeal trauma
Nondisplaced fractures of the thyroid cartilage can be managed conservatively. Displaced or comminuted fractures of the thyroid cartilage should be repaired to restore the endolaryngeal framework and support. Evidence suggests that early repair within 24 to 48 hours of injury leads to improved phonatory outcomes. Repair of fractures using miniplate fixation has gained popularity over previous techniques using sutures and wires.[39,40] Extensive endolaryngeal mucosal injuries are traditionally repaired via thyrotomy, but advancements in optics, magnification, and surgical technique allow transoral repair of some isolated mucosal injuries. Stenting for extensive mucosal injuries or anterior commissure involvement may reduce synechia formation (**Fig. 4**).

Cricoid fractures
Isolated cricoid fractures are rare and can cause rapid airway decompensation. Prompt diagnosis and airway management with tracheostomy are necessary to avoid catastrophic outcomes. Concurrent injury to the recurrent laryngeal nerve is often encountered. Placement of stents allows delayed repair once edema has resolved. Grafting with either rib cartilage or hyoid bone helps to restore patency. Stenting for 4 to 6 weeks is necessary to maintain patency during wound healing.[41]

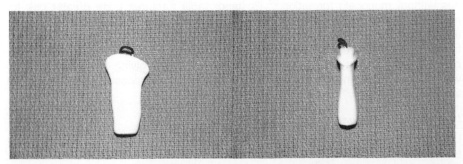

Fig. 4. An example of a laryngeal stent used for extensive endolaryngeal trauma or trauma involving the anterior commissure.

Tracheal injuries

Tracheal trauma including laryngotracheal separation requires prompt diagnosis and early airway management. Tracheostomy below the site of injury is recommended but may not be possible if the injury occurs in the thoracic trachea or bronchus. These cases require intubation with bronchoscopic guidance and should be managed in conjunction with cardiothoracic surgery support.[42] For cervical tracheal injuries and laryngotracheal separation, early management with surgical repair is important. The trachea can be repaired primarily, and stenting is typically not required if the injury occurs below the cricoid.

Esophageal injuries

Prompt diagnosis of cervical esophageal injuries is important for proper management. Minor mucosal injuries identified on esophagoscopy can be managed conservatively. Extensive esophageal injuries should be repaired within the first 24 hours if feasible. Injuries are repaired in a layered fashion and covered with a local muscle flap using strap musculature or omohyoid. Placement of a feeding tube under direct visualization allows for enteral feedings during the healing period. If the injury is not immediately recognized or inflammation precludes closure, external drainage with or without delayed repair may be required.[43]

Vascular Trauma

In 1969 Monson described 3 vascular zones of the neck and advocated exploration of all penetrating neck injuries in zone II.[44] Improvements in imaging techniques and treatment options challenge this dictum and present a "no-zone" approach to vascular injuries within the head and neck with exploration versus evaluation based on presenting signs and symptoms.[45] Hard signs of acute bleeds including expanding hematomas, pulsatile bleeding, or thrill on auscultation require emergent exploration without radiographic evaluation. Injuries to the common carotid artery or internal carotid artery require primary repair, bypass, or stent to avoid neurologic deficits. Injuries to other vascular structures in the head and neck can be repaired or ligated with very little morbidity.

SUMMARY

Knowledge of contemporary management of head and neck trauma is important for the comprehensive otolaryngologist. Injuries related to the soft tissues of the head and neck, craniofacial skeleton, laryngotracheal complex, and vascular structures are complex, and associated injuries are common. Advances in materials, surgical equipment, bioengineering, and computer-aided surgery aim to improve patient outcomes and minimize morbidity. Technologic advancements allow adaptations of surgical techniques and challenge previous held dogma related to patient management. Surgeons should continue to investigate current trends and adopt evidence-based practices into their routine.

CLINICS CARE POINTS

- Head and neck trauma is often multifactorial, and patients benefit from a multidisciplinary approach to care.
- Intervention should focus on restoration of form and function while optimizing cosmetic outcomes whenever possible.

- Technologic advancements in imaging, endoscopy, and biomedical materials have driven advancements in trauma care.
- Computer-assisted surgery including virtual surgical planning, image guidance surgery, and patient-specific implants are subjects of ongoing research and show promise in improving operative outcomes.

FUNDING

None.

CONFLICT OF INTEREST

The authors report no relevant conflict of interest in submitting this article for publication. The views expressed herein are those of the authors and do not reflect the official policy or position of Brooke Army Medical Center, the US Army Medical Department, the US Army Office of the Surgeon General, the US Air Force Office of the Surgeon General, the Department of the Army, the United States Air Force, the Department of Defense, or the US Government.

AUTHOR CONTRIBUTIONS

G.I. Kelts: substantial contributions to the conception or design of the work; acquisition, analysis, and interpretation of data for the work; drafting the work and revising it critically for important intellectual content; final approval of the version to be published; agreement to be accountable for all aspects of the work; T.R. Newberry: substantial contributions to the conception or design of the work; acquisition, analysis, and interpretation of data for the work; revising the work critically for important intellectual content; final approval of the version to be published; final approval of the version to be published; agreement to be accountable for all aspects of the work.

REFERENCES

1. McCusker SB, Schmalbach CE. The otolaryngologist's cost in treating facial trauma: American Academy of otolaryngology–head and neck surgery survey. Otolaryngol Head Neck Surg 2012;146(3):366–7.
2. Cho DY, Willborg BE, Lu GN. Management of traumatic soft tissue injuries of the Face. Semin Plast Surg 2021;35(4):229–37.
3. Gustafsson J, Lidén M, Thorarinsson A. Microsurgically aided upper lip replantation - case report and literature review. Case Reports Plast Surg Hand Surg 2016; 3(1):66–9.
4. Powers DB, Breeze J. Avulsive soft tissue injuries. Atlas Oral Maxillofacial Surg Clin N Am 2019;27(2):135–42.
5. Haller JR. Trauma to the salivary glands. Otolaryngol Clin North Am 1999;32(5):907–18.
6. Mardani M, Arabion H. Surgical management of parotid duct injury using a feeding tube. Ann Maxillofac Surg 2020;10(2):472–4.
7. Lazaridou M, Iliopoulos C, Antoniades K, et al. Salivary gland trauma: a review of diagnosis and treatment. Craniomaxillofac Trauma Reconstr 2012;5:189–96.
8. Shupak RP, Williams FC, Kim RY. Management of salivary gland injury. Oral Maxillofacial Surg Clin N Am 2021;33(3):343–50.

9. Van Sickels JE. Management of parotid gland and duct injuries. Oral Maxillofacial Surg Clin N Am 2009;21(2):243–6.
10. Lam AQ, Tran Phan Chung T, Tran Viet L, et al. The anatomic landmark approach to extratemporal facial nerve repair in facial trauma. Cureus 2022;14(3):e22787.
11. Barrs DM. Facial nerve trauma: optimal timing for repair. Laryngoscope 1991; 101(8):835–48.
12. Gordin E, Lee TS, Ducic Y, et al. Facial nerve trauma: evaluation and considerations in management. Craniomaxillofac Trauma Reconstr 2015;8:1–13.
13. Hoshal SG, Solis RN, Bewley AF. Nerve grafts in head and neck reconstruction. Curr Opin Otolaryngol Head Neck Surg 2020;28:346.
14. Navissano M, Malan F, Carnino R, et al. Neurotube for facial nerve repair. Microsurgery 2005;25:268.
15. Bengur FB, Stoy C, Binko MA, et al. Facial nerve repair: bioengineering approaches in preclinical models. Tissue Eng Part B Rev 2022;28(2):364–78.
16. Jain A, Taneja S, Rai A. What is a better modality of maxillomandibular fixation: bone-supported arch bars or Erich arch bars? A systematic review and meta-analysis. Br J Oral Maxillofac Surg 2021;59(8):858–66.
17. Sauerbier S, Schön R, Otten JE, et al. The development of plate osteosynthesis for the treatment of fractures of the mandibular body - a literature review. J Cranio-Maxillo-Fac Surg 2008;36(5):251–9.
18. Champy M, Loddé JP, Schmitt R, et al. Mandibular osteosynthesis by miniature screwed plates via a buccal approach. J Maxillofac Surg 1978;6(1):14–21.
19. Malhotra K, Sharma A, Giraddi G, et al. Versatility of titanium 3D plate in comparison with conventional titanium miniplate fixation for the management of mandibular fracture. J Maxillofac Oral Surg 2012;11(3):284–90.
20. Mooney S, Gulati RD, Yusupov S, et al. Mandibular condylar fractures. Facial Plast Surg Clin North Am 2022;30(1):85–98.
21. Zide MF, Kent JN. Indications for open reduction of mandibular condyle fractures. J Oral Maxillofac Surg 1983;41(2):89–98.
22. Chrcanovic BR. Surgical versus non-surgical treatment of mandibular condylar fractures: a meta-analysis. Int J Oral Maxillofac Surg 2015;44(2):158–79.
23. Marwan H, Sawatari Y. What is the most stable fixation technique for mandibular condyle fracture? J Oral Maxillofac Surg 2019;77(12):2522.
24. Long S, Spielman DB, Losenegger T, et al. Patterns of facial fractures in a major metropolitan level 1 trauma center: a 10-year experience. Laryngoscope 2021; 131(7):E2176–80.
25. Cole BL, Tran AQ. Controversies in ophthalmology: timing of isolated orbital floor fracture repair. Int Ophthalmol Clin 2022;62(4):63–7.
26. Bly RA, Chang SH, Cudejkova M, et al. Computer-guided orbital reconstruction to improve outcomes. JAMA Facial Plast Surg 2013;15(2):113–20.
27. Schreurs R, Klop C, Maal TJJ. Advanced diagnostics and three-dimensional virtual surgical planning in orbital reconstruction. Atlas Oral Maxillofacial Surg Clin N Am 2021;29(1):79–96.
28. Habib LA, Yoon MK. Patient specific implants in orbital reconstruction: a pilot study. Am J Ophthalmol Case Rep 2021;24:101222.
29. Blumer M, Essig H, Steigmiller K, et al. Surgical outcomes of orbital fracture reconstruction using patient-specific implants. J Oral Maxillofac Surg 2021; 79(6):1302–12.
30. Schreurs R, Wilde F, Schramm A, et al. Intraoperative feedback and quality control in orbital reconstruction: the past, the present, and the future. Atlas Oral Maxillofacial Surg Clin N Am 2021;29(1):97–108.

31. Bevans SE, Moe KS. Advances in the reconstruction of orbital fractures. Facial Plast Surg Clin North Am 2017;25(4):513–35.

32. Sharma P, Rattan V, Rai S, et al. Does intraoperative computed tomography improve the outcome in zygomatico-orbital complex fracture reduction? J Maxillofac Oral Surg 2021;20(2):189–200.

33. Patel SA, Berens AM, Devarajan K, et al. Evaluation of a minimally disruptive treatment protocol for frontal sinus fractures. JAMA Facial Plast Surg 2017;19: 225–31.

34. Choi KJ, Chang B, Woodard CR, et al. Survey of current practice patterns in the management of frontal sinus fractures. Craniomaxillofac Trauma Reconstr 2017; 10:106–16.

35. Choi M, Li Y, Shapiro SA, et al. A 10-year review of frontal sinus fractures: clinical outcomes of conservative management of posterior table fractures. Plast Reconstr Surg 2012;130:399–406.

36. Grayson JW, Jeyarajan H, Illing EA, et al. Changing the surgical dogma in frontal sinus trauma: transnasal endoscopic repair. Int Forum Allergy Rhinol 2017;7: 441–9.

37. Bourdillon AT, Kafle S, Salehi PP, et al. Characterization of laryngotracheal fractures and repairs: a TQIP study. J Voice 2022. S0892-1997(22)00163-1.

38. Schaefer SD. The acute management of external laryngeal trauma. A 27-year experience. Arch Otolaryngol Head Neck Surg. 1992;118(6):598–604.

39. Woo P. Laryngeal framework reconstruction with miniplates. Ann Otol Rhinol Laryngol 1990;99:772–7.

40. Thor A, Linder A. Repair of a laryngeal fracture using miniplates. Int J Oral Maxillofac Surg 2007 Aug;36(8):748–50.

41. Wasif M, Dhanani R, Ghaloo SK, et al. Management of laryngotracheal trauma: a review of current trends and future directions. J Pak Med Assoc 2020;70(Suppl 1):S60–4, 2.

42. Moonsamy P, Sachdeva UM, Morse CR. Management of laryngotracheal trauma. Ann Cardiothorac Surg 2018;7(2):210–6.

43. Sudarshan M, Cassivi SD. Management of traumatic esophageal injuries. J Thorac Dis 2019;11(Suppl 2):S172–6.

44. Monson DO, Saletta JD, Freeark RJ. Carotid vertebral trauma. J Trauma Acute Care Surg 1969;9(12):987–99.

45. Shiroff AM, Gale SC, Martin ND, et al. Penetrating neck trauma: a review of management strategies and discussion of the 'No Zone'approach. Am Surg 2013; 79(1):23–9.

Enhanced Recovery After Surgery for Head and Neck Oncologic Surgery Requiring Microvascular Reconstruction

Curtis Hanba, MD*, Carol Lewis, MD, MPH

KEYWORDS

- ERAS • Head and neck reconstruction • Enhanced recovery after surgery

KEY POINTS

- ERAS protocols can significantly reduce perioperative complications and simultaneously improve patient experience.
- An opportunity exists for the implementation of ERAS across preoperative, intraoperative, and postoperative settings.
- A collaborative effort to implement ERAS protocol will include team members of hospital administration, nurses, physicians, and supporting staff in the inpatient, and outpatient setting.

INTRODUCTION

It has been demonstrated since the 1990's that surgical outcomes can be improved through protocolized perioperative interventions.[1] Since then, multiple surgical societies have engaged in adopting Enhanced Recovery After Surgery (ERAS) Societal recommendations to improve patient satisfaction, decrease the cost of interventions, and improve outcomes. In 2017, ERAS released consensus recommendations detailing the perioperative optimization of patients undergoing head and neck free flap reconstruction. This population was identified as a high resource demand, oftentimes burdened with challenging comorbidity, and poorly described cohort for which a perioperative management protocol could help to optimize outcomes.[2] The following pages aim to further detail perioperative strategies to streamline patient recovery after head and neck reconstructive surgery.

Financial Disclosures: None.
Conflicts of Interest: None.
Department of Otolaryngology-Head and Neck Surgery, MD Anderson Cancer Center, 1515 Holcombe Boulevard, Houston, TX 77030, USA
* Corresponding author.
E-mail address: cjhanba@umn.edu

Otolaryngol Clin N Am 56 (2023) 801–812
https://doi.org/10.1016/j.otc.2023.04.012
0030-6665/23/© 2023 Elsevier Inc. All rights reserved.

PREHAB/REHAB

The head and neck oncologic surgery patient population is a unique and notoriously ill group of individuals. A thorough history and physical can identify many potential barriers to a successful recovery; the preoperative assessment is a critical opportunity to mitigate surgical risk. Not only can significant medical comorbidities be addressed and hopefully mitigated by an appropriate preoperative workup, but it's an excellent time to introduce "prehabilitation." Patients with head and neck cancer manifest significant impairments in nutrition, swallowing, and can often present in a state of cachexia related to systemic inflammation and altered upper aerodigestive anatomy.[3] Perioperative enteral nutrition has been identified to decrease surgical complication and improve quality of life in head and neck cancer patients suffering from systemic malnutrition.[3–5] Swallowing exercises and strength training programs have been identified to decrease treatment-related aspiration and decrease time to the resumption of oral nutrition postoperatively.[6] Consultation with a speech and language pathologist, nutritional support team, and occupational/physical therapist can be critical interventions to avoid unwanted perioperative complications.

Regardless of a primary tumor's location, elderly patients are known to struggle with perioperative nutrition, mobilization, and fatigue. Nearly 15% of head and neck cancers are diagnosed in patients over the age of 70 years, and surgeons need to address the specific needs of this population prior to offering potential interventions.[7] Elderly patients are known to have increased medical complexity and higher hospitalization-related medical complications, although surgical complications tend to be similar among groups. Ozkan and colleagues demonstrated this concept in their 2005 publication assessing a series of patients undergoing free flap reconstruction. Patients with a more complex medical history tended to have more hospitalization-related complications, and their results were independent of a patient's age.[8] Healthy elderly had similar outcomes to healthy young patients. This outcome was further supported by Grammaica's 2015 publication which detailed the recovery of free flap patients after head and neck surgery.[7] The Pre-Operative Assessment of Cancer in the Elderly (PACE) questionnaire was suggested as a screening tool for preoperative assessment by a team of physicians dedicated to assessing geriatric health prior to surgery. The PACE has identified fatigue, a low ability to perform activities of daily living, and low-performance status to independently predict elderly post-surgical complication.

RISK CALCULATORS

Further support for the unique needs of patients with head and neck cancer is detailed through multiple prior appraisals of the American College of Surgeons National Surgical Quality Improvement Program (ACS NSQIP). ACS NSQIP provides risk-adjusted outcomes use to assess the quality of an institution's perioperative care and has created an online risk calculator to aid in the preoperative assessment of postoperative outcomes. Unfortunately, the validity of the ACS NSQIP has not been shown to adequately evaluate postoperative risk in head and neck oncologic surgery.[9–12] More recently, Ma and colleagues demonstrated the algorithm to poorly predict outcomes in the Head and Neck microsurgical population.[13] Interestingly, these shortcomings were anticipated by ACS NSQIP's internal Measurement and Evaluation Committee in 2007 when specialty-specific algorithms were proposed to be superior to a random sampling of procedures across multiple subspecialities.[14] Accordingly, Lewis and colleagues introduced a pilot model to more appropriate stratify perioperative risk in patients undergoing head and neck oncologic surgery in 2016. The authors incorporated 11 preoperative, 6 intraoperative, and 10 postoperative variables largely unique to head and neck free tissue transfer cases and identified smoking, alcohol abuse, and hypertension to correlate with serious postoperative morbidity.[15] Authors suggested preoperative optimization, when possible, to prevent perioperative complications. Similarly, Mascarella and company proposed a revised ACS NSQIP calculator, the Head and Neck Surgery Risk Index (HNSRI), in 2019 and suggested that the addition of head and neck cancer- and surgery-specific parameters could increase the applicability of the NSQIP to identify adverse events with an 80% sensitivity, and 72% specificity.[16] It is critical to understand perioperative risk to appropriately educate a patient on the potential drawbacks of a planned intervention, and to intervene when able to optimize one's health perioperatively. Understanding the specific risk factors of head and neck patients is an essential way to optimize recovery after head and neck oncologic surgery with reconstruction.

The need for preoperative cardiac appraisal in patients undergoing major head and neck surgery is highlighted in a 2010 publication by Nagele and colleagues Authors detailed that roughly 15% of patients manifest elevated troponins postoperatively, with this population suffering prolonged hospitalization and increased 60-day mortality as compared to a matched cohort without troponin elevation.[17] One tool commonly implemented by anesthesiologists and general practitioners during a preoperative cardiac risk assessment is the Revised Cardiac Risk Index (RCRI).[18] The likelihood of perioperative complication increases as more of the mentioned risks are identified: high-risk surgical type, history of ischemic heart disease, history of congestive heart failure (CHF), history of cardiovascular disease (CVD), preoperative insulin use, and preoperative creatinine greater than 2.0 mg/dL. Patients with recent cardiac events, unstable angina, heart failure, high-grade arrhythmias, and valvular heart disease are to be considered very-high risk and consideration should be made for consultation to a cardiologist prior to surgery regardless of the RCRI score. The RCRI has not been assessed for validity in patients undergoing head and neck oncologic surgery, although the information collected can help to triage the necessity for specialized referral and likely contribute to improved perioperative outcomes.

SMOKING CESSATION

Surgeons must pay special attention to a head and neck cancer patient's social history when stratifying surgical risk. For example, smoking is associated with delayed wound healing, vasoconstriction, and skin flap necrosis.[19] Smoking has been associated with postoperative emergency room visitation, hospital admission, and reoperation.[20] Unfortunately, the head and neck cancer population is heavily burdened with tobacco dependence. Tobacco smokers have a 10-fold increased risk in developing head and neck cancer when compared to a nonsmoking population, and nearly 70% of new head and neck cancers may be associated with tobacco and alcohol use.[21] Tobacco use so significantly impacts otolaryngology as a field that the American Academy of Otolaryngology – Head and Neck Surgery released a position statement supporting state and federal legislation and regulatory efforts to reduce tobacco exposure and promote healthy environments to the public.[22] Behavioral interventions and pharmacotherapy can decrease nicotine dependence and studies demonstrate combination therapy to increase the likelihood abstinence long-term.[23] Addressing smoking habits preoperatively is critical to increase the likelihood of successful surgery.

OTHER PREOPERATIVE CONSIDERATIONS

One of the more common complications important to include in an informed consent discussion is the potential for postoperative hematoma. The face, scalp, and neck have a rich blood supply and despite meticulous operative hemostasis this unfortunate surgical complication occurs in 1% to 4% of cases.[24] Risk factors associated with an increased risk for perioperative hematoma include male sex, 4 or more comorbidities, and preoperative anticoagulant use.[24] Some of these risks can be mitigated with appropriate perioperative evaluation and management.

Another comorbidity to evaluate for prior to head and neck surgery, especially in patients previously treated with radiotherapy, is hypothyroidism. Hypothyroidism is associated with an increased bleeding risk related to attributable to biochemical alterations in von Willebrand Factor.[25] The National Comprehensive Cancer Network (NCCN) suggests checking TSH levels every 6 to 12 months in patients who receive neck radiation, and corrective replacement can decrease one's perioperative bleeding risk. Many providers routinely will check this level prior to revision or salvage oncologic surgery. Hypothyroidism has also been associated with delayed wound healing and increased risk of pharyngocutenous fistula after total laryngectomy.[26] Preoperative biochemical optimization is critical in select patients when optimizing postoperative outcomes.

ANTIBIOTICS

Perioperative antibiotic management has been a topic of debate for decades in the otolaryngology literature. Prior to appropriate antibiotic use, patients experienced postoperative wound complications in nearly 70% of cases.[27-29] Seagle's work in the 1970s laid a groundwork for demonstrating perioperative antibiotic utility in the head and neck patient population. The authors demonstrated a reduction in surgical site infection by 32% when cefazolin was compared to placebo perioperatively. Since then, an increased understanding of the microbial burden in the upper aerodigestive tract has identified an increased need for gram-negative coverage. Ampicillin with sulbactam has demonstrated superiority to clindamycin and has largely been adopted as the perioperative antibiotic of choice when undertaking clean contaminated surgery of the head and neck.[30,31] Duration of antibiotic use perioperatively has also been heavily studied. Evidence suggests that courses longer than 48 hours postoperatively yield no additional benefit.[30] When a penicillin allergy exists, combination coverage is most often employed. Patients with a minor reaction to penicillin often receive cefazolin plus metronidazole and severely allergic patients can benefit from levofloxacin plus metronidazole.[32] Conversely, appropriate antimicrobial stewardship efforts have driven inquiry into the necessity of prophylactic antibiotics in clean cases of the head and neck. Substantial evidence supports the avoidance of routine perioperative prophylaxis in clean cases (eg, parotidectomy, neck dissection, endocrine surgery).[33-37] This statement has even proven true for clean revision surgery of the head and neck in a publication published in 2018 by Shkedy and colleagues[34] Despite appropriate perioperative use, patients undergoing head and neck oncologic surgery commonly present postoperatively with delayed surgical site infection; up to 30% of patients receiving free tissue reconstruction manifest postoperative infection.[35,38-40] Bony reconstruction patients have a notoriously high postoperative infection risk. Some authors have advocated for increased and prolonged gram-negative coverage in this population, although data is currently lacking to support this conclusion.[41] A 2022 publication by Beydoun and colleagues introduced a role for topical antibiosis during upper aerodigestive reconstruction suggesting perioperative application to significantly reduce the incidence of postoperative infection.[41]

VENOUS THROMBOEMBOLISM PROPHYLAXIS

Despite a suggested protocolization of perioperative chemoprophylaxis for venous thromboembolism (VTE), this decision is often made on a case-by-case basis in head and neck oncology surgery. One tool useful in determining who may benefit from perioperative prophylaxis is the Caprini score. The Caprini score is a measure of one's perioperative risk of VTE and has been consistently validated in a head and neck surgical patient cohort.[42–45] An increased Caprini score correlates with an increased risk of perioperative VTE, indicating that perioperative chemoprophylaxis is warranted. Notably, the decision to initiate chemoprophylaxis must be weighed against increased risk for perioperative bleeding complications recognized in patients treated with these medications.

POSTOPERATIVE NAUSEA AND VOMITING

Nausea can be a significant challenge to overcome for patients undergoing head and neck oncologic surgery. The combination of perioperative anxiety, anesthetics, and operative stimulus among other factors can lead to postoperative nausea and vomiting in nearly 60% of patients undergoing head and neck surgery.[46,47] Perioperative anti-emetic medication is often advocated for during Head and Neck procedures, although data is a bit conflicted regarding specific medical management recommendations. Silva and company identified young age (<25 years), procedures over 1-h, maxillary procedures, cases that involved inhalation anesthetics, postoperative opioid use, and elevated postoperative pain to have increased risk of PONV. Authors suggested further studies to be conducted prior to recommending a specific prophylactic regiment.[47] Notably, Kainulainen and colleagues have suggested caution when prescribing dexamethasone in a perioperative setting for patients undergoing head and neck microvascular reconstruction. Their 2018 review of 93 patients identified a lack of reduction in PONV, increased insulin use, and similar length of stay when compared to a cohort treated without perioperative steroids.[48,49] These data seemingly contradict The Journal of Anesthesia and Analgesia's recently released 4th edition Consensus Guideline for the Management of Postoperative Nausea and Vomiting.[50] This publication reported that dexamethasone had one of the lower numbers needed to treat in regard to reducing postoperative nausea and vomiting and highlighted the need to identify patients with elevated PONV risk. The Apfel simplified risk score was recommended to determine PONV risk. This instrument considers female sex, history of PONV or motion sickness, nonsmoking status, and postoperative opioid use to identify risk for PONV.[51] The authors suggested that adults with an elevated risk for PONV be treated with combined modality treatment. For example, the authors suggested patients undergoing laryngeal surgery receive PONV prophylaxis with IV ondansetron (4 mg) and dexamethasone (4 mg) 2 hours prior to the end of surgery. However, further inquiry into optimal PONV prophylaxis for other head and neck surgical procedures is warranted.

MULTIMODAL ANALGESIA

Managing pain is a necessary responsibility to facilitate a successful recovery. Pain, which is often cited as one of the leading contributors to tomophobia, is a common manifestation of head and neck cancer. Patient-reported outcome metrics often reflect a provider's ability to adequately manage patient pain perioperatively. Despite a recent significant effort to curtail perioperative narcotic use, nearly 40% of head and neck cancer patients receive opioid medications prior to treatment.[52] Data suggests that multimodal analgesic (MMA) strategies can significantly decrease a patient's need for postoperative narcotics.[2,52–54] MMA protocols target inflammation, and pain, commonly utilizing Acetaminophen, nonsteroidal anti-inflammatory agents (NSAIDs), anticonvulsants, and steroid medications in a prophylactic setting. Kiong and colleagues published the successful implementation of a Head and Neck specific MMA protocol in their work released in 2021. The group demonstrated a preoperative routine consisting of celecoxib 400 mg, tramadol extended release 300 mg, and gabapentin 300 mg, combined with postoperative scheduled doses of the previously mentioned medications to significantly reduce perioperative opioid consumption, decrease ICU utilization, and shorten one's length of stay.[54] Acetaminophen can also reduce narcotic use perioperatively and, when comorbidities allow, is useful as adjunct analgesia in a majority of head and neck surgical procedures.[52]

Some providers may be hesitant to use NSAIDs perioperatively, since these medications have historically been thought to confer an increased bleeding risk perioperatively. A systematic review and meta-analysis performed by Kelley and company concluded that ibuprofen use perioperatively had no influence on bleeding risk when reviewing a population undergoing soft tissue reconstructive procedures.[55] Similarly, the NSAID celecoxib, a selective cyclo-oxygenase (COX) 2 inhibitor with anti-inflammatory and analgesic properties, has demonstrated a well-tolerated safety profile in a number of head and neck surgical procedures.[56] Celecoxib has also demonstrated protective antitumoral properties and was recently studied as a modality to treat premalignant oral lesions.[56–58] Its perioperative use can also reduce the need for narcotic medications and enhance one's recovery.[52]

Gabapentin and pregabalin are anticonvulsant medications often used to treat complex postoperative pain. Some providers advocate that preoperative prophylactic gabapentin use can decrease narcotic usage postoperatively, but this claim is not uniformly supported in the literature.[59–62] Fortunately, gabapentin has a relatively well-tolerated safety profile and has been recognized as the most commonly implemented preoperative intervention in head and neck surgery MMA strategies.[63]

INTRAVENOUS FLUIDS

Perioperative intravenous fluid usage should be used sparingly in head and neck oncologic surgery requiring free tissue transfer. Perioperative fluid administration of more than 5500 mL has been identified to contribute to perioperative complication, with a threshold of 7000 mL contributing more significant risk including death, partial/total flap loss, and increased return to the OR.[64] Goal-directed fluid management strategies have demonstrated efficacy in patients undergoing head and neck surgery with reconstruction and suggest cardiac output monitoring may be a strategy to prevent intraoperative fluid overload.[65] It's generally agreed upon that a net-zero strategy should be implemented when feasible, and early mobilization can significantly reduce perioperative complication.[66,67]

To avoid fluid overload intraoperatively, goal-directed fluid algorithms rely on vasopressors for blood pressure management. Vasopressor use has historically been avoided during microvascular surgery due to a concern for flap ischemia and higher surgical complication. Data however, has suggested otherwise.[68–70] Fang and colleagues studied a population of 4888 patients undergoing free flap reconstruction and identified intraoperative vasopressor use to occur in 85% of cases. They demonstrated similar surgical outcomes between groups, and interestingly, the group identified the vasopressor group to be associated with less postoperative venous congestion than the cohort avoiding vasopressor use (2.1% vs 3.9%).[71] Vasopressor use was not associated with flap loss or pedicle compromise.[71] Authors state, "intraoperative use of vasopressors improves free flap survival" and continue to recommend these medications as needed during complex head and neck microvascular reconstruction.

OTHER POSTOPERATIVE CONSIDERATIONS

Patients undergoing head and neck surgery have unique needs, and unfortunately remain an understudied group.[72] Because of this, many ERAS protocols have been implemented based on data gleaned from non-head and neck surgical services. For example, in Dort and colleagues's 2017 consensus review from the ERAS society, urinary catheter removal was suggested to happen as soon as a patient is likely ready to void on their own, and preferably within 24 hours of surgery. This recommendation was supported by high-quality evidence and given a strong recommendation. Interestingly, the cited literature leaned heavily on intraabdominal surgery patients, a majority undergoing hysterectomy. It will be important to monitor the effects of ERAS implementation in a population specific to head and neck surgery to further justify the accuracy of these initiatives. Regardless, Foley catheter removal can facilitate mobility. A recent retrospective review of 445 patients who underwent head and neck-specific free tissue transfer identified 48h of postoperative immobility to significantly worsen outcomes and increase one's risk of a prolonged hospitalization and pneumonia. The authors suggested avoidance of tracheostomy, and recovery in a unit familiar with head and neck microvascular reconstruction as a way to facilitate early mobilization. Authors proposed a goal of ambulation within 24 hours of surgery.[67] One practical way to help facilitate mobility is it limit invasive monitoring and remove drains when able. Central lines should be used sparingly, arterial lines should be removed when able, and drains should be monitored and removed in timely fashion.

CREATING YOUR OWN ENHANCED RECOVERY AFTER SURGERY PROTOCOL

The interventions and considerations discussed here can significantly improve a patient's recovery (**Box 1**). In all likelihood, most practices already incorporate many of the ERAS protocol components into their perioperative care; formalizing these into a clinical care pathway yields additional benefit for patient recovery. Prasad and colleagues published a guide aimed to address concerns around implementation by detailing useful strategies.[73] First and foremost, a multidisciplinary team must be assembled, including nurses, physicians, support staff, and advanced practice providers who care for patients in each phase of care. This team of providers should then review the components of care that they which to incorporate into their ERAS protocol, weighing which are feasible based on hospital culture and existing resources. Involvement of all levels of providers from each phase of care raises the likelihood of programmatic success through the identification of engaged stakeholders, who will hold accountability among their provider groups and have a continued interest in seeing the program succeed. Moreover, these team meetings provide a forum for multidisciplinary discussions of feasibility such that troubleshooting can occur before attempted implementation. A team lead may be selected in each phase of care to address hurdles as they are identified. Regular team follow-up meetings support the continued engagement of team members and provide dedicated time to debrief on challenges and successes. From a hospital systems standpoint, information technologists and hospital finance specialists can help to monitor the impact of ERAS protocols and can help to identify that desired outcomes are being met. Encouragement early in the process is likely to gather momentum although undoubtably the rewards of an improved patient experience, decreased cost, and improved outcomes can perpetuate enthusiasm toward ERAS implementation.

Box 1
Components of an ERAS pathway

Preoperative
    Preoperative Education – Expected surgical outcomes and anticipated course of treatment
    Prehab/Rehab – Speech and language pathology consultation, nutrition consultation
        Occupational/Physical Therapy
    Medical evaluation - Comorbidity assessment
    Social history modification – Smoking and alcohol cessation
    Multimodal Analgesia

Intraoperative
    Multimodal Analgesia – Scheduled non-narcotics
    VTE Prophylaxis – Caprini score guided risk
    Antibiotic Prophylaxis – Perioperative short-term coverage when appropriate
    PONV evaluation – Consideration of intraoperative anti-emetics
    Goal Directed Fluid Usage – Vasopressor use as necessary, net zero fluid goals

Postoperative
    Recovery in a dedicated free flap unit
    Early mobilization
    Post op rehab – Physical and occupational therapy, speech and language pathology
    involvement
    Multimodal Analgesia – Weaning of perioperative narcotics

---

CLINICS CARE POINTS

- Perioperative antibiotics seems unnecessary when performing clean surgery.

- In clean contaminated cases, 48 hours of Ampicillin with Sulbactam is an appropriate duration of treatment.

REFERENCES

1. Kehlet H. Multimodal approach to control postoperative pathophysiology and rehabilitation. Br J Anaesth 1997;78(5):606–17.
2. Dort JC, Farwell DG, Findlay M, et al. Optimal Perioperative Care in Major Head and Neck Cancer Surgery With Free Flap Reconstruction: A Consensus Review and Recommendations From the Enhanced Recovery After Surgery Society. JAMA Otolaryngol Head Neck Surg 2017;143(3):292–303.
3. Talwar B, Donnelly R, Skelly R, et al. Nutritional management in head and neck cancer: United Kingdom National Multidisciplinary Guidelines. J Laryngol Otol 2016;130(S2):S32–40.
4. Bertrand PC, Piquet MA, Bordier I, et al. Preoperative nutritional support at home in head and neck cancer patients: from nutritional benefits to the prevention of the alcohol withdrawal syndrome. Curr Opin Clin Nutr Metab Care 2002;5(4):435–40.
5. Van Bokhorst-de Van der Schuer MA, Langendoen SI, Vondeling H, et al. Perioperative enteral nutrition and quality of life of severely malnourished head and neck cancer patients: a randomized clinical trial. Clin Nutr 2000;19(6):437–44.
6. Hutcheson KA, Barrow MP, Plowman EK, et al. Expiratory muscle strength training for radiation-associated aspiration after head and neck cancer: A case series. Laryngoscope 2018;128(5):1044–51.
7. Grammatica A, Piazza C, Paderno A, et al. Free flaps in head and neck reconstruction after oncologic surgery: expected outcomes in the elderly. Otolaryngol Head Neck Surg 2015;152(5):796–802.

8. Ozkan O, Ozgentas HE, Islamoglu K, et al. Experiences with microsurgical tissue transfers in elderly patients. Microsurgery 2005;25(5):390–5.

9. Prasad KG, Nelson BG, Deig CR, et al. ACS NSQIP Risk Calculator: An Accurate Predictor of Complications in Major Head and Neck Surgery? Otolaryngol Head Neck Surg 2016;155(5):740–2.

10. Schneider AL, Lavin JM. Publicly Available Databases in Otolaryngology Quality Improvement. Otolaryngol Clin North Am 2019;52(1):185–94.

11. Cao A, Khayat S, Cash E, et al. ACS NSQIP risk calculator reliability in head and neck oncology: The effect of prior chemoradiation on NSQIP risk estimates following laryngectomy. Am J Otolaryngol 2018;39(2):192–6.

12. Arce K, Moore EJ, Lohse CM, et al. The American College of Surgeons National Surgical Quality Improvement Program Surgical Risk Calculator Does Not Accurately Predict Risk of 30-Day Complications Among Patients Undergoing Microvascular Head and Neck Reconstruction. J Oral Maxillofac Surg 2016;74(9):1850–8.

13. Ma Y, Laitman BM, Patel V, et al. Assessment of the NSQIP Surgical Risk Calculator in Predicting Microvascular Head and Neck Reconstruction Outcomes. Otolaryngol Head Neck Surg 2019;160(1):100–6.

14. Birkmeyer JD, Shahian DM, Dimick JB, et al. Blueprint for a new American College of Surgeons: National Surgical Quality Improvement Program. J Am Coll Surg 2008;207(5):777–82.

15. Lewis CM, Aloia TA, Shi W, et al. Development and Feasibility of a Specialty-Specific National Surgical Quality Improvement Program (NSQIP): The Head and Neck-Reconstructive Surgery NSQIP. JAMA Otolaryngol Head Neck Surg 2016;142(4):321–7.

16. Mascarella MA, Richardson K, Mlynarek A, et al. Evaluation of a Preoperative Adverse Event Risk Index for Patients Undergoing Head and Neck Cancer Surgery. JAMA Otolaryngol Head Neck Surg 2019;145(4):345–51.

17. Nagele P, Rao LK, Penta M, et al. Postoperative myocardial injury after major head and neck cancer surgery. Head Neck 2011;33(8):1085–91.

18. Lee TH, Marcantonio ER, Mangione CM, et al. Derivation and prospective validation of a simple index for prediction of cardiac risk of major noncardiac surgery. Circulation 1999;100(10):1043–9.

19. McDaniel JC, Browning KK. Smoking, chronic wound healing, and implications for evidence-based practice. J Wound Ostomy Continence Nurs 2014;41(5):415-E2.

20. Kaoutzanis C, Winocour J, Gupta V, et al. The Effect of Smoking in the Cosmetic Surgery Population: Analysis of 129,007 Patients. Aesthet Surg J 2019;39(1):109–19.

21. Jethwa AR, Khariwala SS. Tobacco-related carcinogenesis in head and neck cancer. Cancer Metastasis Rev 2017;36(3):411–23.

22. "Position Statement: Tobacco Use and Secondhand Smoke." American Academy of Otolaryngology-Head and Neck Surgery (AAO-HNS), 23 Sept. 2021, Available at: https://www.entnet.org/resource/position-statement-tobacco-use-and-secondhand-smoke/. Accessed December 25, 2022.

23. Zwar NA. Smoking cessation. Aust J Gen Pract 2020;49(8):474–81.

24. Shah-Becker S, Greenleaf EK, Boltz MM, et al. Neck hematoma after major head and neck surgery: Risk factors, costs, and resource utilization. Head Neck 2018;40(6):1219–27.

25. Elbers LPB, Fliers E, Cannegieter SC. The influence of thyroid function on the coagulation system and its clinical consequences. J Thromb Haemost 2018; 16(4):634–45.

26. Rosko AJ, Birkeland AC, Bellile E, et al. Hypothyroidism and Wound Healing After Salvage Laryngectomy. Ann Surg Oncol 2018;25(5):1288–95.

27. Dor P, Klastersky J. Prophylactic antibiotics in oral, pharyngeal and laryngeal surgery for cancer: (a double-blind study). Laryngoscope 1973;83(12):1992–8.

28. Raine CH, Bartzokas CA, Stell PM, et al. Chemoprophylaxis in major head and neck surgery. J R Soc Med 1984;77(12):1006–9.

29. Johnson JT, Myers EN, Thearle PB, et al. Antimicrobial prophylaxis for contaminated head and neck surgery. Laryngoscope 1984;94(1):46–51.

30. Vander Poorten V, Uyttebroek S, Robbins KT, et al. Perioperative Antibiotics in Clean-Contaminated Head and Neck Surgery: A Systematic Review and Meta-Analysis. Adv Ther 2020;37(4):1360–80.

31. Weber RS, Raad I, Frankenthaler R, et al. Ampicillin-sulbactam vs clindamycin in head and neck oncologic surgery. The need for gram-negative coverage. Arch Otolaryngol Head Neck Surg 1992;118(11):1159–63.

32. Sobottka I, Wegscheider K, Balzer L, et al. Microbiological analysis of a prospective, randomized, double-blind trial comparing moxifloxacin and clindamycin in the treatment of odontogenic infiltrates and abscesses. Antimicrob Agents Chemother 2012;56(5):2565–9.

33. Chiesa-Estomba CM, Ninchritz E, González-García JA, et al. Antibiotic Prophylaxis in Clean Head and Neck Surgery: An Observational Retrospective Single-Centre Study. Ear Nose Throat J 2019;98(6):362–5.

34. Shkedy Y, Stern S, Nachalon Y, et al. Antibiotic prophylaxis in clean head and neck surgery: A prospective randomised controlled trial. Clin Otolaryngol 2018; 43(6):1508–12.

35. Mitchell RM, Mendez E, Schmitt NC, et al. Antibiotic Prophylaxis in Patients Undergoing Head and Neck Free Flap Reconstruction. JAMA Otolaryngol Head Neck Surg 2015;141(12):1096–103.

36. Bratzler DW, Dellinger EP, Olsen KM, et al. Clinical practice guidelines for antimicrobial prophylaxis in surgery. Am J Health Syst Pharm 2013;70(3):195–283.

37. Vamvakidis K, Rellos K, Tsourma M, et al. Antibiotic prophylaxis for clean neck surgery. Ann R Coll Surg Engl 2017;99(5):410–2.

38. Vila PM, Zenga J, Jackson RS. Antibiotic Prophylaxis in Clean-Contaminated Head and Neck Surgery: A Systematic Review and Meta-analysis. Otolaryngol Head Neck Surg 2017;157(4):580–8 [published correction appears in Otolaryngol Head Neck Surg. 2018 Aug;159(2):402].

39. Wagner JL, Kenney RM, Vazquez JA, et al. Surgical prophylaxis with gram-negative activity for reduction of surgical site infections after microvascular reconstruction for head and neck cancer. Head Neck 2016;38(10):1449–54.

40. Yarlagadda BB, Deschler DG, Rich DL, et al. Head and neck free flap surgical site infections in the era of the Surgical Care Improvement Project. Head Neck 2016;38(Suppl 1):E392–8.

41. Beydoun AS, Koss K, Nielsen T, et al. Perioperative Topical Antisepsis and Surgical Site Infection in Patients Undergoing Upper Aerodigestive Tract Reconstruction. JAMA Otolaryngol Head Neck Surg 2022;148(6):547–54.

42. Shuman AG, Hu HM, Pannucci CJ, et al. Stratifying the risk of venous thromboembolism in otolaryngology. Otolaryngol Head Neck Surg 2012;146(5):719–24.

43. Garritano FG, Andrews GA. Current practices in venous thromboembolism pro-phylaxis in otolaryngology-head and neck surgery. Head Neck 2016;38(Suppl 1):E341–5.

44. Bahl V, Shuman AG, Hu HM, et al. Chemoprophylaxis for venous thromboembo-lism in otolaryngology. JAMA Otolaryngol Head Neck Surg 2014;140(11): 999–1005.

45. Yarlagadda BB, Brook CD, Stein DJ, et al. Venous thromboembolism in otolaryn-gology surgical inpatients receiving chemoprophylaxis. Head Neck 2014;36(8): 1087–93.

46. Eryilmaz T, Sencan A, Camgoz N, et al. A challenging problem that concerns the aesthetic surgeon: postoperative nausea and vomiting. Ann Plast Surg 2008; 61(5):489–91.

47. Silva AC, O'Ryan F, Poor DB. Postoperative nausea and vomiting (PONV) after orthognathic surgery: a retrospective study and literature review. J Oral Maxillo-fac Surg 2006;64(9):1385–97.

48. Kainulainen S, Lassus P, Suominen AL, et al. More Harm Than Benefit of Periop-erative Dexamethasone on Recovery Following Reconstructive Head and Neck Cancer Surgery: A Prospective Double-Blind Randomized Trial. J Oral Maxillofac Surg 2018;76(11):2425–32.

49. Kainulainen S, Törnwall J, Koivusalo AM, et al. Dexamethasone in head and neck cancer patients with microvascular reconstruction: No benefit, more complica-tions. Oral Oncol 2017;65:45–50.

50. Gan TJ, Belani KG, Bergese S, et al. Fourth Consensus Guidelines for the Man-agement of Postoperative Nausea and Vomiting [published correction appears in Anesth Analg. 2020 Nov;131(5):e241]. Anesth Analg 2020;131(2):411–48.

51. Apfel CC, Läärä E, Koivuranta M, et al. A simplified risk score for predicting post-operative nausea and vomiting: conclusions from cross-validations between two centers. Anesthesiology 1999;91(3):693–700.

52. Bobian M, Gupta A, Graboyes EM. Acute Pain Management Following Head and Neck Surgery. Otolaryngol Clin North Am 2020;53(5):753–64.

53. Vu CN, Lewis CM, Bailard NS, et al. Association Between Multimodal Analgesia Administration and Perioperative Opioid Requirements in Patients Undergoing Head and Neck Surgery With Free Flap Reconstruction. JAMA Otolaryngol Head Neck Surg 2020;146(8):708–13.

54. Kiong KL, Vu CN, Yao CMKL, et al. Enhanced Recovery After Surgery (ERAS) in Head and Neck Oncologic Surgery: A Case-Matched Analysis of Perioperative and Pain Outcomes. Ann Surg Oncol 2021;28(2):867–76.

55. Kelley BP, Bennett KG, Chung KC, et al. Ibuprofen May Not Increase Bleeding Risk in Plastic Surgery: A Systematic Review and Meta-Analysis. Plast Reconstr Surg 2016;137(4):1309–16.

56. Giordano T, Durkin A, Simi A, et al. High-Dose Celecoxib for Pain After Pediatric Tonsillectomy: A Randomized Controlled Trial. Otolaryngol Head Neck Surg 2022. https://doi.org/10.1177/01945998221091695. 1945998221091695.

57. Cohen B, Preuss CV. Celecoxib. [Updated 2022 Oct 10]. In: StatPearls [Internet]. Treasure Island (FL): StatPearls Publishing; 2023 Jan-. Available at: https://www.ncbi.nlm.nih.gov/books/NBK535359/.

58. Saba NF, Hurwitz SJ, Kono SA, et al. Chemoprevention of head and neck cancer with celecoxib and erlotinib: results of a phase ib and pharmacokinetic study. Cancer Prev Res 2014;7(3):283–91.

59. Gill AS, Virani FR, Hwang JC, et al. Preoperative Gabapentin Administration and Its Impact on Postoperative Opioid Requirement and Pain in Sinonasal Surgery. Otolaryngol Head Neck Surg 2021;164(4):889–94.

60. Rai AS, Khan JS, Dhaliwal J, et al. Preoperative pregabalin or gabapentin for acute and chronic postoperative pain among patients undergoing breast cancer surgery: A systematic review and meta-analysis of randomized controlled trials. J Plast Reconstr Aesthet Surg 2017;70(10):1317–28.

61. Hah J, Mackey SC, Schmidt P, et al. Effect of Perioperative Gabapentin on Postoperative Pain Resolution and Opioid Cessation in a Mixed Surgical Cohort: A Randomized Clinical Trial. JAMA Surg 2018;153(4):303–11 [published correction appears in JAMA Surg. 2018 Apr 1;153(4):396] [published correction appears in JAMA Surg. 2022 Jun 1;157(6):553].

62. Ladich EM, Zhou KQ, Spence DL, et al. Opioid-Sparing Anesthesia: Gabapentin and Postoperative Pain. J Perianesth Nurs 2022;37(6):966–70.

63. Go BC, Go CC, Chorath K, et al. Multimodal Analgesia in Head and Neck Free Flap Reconstruction: A Systematic Review. Otolaryngol Head Neck Surg 2022; 166(5):820–31.

64. Ettinger KS, Arce K, Lohse CM, et al. Higher perioperative fluid administration is associated with increased rates of complications following head and neck microvascular reconstruction with fibular free flaps. Microsurgery 2017;37(2):128–36.

65. Tapia B, Garrido E, Cebrian JL, et al. Impact of Goal Directed Therapy in Head and Neck Oncological Surgery with Microsurgical Reconstruction: Free Flap Viability and Complications. Cancers 2021;13(7):1545.

66. Bellamy MC. Wet, dry or something else? Br J Anaesth 2006;97(6):755–7.

67. Twomey R, Matthews TW, Nakoneshny S, et al. Impact of Early Mobilization on Recovery after Major Head and Neck Surgery with Free Flap Reconstruction. Cancers 2021;13(12):2852.

68. Monroe MM, McClelland J, Swide C, et al. Vasopressor use in free tissue transfer surgery. Otolaryngol Head Neck Surg 2010;142(2):169–73.

69. Harris L, Goldstein D, Hofer S, et al. Impact of vasopressors on outcomes in head and neck free tissue transfer. Microsurgery 2012;32(1):15–9.

70. Taylor RJ, Patel R, Wolf BJ, et al. Intraoperative vasopressors in head and neck free flap reconstruction. Microsurgery 2021;41(1):5–13.

71. Fang L, Liu J, Yu C, et al. Intraoperative Use of Vasopressors Does Not Increase the Risk of Free Flap Compromise and Failure in Cancer Patients. Ann Surg 2018; 268(2):379–84.

72. Svider PF, Blasco MA, Raza SN, et al. Head and Neck Cancer. Otolaryngol Head Neck Surg 2017;156(1):10–3.

73. Prasad A, Chorath K, Barrette LX, et al. Implementation of an enhanced recovery after surgery protocol for head and neck cancer patients: Considerations and best practices. World J Otorhinolaryngol Head Neck Surg 2022;8(2):91–5.

Virtual Surgical Planning in Head and Neck Reconstruction

Evan A. Jones, MD, Andrew T. Huang, MD*

KEYWORDS

- Virtual surgical planning • Head and neck reconstruction
- Computer-assisted design • Microvascular free tissue transfer

KEY POINTS

- Virtual surgical planning is a multistep process that encompasses preoperative modeling and manufacturing to use intraoperative cutting guides and patient-specific reconstructive materials.
- Virtual surgical planning can aid the head and neck reconstructive surgeon in the management of complex osseous deformities by facilitating conceptualization, shortening operative time, and improving outcomes.
- Virtual surgical planning enables both the ablative and reconstructive surgeons to visualize and optimize oncologic, esthetic, and functional goals.

INTRODUCTION

Head and neck reconstructive roots are intertwined with the innovative minds of surgeons, scientists, and engineers. Numerous autologous and synthetic media have been grown in this manner from concept to practice. Today, before entering the operating room, surgeons can avail themselves not only with clinical and radiographic information to envision their surgical steps but also with virtually engineered plans and tools to recreate the form and function of the native facial skeleton as closely as possible. Virtual surgical planning (VSP) with computer-assisted design and computer-assisted manufacturing (CAD/CAM) has transformed head and neck reconstruction.

HISTORY

The intricacies of reconstructive options for head and neck defects are beyond the scope of this article; however, historical perspective is warranted to appreciate the

Department of Otolaryngology–Head and Neck Surgery, Baylor College of Medicine, 1977 Butler Boulevard, Suite E5.200, Houston, TX 77030, USA
* Corresponding author.
E-mail address: andrew.huang@bcm.edu

Otolaryngol Clin N Am 56 (2023) 813–822
https://doi.org/10.1016/j.otc.2023.04.013
0030-6665/23/© 2023 Elsevier Inc. All rights reserved.

development of VSP. Reconstruction of the facial skeleton, especially the maxillomandibular complex, has evolved from the use of avascular, allogeneic, or synthetic options such as bone grafts, prosthetics, natural elements, metals, and meshes into predominantly autologous fasciocutaneous, osseous, and osteocutaneous tissues through microvascular free tissue transfer (MVFTT).[1] Since its inception for reconstruction of the head and neck in the 1950s, MVFTT has used numerous donor sites depending on the tissue requirement of the deformity with composite donor sites of the iliac crest, scapula, rib, and fibula being reported.[1–3]

Traditionally, surgical planning for MVFTT head and neck reconstruction relied less on radiography, computed tomography (CT), and photography, and more on intraoperative assessment of the resultant defect. For composite deformities of skin, soft tissue, and bone, the act of insetting fasciocutaneous tissue and fixating autologous bone or cranioplasty mesh relied on in situ assessment of the deformity for titanium hardware conformation and/or creating osteotomy templates for bony contouring for maxillomandibular reconstruction. In the case of exophytic tumors, large resections, or extensive trauma, these in situ practices can be difficult or impossible given the disrupted topography of the anatomy.[4] In addition, the intraoperative decision-making to become facile and accurate can have a steep learning curve, predisposing to human error and adding substantial operative time.[5]

To mitigate intraoperative inaccuracies, improve reconstructed bone contour, improve bone-to-bone contact for union, and decrease operating room time, VSP protocols were created. The first to use VSP was orthopedic and maxillofacial surgeons in attempt to reconstruct osseous deformities with similarly solid prosthetic materials.[6] VSP protocols blossomed from there with the goal to translate three-dimensional (3D) reconstructed images, usually from CT scans, for use in CAD/CAM processes. The first generation included software that allowed for 3D printing of patient-specific maxillomandibular models, first described by oral and maxillofacial surgeons in 1987.[7,8] These models enabled surgeons to preoperatively conform reconstructive plates and then sterilize them for operative use to potentially improve accuracy and decrease operative time. In the second generation of VSP, software development improved to include not only patient-specific pre-bent titanium reconstruction plates but also 3D printing of the planned donor autologous bone with preoperative manufacturing of cutting guides or jigs to reduce intraoperative error and operative time (**Fig. 1**). For the current third generation of VSP, advances in stereolithography, patient-specific titanium reconstruction plate design (eg, milled or additively manufactured plates), along with the ability to preoperatively plan screw fixation holes and osseointegrated dental implant placement through predrilled cylinders have allowed for further improvement in operative efficiency and reconstructive accuracy.

TECHNIQUE

VSP is a multistep process of data acquisition, data integration, design, planning, and manufacturing. First, the patient must obtain high-quality CT scans of both the primary resection site and the potential donor site with a recommended maximum slice increment of 1.0 mm within 6 weeks of surgery.[9] The CT data along with key information regarding the proposed intervention (position of the vascular pedicle and flap harvest site) are delivered to a commercial VSP provider whose engineers generate a virtual anatomic model.[9,10] After modeling is complete, the surgeons and engineer review digital renderings of the anatomy to plan both the resection and reconstruction. This planning meeting is a shared screen experience to define resection margins with the ablative surgeon at which point the reconstructive surgeon can then determine

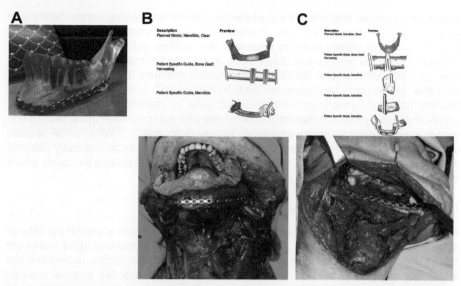

Fig. 1. Earlier generations of VSP ushered in stereolithography with creation of preoperative models for surgical planning. (*A*) First-generation VSP used printed mandible models allowing preoperative bending of titanium reconstruction plates for intraoperative use. (*B*, *C*) Second-generation VSP allowed for donor and recipient cutting guide fabrication, but still relied on the use of generic titanium plates requiring preoperative bending.

prosthetic shape/contour in the setting of cranioplasty (**Fig. 2**), or cutting/shaping osteotomy location, cutting guide preferences (slotted/flanged; 3D printed titanium/ plastic), and reconstructive plate design and modifications for maxillomandibular reconstruction (**Figs. 3 and 4**). Specific titanium hardware modifications could include

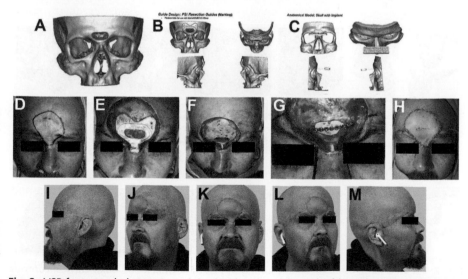

Fig. 2. VSP for extended resection of the forehead and frontal table with PEEK cranioplasty and radial forearm free flap reconstruction. (*A–C*) VSP plan with resection guide and implant. (*D–H*) Intraoperative photos demonstrating the defect and patient-specific implant in place. (*I–M*) Two-month postoperative result.

screw hole number and intervening distances, screw angulation, screw depth, and osseointegrated dental implant position.[9,11] The planning meeting enables manufacturing of patient-specific materials (eg, cutting guides, fixation hardware, prosthetics) for the primary and donor sites, which can be made from synthetic polymer (polyetheretherketone [PEEK]) or low-profile titanium. Patient-specific reconstructive plates can be designed and manufactured using contralateral facial skeletal mirroring, generic population-based data, or statistical and artificial intelligence predictive models to facilitate optimal esthetic outcome even in the face of disrupted anatomy from extensive oncologic disease or trauma.[10,12] When a VSP session uses CT angiography, fasciocutaneous perforator location can be precisely planned into the reconstructive design, facilitating skin and soft tissue paddle inclusion, which is especially pertinent for composite deformities.[13,14]

BENEFITS OF VIRTUAL SURGICAL PLANNING

Patient-specific titanium plates are made either by additive laser stereolithography or milled from solid titanium.[9,14,15] These milled and additively manufactured plates are stronger and more durable than standard bent reconstructive plates, decreasing the incidence of plate fracture in both laboratory and retrospective patient analysis showing plate fracture reduction from 9% to 0%.[16,17] The strength and potential to position these plates in more difficult locations is further augmented by the ability to plan obliquely oriented screw holes up to 15°, increased or reduced screw hole intervening distances, and the manufacture of nonlinear designs, that is, mesh or dog-bone shapes.[9] Taken together, these modifications can facilitate the placement of screws into smaller or more difficult to access locations.

A significant change to practice resulting from the wide adoption of VSP includes streamlined dental rehabilitation and customization of alternative donor sites. Before the broad utilization of VSP, high-volume surgical practices had published reports on osseointegrated dental implantation during primary ablation and reconstructive

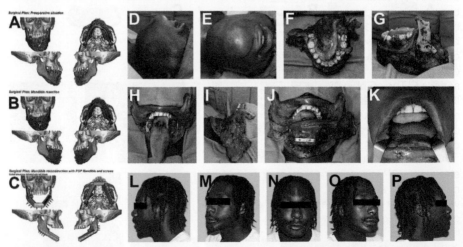

Fig. 3. VSP of a large osteosarcoma resulting in loss of normal mandibular cortical contour making intraoperative bending of a reconstruction plate difficult. (*A–C*) VSP session showing the planned resection and reconstruction with milled titanium reconstruction plate. (*D–K*). Intraoperative views of the surgical resection and reconstruction. (*L–P*) One-year post-operative result.

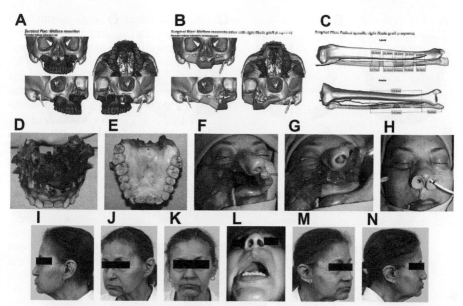

Fig. 4. VSP of a total palatectomy reconstruction. (*A–C*) VSP session showing a complex ome-goid five-segment fibula reconstruction. (*D–H*) Intraoperative views of the surgical resection and reconstruction. (*I–N*) One year postoperative result.

surgery.[18] VSP did not initiate this concept; however, it enabled systematic implementation. Placing implants at the time of reconstruction improves the efficiency of osseointegration and shortens the time to dental prosthesis delivery (approximately 4–6 weeks).[19] With virtually planned osseous reconstruction, implant location can be selected carefully considering vascular anatomy, bony anatomy with appropriate bone stock, osteotomy location, fixation screw placement, and final geometry. Placement of the implants can even be done before cutting osteotomies or removing the bone from its vascular pedicle.[19] Placing implants with VSP while the tissue remains on its native vascular supply improves efficiency and accuracy of dental rehabilitation, decreases ischemia duration, and prevents implant interaction with reconstructive screws.[20] The combination of VSP techniques with careful planning has even afforded the reconstructive surgeon the opportunity to simultaneously reconstruct the maxillo-mandibular complex and deliver a provisional denture prosthetic at the time of the index surgery for an immediate cosmetic benefit—the so-called "jaw in a day" procedure (**Fig. 5**).

Although the fibula is the most used bony MVFTT donor site in head and neck reconstruction, VSP is not limited to use with this flap. VSP has shown utility in designing models with scapular tip and iliac crest reconstructions.[21–23] The application to various donor sites enables the reconstructive surgeon to weigh the pros and cons of each site (ie, bone contour, cortical thickness, soft tissue attachments, volume of reconstruction) with the confidence that an intricate and successful reconstruction can be achieved with VSP and good surgical technique. VSP also serves as a tool to improve pattern of practice in determining esthetic goals and the procedures necessary to achieve them.[24] This is especially pertinent in cranial reconstruction and cranioplasty where the VSP techniques have been shown to afford accuracy to less than 2 mm in PEEK implant placement, improving outcome.[25]

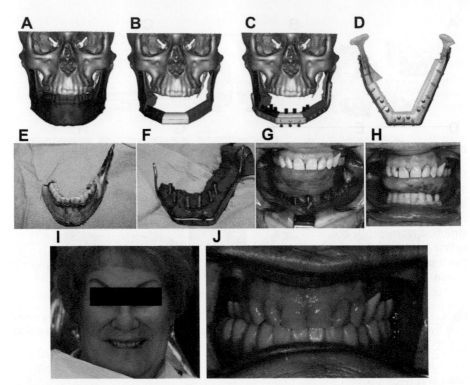

Fig. 5. VSP of "jaw in a day" procedure. (*A–D*) Planned segmental mandibulectomy, three-segment fibula, and guided osseointegrated dental implants. (*E–H*) Intraoperative photos of the resected specimen, prepared flap with cylinders, and provisional prosthesis in place. (*I, J*) One-year outcome with permanent fixed prosthesis in place.

RECONSTRUCTIVE OUTCOMES

The operative impact of VSP has been commented on in numerous publications from opinion pieces to systematic reviews. A recent systematic review and meta-analysis of 12 cohort studies including 355 patients comparing computer-assisted mandibular reconstruction versus freehand reconstruction showed decreased total operative time by 80 minutes, ischemic time by 35 minutes, and length of stay by 2 days. The decreased total and ischemic operative times are attributed to having a set plan and guides for osteotomies that reduce surgical decision-making time as well as manufactured plating that reduces physical work time. Complication rates between groups were nonsignificant.[5] Although VSP objectively reduces operative times, questions remain regarding the impact on improvement of reconstructive accuracy. Based on the meta-analysis and systemic review, there do not seem to be significant differences in reconstructive accuracy; however, accuracy was less frequently reported and more variably measured.[5] Additional studies have evaluated objective measurements with postoperative imaging. One retrospective study of 42 patients evaluated measurements between anatomic landmarks with patient-specific milled or additively manufactured plates versus pre-bent reconstructive plates on a 3D printed model and found no difference between the groups.[16] On the other hand, a study from a high-volume MVFTT center including 90 patients showed significantly improved bone-to-bone contact resulting in decreased rates of bony malunion or nonunion with VSP;

however, the improved bony union did not significantly decrease complication rates between groups.[26] Although the improved bony contact did not change esthetic outcome or complications identified, it ought to be appreciated in the head and neck oncologic setting as improved bony union and faster healing may facilitate timely initiation of adjuvant oncologic therapy. Altogether, VSP has been demonstrated to improve surgical efficiency without increasing complications but can be considered equivalent to traditional methods in terms of accuracy in experienced hands.

COST AND FUTURE IMPROVEMENTS

A discussion regarding VSP would be incomplete without evaluating cost and necessary manufacturing time. A cost analysis article published in 2015 showed that VSP averaged $7000 when a patient-specific plate was used and approximately $5000 with a pre-bent plate.[27] This is considerably higher than a standard generic reconstruction plate which costs $665 at the time of publication. It is a striking disparity at first glance, however, when operating room utilization costs and decreased operative time are considered the cost disparity all but evaporates with a conservative estimate for operative cost per minute of $47.50.[27] Considering this, the utilization of VSP is approximately cost neutral and some would argue is cost-effective as some operating room dollar per minute estimates have been published at nearly double this rate.[28]

Owing to the need to process the anatomic imaging, schedule and perform a VSP session, and manufacture patient-specific materials, the turnaround time for delivery and surgery coordination can take anywhere from 1 to 3 weeks.[29] In the setting of head and neck cancer, this wait time can be anxiety provoking to the patient, and worse, could mean the difference between an operable and inoperable tumor. As surgeons and manufacturers become more experienced with the VSP process, and as it becomes even more widespread in its use, this delivery time should continue to decrease. A more important long-term solution in reducing costs and manufacturing time, however, would be the development of in-house VSP systems and increased commercial global printing centers.

Criticisms of VSP in head and neck cancer reconstruction are inflexibility on the day of surgery and loss of familiarity with traditionally planned surgery. Reported evidence suggests that most tumor resections in which VSP is used do not require resection modification on the day of surgery and the resection margins are cleared at similar rates when using VSP or conventional methods; however, exceptions may arise necessitating abandonment of the plan.[29,30] For this reason, manufacturers can produce multiple cutting guides with different slots if rapid progression is anticipated.[31]

SUMMARY

VSP is a revolutionary tool for the head and neck reconstructive surgeon. As with any tool, there are strengths and weaknesses. The strengths include shorter operative time, shorter reconstructive time, shorter ischemic time, streamlined dental rehabilitation, facilitation of complex reconstruction, non-inferior and possibly superior accuracy, and increased durability. The weaknesses are increased up-front costs, potential delays to operative management while awaiting products, limited flexibility on the day of surgery, and loss of familiarity with conventionally planned surgery.

CLINICS CARE POINTS

- Virtual surgical planning (VSP) is a safe tool that maintains oncologic resection integrity and facilitates reconstruction.
- VSP shortens ischemic, reconstructive, and total operating time in head and neck microvascular free tissue transfer.
- VSP enables stream-lined dental rehabilitation which may improve quality of life for patients with head and neck cancer.
- VSP delays time from initial contact to operative management when compared with traditionally planned surgery as it requires high-quality computed tomography scans, a planning meeting, and device manufacturing (cutting guides and reconstructive plates).
- VSP maintains and may improve surgical accuracy when compared with traditionally planned head and neck reconstructive surgery.
- VSP enables preoperative planning and comfort with complex donor and defect sites for osseous reconstruction.
- VSP is at least cost-neutral when compared with traditional surgical planning.

DISCLOSURE

None.

REFERENCES

1. Kumar BP, Venkatesh V, Kumar KAJ, et al. Mandibular Reconstruction: Overview. J Maxillofac Oral Surg 2016;15(4):425–41.
2. Swartz WM, Banis JC, Newton ED, et al. The osteocutaneous scapular flap for mandibular and maxillary reconstruction. Plast Reconstr Surg 1986;77(4):530–45.
3. Hidalgo DA. Fibula free flap: A new method of mandible reconstruction. Plast Reconstr Surg 1989;84(1):71–9.
4. Largo RD, Garvey PB. Updates in head and neck reconstruction. Plast Reconstr Surg 2018;141(2):271E–85E.
5. Powcharoen W, Yang WF, Yan Li K, et al. Computer-Assisted versus Conventional Freehand Mandibular Reconstruction with Fibula Free Flap: A Systematic Review and Meta-Analysis. Plast Reconstr Surg 2019;144(6):1417–28.
6. Hoang D, Perrault D, Stevanovic M, et al. Surgical applications of three-dimensional printing: A review of the current literature & how to get started. Ann Transl Med 2016;4(23):1–19.
7. Brix F, Lambrecht JT. Preparation of Individual Skull Models Based on Computed Tomographic Information. Fortschr Kiefer Gesichtchir 1987;32:74.
8. Lambrecht JT, Brix F. Individual skull model fabrication for craniofacial surgery. Cleft Palate J 1990;27(4):382–5.
9. Wilde F, Hanken H, Probst F, et al. Multicenter study on the use of patient-specific CAD/CAM reconstruction plates for mandibular reconstruction. Int J Comput Assist Radiol Surg 2015;10(12):2035–51.
10. Singh GD, Singh M. Virtual surgical planning: Modeling from the present to the future. J Clin Med 2021;10(5655):1–18.
11. Rodby KA, Turin S, Jacobs RJ, et al. Advances in oncologic head and neck reconstruction: Systematic review and future considerations of virtual surgical

planning and computer aided design/computer aided modeling. J Plast Reconstr Aesthetic Surg 2014;67(9):1171–85.

12. Nwagu U, Swendseid B, Ross H, et al. Maxillectomy Reconstruction Revision Using Virtual Surgical Planning and Intraoperative Navigation. Laryngoscope 2021; 131(10):E2655–9.

13. Garvey PB, Chang EI, Selber JC, et al. A prospective study of preoperative computed tomographic angiographic mapping of free fibula osteocutaneous flaps for head and neck reconstruction. Plast Reconstr Surg 2012;130(4):6–13.

14. Parras D, Ramos B, Haro JJ, et al. Virtual surgical planning for mandibular reconstruction: Improving the fibula bone flap. Lect Notes Comput Sci 2017;10208 LNCS:282–91.

15. Tarsitano A, Battaglia S, Crimi S, et al. Is a computer-assisted design and computer-assisted manufacturing method for mandibular reconstruction economically viable? J Cranio-Maxillofacial Surg 2016;44(7):795–9.

16. Zeller AN, Neuhaus MT, Weissbach LVM, et al. Patient-Specific Mandibular Reconstruction Plates Increase Accuracy and Long-Term Stability in Immediate Alloplastic Reconstruction of Segmental Mandibular Defects. J Maxillofac Oral Surg 2020;19(4):609–15.

17. Kasper R, Winter K, Pietzka S, et al. Biomechanical In Vitro Study on the Stability of Patient-Specific CAD/CAM Mandibular Reconstruction Plates: A Comparison Between Selective Laser Melted, Milled, and Hand-Bent Plates. Craniomaxillofac Trauma Reconstr 2021;14(2):135–43.

18. Urken ML, Buchbinder D, Costantino PD, et al. Oromandibular reconstruction using microvascular composite flaps: Report of 210 cases. Arch Otolaryngol Head Neck Surg 1998;124(1):46–55.

19. Allen RJ, Shenaq DS, Rosen EB, et al. Immediate dental implantation in oncologic jaw reconstruction: Workflow optimization to decrease time to full dental rehabilitation. Plast Reconstr Surg - Glob Open 2019;7(1):1–4.

20. Runyan CM, Sharma V, Staffenberg DA, et al. Jaw in a day: State of the art in maxillary reconstruction. J Craniofac Surg 2016;27(8):2101–4.

21. Foley BD, Thayer WP, Honeybrook A, et al. Mandibular reconstruction using computer-aided design and computer-aided manufacturing: An analysis of surgical results. J Oral Maxillofac Surg 2013;71(2):e111–9.

22. Sheehan CC, Haskins AD, Huang AT, et al. Cephalometric and Functional Mandibular Reconstructive Outcomes Using a Horizontal Scapular Tip Free Flap. Otolaryngol Head Neck Surg 2021;165(3):414–8.

23. Kass JI, Prisman E, Miles BA. Guide design in virtual planning for scapular tip free flap reconstruction. Laryngoscope Investig Otolaryngol 2018;3(3):162–8.

24. Edward I, Chang MD, Mark W, et al. Cephalometric analysis for microvascular head and neck reconstruction. Head Neck 2012;34(11):1607–14.

25. Wandell A, Papanastassiou A, Tarasiewicz I, et al. What is the Accuracy of PEEK Implants for Cranioplasty in Comparison to Their Patient Specific Surgical Plan? J Oral Maxillofac Surg 2022;81(1):24–31.

26. Chang EI, Jenkins MP, Patel SA, et al. Long-Term Operative Outcomes of Preoperative Computed Tomography-Guided Virtual Surgical Planning for Osteocutaneous Free Flap Mandible Reconstruction. Plast Reconstr Surg 2016;137(2): 619–23.

27. Zweifel DF, Simon C, Hoarau R, et al. Are virtual planning and guided surgery for head and neck reconstruction economically viable? J Oral Maxillofac Surg 2015; 73(1):170–5.

28. Haddock NT, Monaco C, Weimer KA, et al. Increasing bony contact and overlap with computer-designed offset cuts in free fibula mandible reconstruction. J Craniofac Surg 2012;23(6):1592–5.
29. Knitschke M, Bäcker C, Schmermund D, et al. Impact of planning method (Conventional versus virtual) on time to therapy initiation and resection margins: A retrospective analysis of 104 immediate jaw reconstructions. Cancers 2021; 13(12):1–16.
30. Kholaki O, Saxe BJ, Williams FC, et al. Does the Use of a Wrap in Three-Dimensional Surgical Planning Influence the Bony Margin Status of Benign and Malignant Neoplasms of the Oral, Head and Neck Region? An Initial Investigation. Oral Surg Oral Med Oral Pathol Oral Radiol 2021;131(4):e140.
31. Efanov JI, Roy AA, Huang KN, et al. Virtual surgical planning: The Pearls and pitfalls. Plast Reconstr Surg - Glob Open 2018;6(1):1–10.

Practice Trends and Evidence-Based Practice in Microvascular Reconstruction

Candace A. Flagg, MD[a],*, Jayne R. Stevens, MD[a],
Steven Chinn, MD, MPH[b,c]

KEYWORDS

- Microvascular • Reconstruction • Free flap

KEY POINTS

- A multitude of surgical techniques is available so that microvascular and free flap reconstruction can be individualized to each patient.
- Admission to a unit familiar with care of patients undergoing microvascular reconstruction requiring attention to complex perioperative factors and frequent serial free flap evaluations are key to postoperative care.
- Free flaps that fail usually do so within the first 48 hours postoperatively but fortunately there are several surgical rescue techniques to restore function.
- Surgeons should be aware of potential risk factors (age, tobacco use, previous radiation, and so forth) but still offer microvascular reconstruction if in the patient's best interest.

INTRODUCTION

Microvascular and free flap reconstruction is now a mainstay of surgical treatment for a variety of patients. From cancer to trauma and across all ages, otolaryngology surgeons have the unique opportunity to restore form and function to the head and neck in ways that accentuate our understanding and respect for such delicate and complex anatomy. There are several prevailing principles to microvascular reconstruction. During the decades since the first use of microvascular reconstruction in the head and neck, there are now also finer details of preoperative planning, surgical technique,

Funding: None.
[a] Department of Otolaryngology–Head and Neck Surgery, San Antonio Uniformed Services Health Education Consortium, JBSA-Fort Sam Houston, TX, USA; [b] Department of Otolaryngology-Head and Neck Surgery, University of Michigan, 1500 East Medical Center Drive, Ann Arbor, MI 48109, USA; [c] Rogel Cancer Center, University of Michigan, 1500 East Medical Center Drive, Ann Arbor, MI 48109, USA
* Corresponding author. Department of Otolaryngology–Head and Neck Surgery, San Antonio Uniformed Services Health Education Consortium, 3551 Roger Brooke Drive, JBSA-Ft Sam Houston, TX 78234.
E-mail address: cflagg150@gmail.com

and postoperative care that have evolved.[1] In this article, we present a collection of up-to-date and evidence-based practice trends surrounding microvascular reconstruction.

DISCUSSION
Microvascular Surgical Techniques

Arterial and venous anastomosis

A wide variety of vessels can be considered for the purpose of microvascular reconstruction. Typical arterial options include branches of the external carotid artery—the superior thyroid, facial, or lingual arteries—as well as the transverse cervical artery. If these branches are not adequate, the main trunk of the external carotid, dorsal scapular arteries, or internal thoracic arteries can also be considered for anastomosis. For venous reconstruction, the internal jugular, external jugular, or common facial vein can be used. There remains debate within the microsurgical community on 1 versus 2 venous anastomoses. The argument for 2 venous anastomoses is that they may allow for increased venous outflow and is a protective measure in the event one vein kinks.[2,3] However, empirically derived flow data looking at this question identified greater blood velocity in 1 venous anastomosis compared with 2.[4]

Donor artery and vein size should be within 1.5 to 2 times that of the recipient vessel to perform end-to-end anastomosis.[1] Otherwise, end-to-side anastomosis is wise.[5] Venous couplers are available for and can ease creation of end-to-side anastomoses, which, as discussed below, have been shown to be more successful than sutured end-to-side anastomoses.[3] In terms of venous function, Stewart and colleagues found that there was no significant difference between end-to-end versus end-to-side anastomoses. They noted that free flaps with end-to-side anastomoses had a higher failure rate but this was thought to be multifactorial rather than solely related to the type of anastomosis.[3]

Patients with vessel-depleted necks secondary to previous neck dissection or radiation therapy can be particularly challenging cases. Surgeons can use the dorsal scapular or internal mammary arteries that are often out of the field of radiotherapy.[5,6] Contralateral anastomoses can also be achieved with great success rates (96%–99%). Vein grafts may be necessary for patients with inadequate vessels, inadequate pedicle length, or as a salvage method after thrombosis or vessel injury. Surgeons may opt for interposition, transposition, arteriovenous loop, or transposition arteriovenous loop grafting.[7] Some studies have reported an increased risk of complications/flap failure with the use of vein grafts while others have not. Maricevich and colleagues reported increased free flap failure in patients with vein grafts and suggest that this is because of an increased risk of vein kinking/twisting. They also raise a key point: patients undergoing vein grafts are typically more complex cases because they have undergone previous radiation, neck dissection, or free flap surgery, and found that some failures were more likely because of surgeon error (intraoperative vessel injury or placement of external compressive dressings) rather than the presence of a vein graft.[8] Seim and colleagues completed a retrospective multi-institutional review of more than 3000 head and neck free flap cases and found no difference in outcomes between patients receiving a vein graft or otherwise.[9]

Couplers versus hand-sewn techniques

Vessel couplers are more often used for venous anastomoses given the increased pliability of veins compared with arteries. Coupler use for arterial anastomosis has been controversial and, historically, is not favored over hand-sewn techniques because arterial walls are thicker, leading to more difficulty preparing and positioning the vessel walls on the coupler. This may be especially true in the postradiotherapy patient. More recently, however, some authors have experienced good success with arterial couplers if both the donor and recipient vessels are larger than 1 mm or the coupler is at least 2.5 mm, the discrepancy in vessel size is no more than a 1.5:1 ratio, and no fibrosis or atherosclerotic plaques are present. Some authors report that hand-sewn anastomoses are advantageous because there is less risk of postoperative thrombosis but others say this is the advantage of using couplers because they can prevent suturing the vessel back wall and placement of uneven sutures.[10,11]

Operative time
The total time a patient spends in the operating room is, of course, multifactorial. Still, there are certain factors that surgeons should keep in mind. For example, a patient's surgical indication in and of itself can be predictive of operative time. Surgical indications listed from longer to shorter times include malignant neoplasm, nonhealing wound, trauma, benign neoplasm, nonfunctional larynx, osteoradionecrosis, fistula repair, and velopharyngeal insufficiency. Performing a neck dissection and especially the addition of a free flap also adds a significant amount of time to total operative time. In general, radial forearm free flaps are considered the quickest free flaps to complete, whereas fibular free flaps are the longest.[12] Longer operative times (greater than 10 hours) are associated with increased risk of postoperative complications.[13]

Anesthetic and Airway Considerations

Intubation
Intubation is a critical time. The anesthesia team should be prepared for a difficult airway, especially if patients have undergone previous neck surgery or radiation. Intubation routes include oral (to include retromolar technique) and nasal; and use of fiberoptic endoscopes to facilitate intubation is often helpful. Submental intubation can also be considered but is more often used in cases of maxillofacial trauma than head and neck microvascular reconstructive cases. Tracheostomy may also be a planned step of the surgery and is discussed in more detail within the 'Tracheostomy' section below.[14]

Anesthetic options
Ultimately, the anesthesia team will likely use the agents they are most familiar/comfortable with; however, from a surgical standpoint, there are some key factors to note. Sevoflurane possesses endothelial protective effects and has been shown to reduce ischemia-reperfusion injury during microvascular surgery.[15,16] However, patients undergoing total intravenous anesthesia may require less intraoperative fluids and have less pulmonary complications.[14,17] Remifentanil allows for adequate intraoperative analgesia and causes vasodilation, which can be helpful in microvascular surgery. Precedex is an alpha-2 agonist and as such may cause vasoconstriction. Research is limited but surprisingly there are a few studies that suggest the use of precedex perioperatively does not compromise flap survival. In addition, it can be used during the perioperative transition as a sedative in the intensive care unit (ICU) for patients left intubated after their procedure.[14,18,19]

Intraoperative monitoring
In addition to standard blood pressure, pulse oximetry, electrocardiogram, temperature, and end-tidal carbon dioxide monitors, it is beneficial to have central venous pressure or invasive arterial blood pressure monitoring. Clinically, the surgical and anesthesia teams can also assess the patient via urine output, arterial blood gases, and estimated blood loss.[14] Intraoperative fluids should be administered judiciously. Intraoperative

intravenous fluids exceeding 5.5 L increases the risk of postoperative complications in general, and fluids exceeding 7 L increases the risk of a major postoperative complication.[20] Funk and colleagues established an additional measure for intraoperative fluid administration by the use of cardiac output monitoring—fluids titrated to maintain a certain cardiac index and stroke volume index ultimately led to less fluid administration while improving patient hemodynamics. Patients also went on to require less resuscitation in the 24 hours following surgery.[21] In the early postoperative period, fluids should ideally be limited to no more 130 mL/kg within the first 24 hours.[22]

Tracheostomy

Tracheostomy is advantageous for several reasons—creation of a definitive airway, decreased sedation requirements, ease of access, improved pulmonary toilet, decreased airway resistance, and an existing airway should further procedures be required.[23] There are certain patient factors for which tracheostomy should be considered, including history of obstructive sleep apnea, morbid obesity, poor pulmonary function, or if the patient is expected to undergo multiple procedures. Surgical factors, such as the size or site of resection, degree of airway edema at the end of a case, or obstructive bulk from a free flap should also influence the surgical team to consider tracheostomy.[23]

If reasonable, though, it is worthwhile sparing patients from tracheostomy because many have negative experiences such as discomfort, trouble with routine care, sleep disruption, or the inability to communicate.[24] Interestingly, Madgar and colleagues found that patients spared from elective tracheostomy were generally younger (better pulmonary reserve), had higher body mass index (better nutrition status), and had shorter hospital stays (avoidance of decannulation process/waiting for discharge tracheostomy materials). They did not find a statistically significant difference in those undergoing a neck dissection but clinically they suggest that completion of a bilateral neck dissection may warrant tracheostomy because these patients are at higher risk of airway compromise.[23]

Monitoring and Troubleshooting

Hospital admission

Microvascular free flap patients each require several days of postoperative monitoring to ensure proper recovery. There is a wide range of practice pattern variation depending on the capabilities of each individual hospital, so while the ICU is generally the most common place of admission following free flap surgery, highly specialized step-down or medical floors may be noninferior, or even preferable.[24–27]

General hospital care

There are several aspects of hospitalization and recovery that should be monitored closely to optimize wound healing and overall outcomes. One of these aspects is patient temperature. Patients are at risk of hypothermia for many reasons: long operative time, multiple exposure sites to room air, and cool IV fluid administration. Hypothermia must be prevented to decrease flap failure, local vasoconstriction, and delayed wound healing.[14]

Many surgeons use antiplatelet medications to optimize outcomes and decrease the risk of thrombosis. Heparin, low molecular weight heparin, aspirin, dextran, and prostaglandin E1 have all been used for postoperative anticoagulation. Low molecular weight heparin may be the safest choice because there are less systemic side effects than IV heparin, less risk of gastrointestinal bleeding as compared with aspirin, and is just as effective as aspirin. Preference for systemic anticoagulation depends on the institution, however, because some still favor aspirin.[15,25]

In addition to antiplatelet medications, many other medications may affect free flap outcomes as well. Vasopressors are thought to compromise flap perfusion but this may depend on the exact vasopressor used. Noradrenaline, for example, has been shown to maintain flap perfusion. Dexamethasone or even mannitol can reduce flap edema, as well as keeping the patient's head of bed elevated.[14] Ampicillin-sulbactam is a good choice for antibiotic coverage because it lowers the odds of skin/soft tissue infection. Clindamycin has been associated with a higher risk of postoperative infection when used for a prolonged period, and so should be combined with other antibiotics, such as metronidazole or gentamicin, if necessary. Regardless of choice, there is no known benefit to antibiotic coverage for free flap patients beyond postoperative day 7.[15,26]

Oral feeding is generally thought to increase the risk of fistula formation but it may be a reasonable consideration in patients who can tolerate an oral diet because some authors have had success with early oral feeding without any increased risk of fistula formation. Otherwise, tube feeding should be started within 24 hours of surgery.[15] Nutrition is just one of many elements covered in most institutions' enhanced recovery after surgery (ERAS) protocols. Although ERAS protocols were first developed in other surgical specialties, the concept of creating a multidisciplinary pathway to improve surgical outcomes and facilitate recovery has been increasingly adopted within head and neck surgery. Dort and colleagues' publication in 2017 is a consensus-based protocol from existing medical literature designed to provide protocols specifically for patients undergoing head and neck surgery with free flap reconstruction.[28]

Flap checks and anastomotic thrombosis

Most flaps that fail do so within the first 48 to 72 hours. Therefore, frequent flap checks are of the utmost importance. Flap checks usually occur hourly for the first 24 to 48 hours, then every 2 hours for following 2 to 3 days, with tapering afterward.[15,29] Shen and colleagues completed a systematic review on free flap monitoring and salvage, including flaps of the head/neck and elsewhere. They found that most flaps can be successfully salvaged within the first 48 hours following surgery—94% success at 24 hours and 83% success at 48 hours. Successful salvage rate drops significantly with only 12% success at 72 hours after surgery and none at 96 hours.[30]

Flap check physical examinations have several components: inspection of warmth and color, blood return on pinprick, and often assessment with both implantable/internal and external Doppler (**Table 1**). Color duplex ultrasound, near infrared spectroscopy, microdialysis, and laser Doppler flowmetry are newer technologies that may also be available for flap surveillance. Nurses are the primary team members completing flap checks, and although physician participation is still integral, having a reliable nursing staff helps relieve physicians of the otherwise burdensome time commitment required to complete such frequent assessments.[15,29,31–33]

Each step of the flap check is essential and designed to assess the patency of both venous and arterial anastomoses. Venous obstruction or thrombosis will usually occur within the first 48 hours postoperatively and is more common than arterial thrombosis because veins bend easily, are more compressible, and are more susceptible to infection, hematoma, or fistula formation. Decreased venous outflow/thrombosis causes a purple or mottled appearance, epidermolysis, edema, and quick return of dark blood on pinprick testing. Arterial thrombosis, however, can be related to a hypercoagulable state (common in patients with cancer) and most frequently occurs within the first 24 hours postoperatively.[11,15]

For either venous or arterial thrombosis, surgeons have multiple treatment options to consider. Mechanical thrombectomy can be performed by reopening the anastomosis, performing a direct thrombectomy, or use of Fogarty catheters. Chemical thrombolysis

Table 1		
Important elements for examination in postoperative monitoring of free flaps		
Elements of Flap Examination	**Normal Examination**	**Abnormality and Potential Causes**
Palpation	Soft	Firm—Potential underlying hematoma
Color	Flesh toned	Pale—Arterial compromise Mottled—Venous congestion Ecchymosis (throughout or in specific area)—Venous congestion/compromise, either at anastomosis or in microvascular bed
Response to pinprick with fine needle	Bright red blood (variable timing depending on flap origin, RFFF in 1–5s, 5–10s for ALT)	Absent bleeding—Arterial compromise Dark brisk bleeding—Venous compromise
Temperature	Warm	Cold—Arterial compromise
Arterial signal (implantable Doppler or on skin paddle)	Present	Absent—Anastomotic thrombus, compression in tunnel

is also an option and involves administration of streptokinase, urokinase, or tissue plasminogen activator.[11,14] Leeches, also known as *Hirudo medicinalis*, can be used as salvage treatment if congestion occurs after venous reanastomosis. Leeches release a substance called hirudin, which has anticoagulative properties and allows for better venous outflow. Leeches remove up to 15 cc of blood per meal but additional bloody oozing continues for up to 3 days following removal from the patient. It should be noted that patients require antibiotic coverage while leeches are in use.[29] Recently, intradermal flap injections with bivalirudin or subcutaneous heparin have shown promise as an alternative to leeching.[34,35]

Efficiency Considerations

Two-team approach

Most free flaps and microvascular reconstruction procedures are carried out using a 2-team approach (**Fig. 1**). Operating in this fashion is advantageous for many reasons. First, it allows one team to focus solely on the ablative aspect without concerning themselves with the difficulty of reconstruction. For example, head and neck cancer surgeons can consider what margins are oncologically sound without worry of resecting essential structures. In the same way, the reconstructive team's main goal is to restore form and function as best as possible without concern of oncologic outcome. Operating in 2 teams also reduces operative time because the 2 teams are working simultaneously. Furthermore, it allows for shared responsibility postoperatively for flap checks, rounding, decision-making, and follow-up visits after the patient is discharged.[25,36,37] Recent cost analyses have shown that 2-team approaches also save time and overall operating costs with reduced intraoperative fluid, thus reducing the risk of flap failure or patient complications.

Quality Recommendations

Fortunately, microvascular free flap success rates are greater than 95%, with some authors quoting up to 99% success.[26,29] Advances in equipment and surgical training

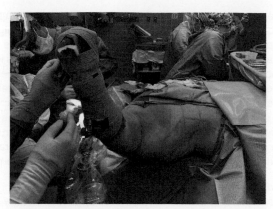

Fig. 1. Example of 2-team approach to ablation and reconstruction—one team works at the head of the patient and the reconstruction team prepares to elevate scapular system free flap, utilizing the SPIDER limb positioner.

have made this possible but even still flap failure remains a devastating complication. There is a litany of different risk factors that may portend worse outcomes or lead to postoperative complications for free flap patients, although the degree to which each of these risks matters is debated in previous literature. These risks are reviewed here.

Preoperative risk factors

Age, previous chemotherapy or radiotherapy, smoking status, tumor stage, peripheral vascular disease, and other medical comorbidities have all been proposed as risks to undergoing microvascular surgery. Specifically for elderly, hypertensive, or postradiotherapy patients, vessels may be more fibrotic and prone to tearing.[10] Tam and colleagues found that patients with preexisting coagulopathy or high alcohol consumption had a higher risk of postoperative infection, hematoma formation, and unplanned return to the operating room for flap failure.[38] Active smokers may also be at an increased risk for flap failure secondary to thrombocytosis, more activation of the sympathetic nervous system, and hypoxia.[29] Leung and colleagues found an inverse correlation between albumin levels and the risk of wound dehiscence, salivary leakage, pulmonary effusion, cardiac complications, and number of days to suture removal. This suggests that patients may benefit from preoperative nutritional screening/intervention to improve the quality of their postoperative course.[26,39]

All these factors seem intuitive; however, there has been much debate surrounding the evidence with which each has been deemed a "risk." For example, Goh and colleagues reported that there were significantly more medical complications (related to patient comorbidities and tumor stage) in elderly patients aged older than 65 years but age alone was not an independent risk factor for free flap failure.[40] Clark and colleagues found the opposite—age over 65 years *was* a notable predictor of complications after free flap procedure, along with ASA class III or IV, current tobacco use, and preoperative anemia (Hgb <11 g/dL).[22] Several other studies also support the notion that age may not be as big a risk it was once thought. In several studies, advanced age had no implications on flap outcomes; however, the elderly did require longer postoperative care and as expected had more perioperative medical issues. In addition, smoking status, alcohol use, diabetes, preoperative stroke, preoperative myocardial infarction, and the presence of peripheral vascular disease have also been found not to influence free flap complications.[41,42]

Another notable potential risk factor is preoperative radiotherapy. Bourget and colleagues describe that while previously irradiated patients are at higher risk of reoperation and postoperative complications, their flap success rate was still 96%, meaning that previous radiotherapy alone is not enough to avoid free flaps in these patients. They also identified larger flap size and postoperative infection as the 2 strongest predictors for complications in previously irradiated patients.[42] le Nobel and colleagues completed a retrospective case series of 304 head and neck free flap reconstructions and reported the only statistically significant predictors of postoperative complications were advanced tumor stage and pharyngoesophageal reconstruction. After controlling for tumor stage and defect type, preoperative chemoradiotherapy and radiotherapy alone did not influence complication rates in their free flap patients.[41]

Intraoperative and surgeon-related risks factors

Intraoperative factors leading to increased risk of flap failure include prolonged operative time and excessive fluid administration, as stated earlier.[13,22] Surgeons should be mindful that longer vascular pedicles tunneled under soft tissue may pose a higher risk for flap failure. It is important to stay attentive to head positioning intraoperatively because the head may be positioned in a manner conducive to adequate vessel flow during the procedure; however, if this position changes postoperatively, the vascular pedicle can become disrupted/kinked and lead to occlusion.[29]

SUMMARY

Microvascular and free flap reconstruction are key elements to many different patients' treatment. There are multiple vessels that can be used to achieve functional anastomosis, and vessel couplers or vein grafts are useful adjuncts. Surgeons should anticipate operative time, have preferred routes of intubation and anesthetic agents in mind, monitor intraoperative vitals and fluids, and develop alternate plans should intraoperative complications develop. The 2-team approach is very helpful and allows for shared responsibility in the operating room and in the acute postoperative period. Flap checks are essential, and the surgical team must be ready to reoperate to salvage a failing anastomosis/flap. Practice trends vary by institution, and there is much debate surrounding the weight of preoperative or intraoperative risk factors; however, patients in need of microvascular reconstruction should be offered such with the appropriate counseling.

CLINICS CARE POINTS

- Consider all reasonable vessels for microvascular anastomosis and be prepared to use an alternate or contralateral vessel if needed. Vessel couplers and vein grafts are also helpful adjuncts.

- Most patients are admitted to the ICU following microvascular surgery but specialized medical floors with highly trained nurses may also be available and are noninferior.

- Avoid hypothermia, treat with anticoagulation (low molecular weight heparin or aspirin) and antibiotics (ampicillin-sulbactam), and start oral/tube feeding within 24 hours after surgery.

- Physical examination, Doppler equipment, and newer technologies are used during flap checks to increase our sensitivity in recognizing flap failure, for which mechanical thrombectomy or chemical thrombolysis are performed.

> • Age, tobacco/alcohol use, medical comorbidities, and earlier chemoradiotherapy are all inconsistent risk factors for poor surgical outcomes. Although important to keep in mind, decide to operate based on the patient's best interest.

CONFLICT OF INTEREST

The authors report no relevant conflict of interest in submitting this article for publication. The view(s) expressed herein are those of the author(s) and do not reflect the official policy or position of Brooke Army Medical Center, the US Army Medical Department, the US Army Office of the Surgeon General, the Department of the Army, the Department of Defense, the US Government, or the University of Michigan.

AUTHOR CONTRIBUTIONS

C.A. Flagg: Substantial contributions to the conception or design of the study; Acquisition, analysis, and interpretation of data for the study; Drafting the work and revising it critically for important intellectual content; Final approval of the version to be published; Agreement to be accountable for all aspects of the study; J.R. Stevens: Substantial contributions to the conception or design of the study; Acquisition, analysis, and interpretation of data for the study; Revising the work critically for important intellectual content; Final approval of the version to be published; Agreement to be accountable for all aspects of the study; S. Chinn: Acquisition, analysis, and interpretation of data for the study; Revising the work critically for important intellectual content; Final approval of the version to be published; Agreement to be accountable for all aspects of the study.

REFERENCES

1. Panje WR, Krause CJ, Bardach J, et al. Reconstruction of intraoral defects with the free groin flap. Arch Otolaryngol 1977;103(2):78–83.
2. Onoda S, Masahito K. Microsurgery for head and neck reconstruction. J Craniofac Surg 2020;31:1441–4.
3. Stewart M, Hammond P, Khatiwala I, et al. Outcomes of venous end-to-side microvascular anastomoses of the head and neck. Laryngoscope 2021;131: 1286–90.
4. Hanasono MM, Kocak E, Ogunleye O, et al. One versus two venous anastomoses in microvascular free flap surgery. Plast Reconstr Surg 2010;126(5):1548–57.
5. Gschossmann JD, Balk M, Rupp R, et al. Results of contralateral anastomosis of microvascular free flaps in head and neck reconstruction. Ear Nose Throat J 2022;0(0):1–10.
6. Rosko AJ, Ryan JT, Wizauer EJ, et al. Dorsal scapular artery as a recipient vessel in the vessel-depleted neck during free tissue transfer in head and neck reconstruction. Head Neck 2017;39(7):E72–6.
7. Langdell HC, Shammas RL, Atia A, et al. Vein Grafts in Free Flap Reconstruction: Review of Indications and Institutional Pearls. Plast Reconstr Surg 2022;149(3): 742–9.
8. Maricevich M, Lin LO, Liu J, et al. Interposition Vein Grafting in Head and Neck Free Flap Reconstruction. Plast Reconstr Surg 2018;142(4):1025–34.
9. Seim NB, Old M, Petrisor D, et al. Head and neck free flap survival when requiring interposition vein grafting: A multi-instiutional review. Oral Oncol 2020;101: 104482.

10. Wang Y-J, Wang X-L, Jin S, et al. Meta-analysis of arterial anastomosis techniques in head and neck free tissue transfer. PLoS One 2021;16(4):e0249418.

11. Hathorn T, Nickel C, Sharma A, et al. How do I salvage that flap?; An evidence-based [rimer on salvage techniques for head & neck microvascular free flaps. Oral Oncol 2022;136(2023):1–10.

12. Sweeny L, Rosenthal EL, Light T, et al. Outcome and cost implications of microvascular reconstructions of the head and neck. Head Neck 2019;41:930–9.

13. Lin Y, He J-f, Zhang X, et al. Intraoperative factors associated with free flap failure in the head and neck region: a four-year retrospective study of 216 patient and review of the literature. J Oral Maxillofac Surg 2018;48:447–51.

14. Goswami U, Jain A. Anaesthetic implications of free-flap microvascular surgery for head and neck malignancies – A relook. J Anaesthesiol Clin Pharmacol 2021;37:499–504.

15. Vincent A, Sawhney R, Ducic Y. Perioperative care of free flap patients. Semin Plast Surg 2019;33:5–12.

16. Claroni C, Torregiani G, Covotta M, et al. Protective effect of sevoflurane preconditioning on ischemia-reperfusion injury in patients undergoing reconstructive plastic surgery with microsurgical flap, a randomized controlled trial. BMC Anesthesiol 2016;16(1):66.

17. Chang YT, Wu CC, Tang TY, et al. Differences between Total Intravenous Anesthesia and Inhalation Anesthesia in Free Flap Surgery of Head and Neck Cancer. PLoS One 2016;11(2):e0147713.

18. Rajan S, Moorthy S, Paul J, et al. Effect of dexmedetomidine on postoperative hemodynamics and outcome of free flaps in head and neck reconstructive surgeries. Open J Anesthesiol 2016;10:12–8.

19. Nunes S, Berg L, Raittinen LP, et al. Deep sedation with dexmedetomidine in a porcine model does not compromise the viability of free microvascular flap as depicted by microdialysis and tissue oxygen tension. Anesth Analg 2007;105(3):666–72.

20. Ettinger KS, Arce K, Lohse CM, et al. Higher perioperative fluid administration is associated with increased rates of complications following head and neck microvascular reconstruction with fibular free flaps. Microsurgery 2017;37:128–36.

21. Funk D, Bohn J, Mutch W, et al. Goal-directed fluid therapy for microvascular free flap reconstruction following mastectomy: A pilot study. Plast Surg (Oakv) 2015;23(4):231–4.

22. Clark JR, McCluskey SA, Hall F, et al. Predictors of morbidity following free flap reconstruction for cancer of the head and neck. Head Neck 2007;29(12):1090–101.

23. Madgar O, Livneh N, Dobriyan A, et al. Airway management following head and neck microvascular reconstruction: is tracheostomy mandatory? Braz J Otorhinolaryngol 2022;88(Suppl 4):S44–9.

24. Rogers SN, Russell L, Lowe D. Patients' experiences of temporary tracheostomy after microvascular reconstruction for cancer of the head and neck. Br J Oral Maxillofac Surg 2017;55:10–6.

25. Sayre KS, Kovatch KJ, Hanks JE, et al. Current practices in microvascular reconstruction by oral and maxillofacial surgeons. J Oral Maxillofac Surg 2021;79:1963–9.

26. Kinzinger MR, Bewley AF. Perioperative care of head and neck free flap patients. Curr Opin Otolaryngol Head Neck Surg 2017;25:405–10.

27. Panwar A, Smith R, Lydiatt D, et al. Vascularized tissue transfer in head and neck surgery: Is intensive care unit-based management necessary? Laryngoscope 2016;126:73–9.

28. Dort JC, Farwell DG, Findlay M, et al. Optimal Perioperative Care in Major Head and Neck Cancer Surgery With Free Flap Reconstruction: A Consensus Review and Recommendations From the Enhanced Recovery After Surgery Society. JAMA Otolaryngol Head Neck Surg 2017;143(3):292–303.

29. Wang W, Ong A, Vincent AG, et al. Flap failure and salvage in head and neck reconstruction. Semin Plast Surg 2020;34:314–20.

30. Shen AY, Lonie S, Lim K, et al. Free flap monitoring, salvage, and failure timing: A systematic review. J Reconstr Microsurg 2021;37(3):300–8.

31. Cannady SB, Hatten K, Wax MK. Postoperative controversies in the management of free flap surgery in the head and neck. Facial Plast Surg Clin North Am 2016; 24(3):309–14.

32. Hayler R, Low T-H, Fung K, et al. Implantable doppler ultrasound monitoring in head and neck free flaps: Balancing the pros and cons. Laryngoscope 2021; 131:E1854–9.

33. Starr NC, Slade E, Gal TJ, et al. Remote monitoring of head and neck free flaps using near infrared spectroscopic tissue oximetry. Am J Otolaryngol Head Neck Surg 2021;42(1):102834.

34. Harun A, Kruer R, Lee A, et al. Experience with pharmacologic leeching with bivalirudin for adjunct treatment of venous congestion of head and neck reconstructive flaps. Microsurgery 2018;38(6):643–50.

35. Perez M, Sancho J, Ferrer C, et al. Management of flap venous congestion: the role of heparin local subcutaneous injection. J Plast Reconstr Aesthet Surg 2014;67(1):48–55.

36. Torabi SJ, Chouairi F, Dinis J, et al. Head and neck reconstructive surgery: Characterization of the one-team and two-team approaches. J Oral Maxillofac Surg 2020;78:295–304.

37. Kovatch KJ, Hanks JE, Stevens JR, et al. Current practices in microvascular reconstruction in otolaryngology-head and neck surgery. Laryngoscope 2019; 129(1):138–45.

38. Tam S, Weber RS, Liu J, et al. Evaluating unplanned returns to the operating room in head and neck free flap patients. Ann Surg Oncol 2020;27:440–8.

39. Leung JS, Seto A, Li GK. Association between preoperative nutritional status and postoperative outcome in head and neck cancer patients. Nutr Cancer 2017;69: 464–9.

40. Goh CS, Kok YO, Yong CP, et al. Outcome predictors in elderly head and neck free flap reconstruction: A retrospective study and systematic review of the current evidence. J Plast Reconstr Aesthet Surg 2018;71(5):719–28.

41. le Nobel GJ, Higgins KM, Enepekides DJ. Predictors of complications of free flap reconstruction in head and neck surgery: Analysis of 304 free flap reconstruction procedures. Laryngoscope 2012;122(5):1014–9.

42. Bourget A, Chang JTC, Wu DB, et al. Free flap reconstruction in the head and neck region following radiotherapy: a cohort study identifying negative outcome predictors. Plast Reconstr Surg 2011;127(5):1901–8.

Optimizing Function and Appearance After Head and Neck Reconstruction
Measurement and Intervention

Evan M. Graboyes, MD, MPH[a,b], Carly E.A. Barbon, PhD[c,*]

KEYWORDS

- Head and neck cancer • Dysphagia • Body image • Disfigurement • Mental health
- Survivorship

KEY POINTS

- Patients with head and neck cancer (HNC) often present with dysphagia before and after surgical reconstruction warranting use of validated clinician-and patient-reported measures for functional outcomes tracking.
- Immediate postoperative rehabilitation should be considered after reconstruction and prior to adjuvant treatments.
- Body image distress (BID) among patients with HNC should be assessed using validated patient-reported outcome measures such as Performance Status Scale for Head and Neck Cancer.
- Evidence-based strategies to manage BID among HNC survivors are lacking. Building a renewed image after head and neck cancer treatment is a brief telemedicine-based cognitive behavioral therapy that has been effective at reducing BID among HNC survivors in small trials.

INTRODUCTION

Standard of care treatment of head and neck cancer (HNC) often involves combinations of surgery, radiation, and chemotherapy to cosmetically and functionally critical areas such as the face, lips, tongue, teeth, jaw, and throat. As a result of these treatments, HNC survivors suffer debilitating acute and long-term treatment toxicities including difficulty swallowing, facial disfigurement, impaired smiling, and challenges

[a] Department of Otolaryngology-Head and Neck Surgery, Medical University of South Carolina, 135 Rutledge Avenue, MSC 550, Charleston, SC 29425, USA; [b] Department of Public Health Sciences, Medical University of South Carolina; [c] Department of Head & Neck Surgery, University of Texas MD Anderson Cancer Center, Unit 1445, 1515 Holcombe Boulevard, Houston, TX 77030-400, USA
* Corresponding author.
E-mail address: cbarbon@mdanderson.org

Otolaryngol Clin N Am 56 (2023) 835–852
https://doi.org/10.1016/j.otc.2023.04.017
0030-6665/23/© 2023 Elsevier Inc. All rights reserved.

speaking. An estimated 50% of patients present with dysphagia after HNC treatment[1,2] and rank the ability to swallow after treatment as a top priority outside of cure and survival.[3] Resection and reconstruction of head and neck malignancies heavily impact the ability to swallow, maintain proper nutrition/hydration, and communicate due to alterations in structural anatomy of the head and neck. For example, treatment of oral cavity cancers typically involves deficits related to lingual manipulation and mastication of complex solids, limiting oral intake related to efficiency of the oral phase of swallowing. Alternatively, reconstruction for oro- and hypopharyngeal cancer impacts pharyngeal swallow function, driven by pharyngeal inefficiency and/or penetration/aspiration. Swallowing-specific deficits are related to the presence, type, and size of reconstruction.[4,5] The aforementioned deficits can contribute to below optimal quality of life (QOL), particularly for patients with reconstruction.[6,7]

HNC treatment-related toxicities occur in highly visible, socially significant parts of the body and limit basic daily activities such as eating, engaging in conversation, being understood by others, and participating in social interactions.[8–10] It is estimated that 75% of HNC survivors express body image concerns[11] and up to 28% have clinically significant body image-related distress (BID).[12,13] Among HNC survivors, BID is a source of devastating psychosocial morbidity and functional impairment, contributing to a 6 fold increase in moderate–severe depressive symptoms, an 8 fold increase in moderate–severe anxiety symptoms, social isolation, stigmatization, and decreased QOL.[8–10,12–16]

Because of their prevalence and morbidity, it is critical for members of the multidisciplinary head and neck oncology team to have an up-to-date and evidence-based approach to assessing and managing swallowing function and appearance-related concerns among HNC survivors. This study highlights the current state of science regarding (1) the measurement of swallowing-related impairment among patients with HNC; (2) strategies to address swallow-related impairment; (3) tools to assess BID and appearance-related concerns for patients with HNC; and (4) interventions to manage BID among HNC survivors.

MEASUREMENT OF FUNCTIONAL OUTCOMES AND QUALITY OF LIFE AMONG PATIENTS WITH HEAD AND NECK CANCER
Clinician-Graded Outcome Measures

Clinician-graded measures are helpful to establish baseline function and aid the speech-language pathologist (SLP) in rehabilitation planning and monitoring of function after dysphagia intervention. The modified barium swallow study (MBS) is a widely used examination to capture swallow function. Traditionally viewed as the gold standard to evaluate swallowing, it is adopted as an endpoint measure in multiple HNC trials. Pre- and postoperative objective swallow function using the MBS is not only vital to identifying benefit of rehabilitation, but to grade and characterize swallow function. During the MBS, SLPs use measurement protocols to determine.

1. *Dysphagia severity.* Using the Dynamic Imaging Grade of Swallowing Toxicity (DIGEST) method allows clinicians to grade pharyngeal swallow impairment as a toxicity of cancer. DIGEST grading uses a decision tree to summarize markers of swallowing safety (penetration/aspiration) and efficiency (pharyngeal bolus residue) which is then summarized into an overall severity grade of impairment on a 5-point scale, aligned with the National Cancer Institute's CTCAE toxicity framework.[17,18]

2. *Physiologic drivers of swallow impairment.* The Modified Barium Swallow Impairment Profile (MBSImP) is a standardized approach to assessment and reporting of swallow physiology based on the MBS.[19,20] The MBSImP provides a summary

of overall impairment for 3 phases of the swallow: oral, pharyngeal, and esophageal. For example, MBSImP breaks down the critical components of swallowing to determine the underlying drivers of impairment. Secondary analysis of MBS using MBSImP and DIGEST identify *focal injury* associated with swallow impairment in patients with oropharynx cancer after surgery in contrast to low-level *diffuse impairment* more associated with RT.[21] Overall, surgical impairments were associated with pharyngeal contraction and propulsive forces placed on the bolus, contributing to swallow inefficiency (ie, retained bolus residue in the pharynx). In contrast, RT-based impairments were associated with impaired laryngeal closure, contributing to impaired swallow safety (penetration/aspiration).

3. *Benefit of postural or compensatory adaptations* to alter the swallow pattern. Objective view of the swallow in real time allows clinicians to trial maneuvers or swallow strategies in real time to determine immediate benefit of strategy adoption versus whether the swallow is refractory to strategies.

4. *Rehabilitative targets* based on impairment and surgical site. Grading of swallow impairment by safety and efficiency paired with identification of underlying pathophysiologic drivers of dysfunction will drive the therapeutic planning process. For example, the SLP may target airway closure and cough strength to mitigate penetration/aspiration using the expiratory muscle strength trainer (EMST) and exercises that target hyolaryngeal elevation.

Components 1 to 4 noted above provide clinicians the ability to make evidence-based recommendations for swallowing strategies, compensations, and treatment for patients.

Another form of objective measures of swallow function are clinician-graded tools that capture markers of baseline and postoperative anatomic function and functional outcomes, such as diet. For example, the Performance Status Scale for Head and Neck Cancer (PSS-HN) is a 3-item instrument rated by semi-structured clinician interview for normalcy of diet (scores range from 0: nonoral nutrition to 100: full oral diet without restriction), public eating (0: always eats alone; 100: no restriction of place, food or companion) and understandability of speech (0: never understandable; 100: always understandable).[22] Contemporary data have identified post-treatment functional status (via PSS-HN) as a strong prognostic marker of survival in HNC patients,[23] whereas other studies have successfully implemented PSS-HN to monitor change in postoperative understanding of speech.[24] Use of the PSS-HN provides a valid, consistent, and efficient method to track function and identify change in status for communication and swallow outcomes.

Patients treated for tongue cancer are left with limited range of motion (ROM) pending the site, size, and nature of the defect and reconstruction. Measures of lingual range of motion are recommended, particularly for oral cavity cancer patients whose surgical resection can result in impaired speech intelligibility, dysphagia, and decreased QOL in survivorship.[6,25,26] Tongue protrusion, lateralization, and tongue tip elevation are globally lower in postoperative tongue patients and significantly correlated with swallow-related QOL and functional status.[27,28] The Tongue ROM[29] is a validated tool that is useful in functional prediction and monitoring of lingual function, particularly in postoperative oral cancer patients and those with late-radiation-associated dysphagia[30] who present with latent hypoglossal neuropathies.[31,32]

See **Table 1** for additional clinician-graded measures.

Patient-Reported Measures

Although clinician-graded outcomes are an invaluable contribution to a clinical assessment, the use of patient-reported outcome measures (PROMs) is growing as

Table 1
Suggested clinician- and patient-reported outcome measures for functional outcomes tracking

Functional Outcome	Outcome Type	1st Author (Year)	Description	Score	Validation
Function					
Performance Status Scale for Head & Neck Cancer (PSS-HN)	CRO	List et al,[22] 1996	Three-item instrument rated via semi-structured interview for normalcy of diet, public eating and understanding of speech	Diets score range from most restricted (nothing by mouth; NPO: 0) to least restricted (full, unrestricted diet: 100). Understandable of speech and eating in public are graded from 0 (never understandable/always eats alone) to 100 (always understandable/no restrictions of place, food or companion).	Correlated PSS-HN with FACT-HN subscales to determine convergent and discriminant validity. High correlation between PSS-HN normalcy of diet and eating in public subscales with head and neck subscale (HNS) of FACT-H&N (r = 0.42–0.66, respectively)[a]
Tongue range of motion (L-ROM)	CRO	Lazarus et al,[42] 2013	Includes measures of 4 global movements; protrusion, lateralizations (left, right) and elevations scores	Four measures range from 0 to 100 in (in increments of 25). Total score for tongue ROM is defined as: the sum of all 4 components divided by 4, creating in overall score ranging from 0 to 100. Healthy subjects average 100, whereas oral cavity cancer patients average 88.6	Tongue ROM significantly correlated with MDADI (0.48); tongue strength (−0.43)[b]

Speech				
Speech handicap index (SHI)	PROM	Rinkel et al,[95] 2018	30-item instrument that measures self-reported speech function and psychosocial function related to speech	Scores range from 0 to 120 with higher scores indicating higher speech-related impact	Internal consistency (Cronbach's alpha) = 0.98; tests-retest reliability (ICC) = 0.92
Quality of life					
MD Anderson Dysphagia Inventory (MDADI)	PROM	Chen et al,[34] 2001	20 item-self-administered questionnaire to assess the impact of dysphagia on QOL	Global composites and 3 subscales (emotional, functional, and physical). Composite scores range from 20 (low function) to 100 (high function)	Overall internal consistency (Cronbach's alpha) = 0.96 tests-retest reliability (ICC) = 0.69–0.88
Multi-symptom					
MD Anderson Dysphagia Inventory for Head and Neck Cancer (MDASI-HN)	PROM	Rosenthal et al,[96] 2014	Multi-symptom PRO instrument measuring severity or burden of cancer-related symptoms and their interface with or effect on patients' daily infection. Includes 13 core MDASI items, and interference items	Each symptoms item rated on a scale from 0 (not at all) to 10 (as bad as you can imagine), respectively	Internal consistency (Cronbach's alpha) > 0.88
FACE-Q	PROM	Cracchiolo et al,[66] 2019	14 independently functioning scales that measures appearance, health-related QOL, function an patient experience of care	Each scale provide a score from 0 to 100, with higher scores indicating better outcome	Internal consistency (Cronbach's alpha) > 0.87; tests-retest reliability (ICC) 0.86, 0.96

The above includes a nonexhaustive list of suggested measurement tools for functional outcomes tracking.

Abbreviations: CRO, clinician-reported/graded outcome; FACT-HN, functional assessment of cancer therapy—head & neck; PROM, patient-reported outcome measure; QOL, quality of life.

[a] Spearman correlation.

[b] Pearson correlation coefficient.

a method to monitor the patient's own perspective regarding outcomes and functional status.[33] The MD Anderson Dysphagia Inventory (MDADI) is a self-administered questionnaire that captures swallowing-specific QOL in patients with HNC.[34] The MDADI has become one of the most commonly published functional endpoints in clinical studies,[35–37] and is used across HNC populations to establish and/or monitor swallowing-related QOL.[38] The MDADI is a relatively quick way to understand the impact dysphagia has on a patient's QOL and a 10 point difference in scores represents a clinically meaningful difference in swallow function,[39] providing clinicians a valid and reliable tool to monitor longitudinal QOL and change in status.

See **Table 1** for additional patient-reported outcome measures.

DYSPHAGIA REHABILITATION AMONG PATIENTS WITH HEAD AND NECK CANCER

Just as the approach to functional reconstruction of the oral cavity involves climbing the reconstructive ladder,[40] SLPs approach rehabilitation in similar ways. Specific to lingual rehabilitation, goal setting is stepwise in nature and depends on postoperative function. First, lingual range of motion and strength contribute to high level lingual function such as diet advancement and overall speech intelligibility, whereas precision and control of the tongue are key drivers for precision of speech, range of diet, and eating in public (per PSS-HN).[28] Further, patients who receive early intensive rehabilitation after oral cavity surgery have shorter length of stay in the acute care hospitals.[41]

Rehabilitation can take many forms, and SLPs have a variety of tools in their clinical toolbox to aid in communication and swallowing rehabilitation. Interventions may include swallowing and range of motion exercises, diet modification, lymphedema management, compensatory maneuvers, manual therapy, device-facilitated exercises, and skill-based training. Key rehabilitation options are reviewed but not limited to those discussed below.

Swallowing Exercises

Initiation of swallowing exercises for pharyngeal function is important for patients who may pursue postoperative radiotherapy and promotes practice of swallowing in the setting of a prolonged period without oral intake. Patients who will not pursue radiotherapy will likely present with a functional swallow in the absence of radiation-induced tissue damage, extensive oropharyngeal reconstruction, or neurogenic causes of dysphagia.

Lingual Range of Motion and Manual Therapy

Lingual range of motion after oral cavity reconstruction may be limited by lingual tethering and the location and nature of the defect. Limited ROM negatively impacts critical oral cavity function such as bolus formation, bolus transit, and oral cavity clearance. For example, patients unable to sweep the hard palate or reach oral cavity sulci with the tongue present with diffuse oral cavity residue particularly with foods beyond the complexity of a puree consistency, requiring various modifications (ie, finger sweep to clear oral sulci that cannot be reached by the native tongue, specific bolus placement, and head tilts to facilitate passive movement of a liquid bolus). Functional ROM is therefore key for advancing diet complexity and QOL.[28]

Optimization of range of motion using biofeedback techniques (eg, lingual protrusion, lateralization in front of a mirror) will help the patient visualize tongue status and location in space, aid in goal setting (eg, targeting beyond central incisors), and awareness of their new anatomy. Initiation of an oral diet with clearance from the microvascular reconstructive or plastic surgeon is optimal for both oral and pharyngeal phases of the swallow. Beginning to take an oral diet prevents disuse atrophy and promotes lingual range of motion and bolus manipulation to further work against postoperative edema. Patients tend to shift the bolus to the native tongue after partial/hemiglossectomy to garner control over the bolus. Although this strategy is useful in the acute postoperative phase, it may promote habituation of preferential chewing. Masticatory impairments contribute to patient-initiated diet downgrading driven by frustration surrounding inefficient bolus preparation and aforementioned oral stasis. Further, incorporation of intra-oral lingual manipulation aids in extension of lingual ROM and may dampen extent of lingual tethering.

Lingual Strength

Evidence supports the importance of lingual strength after partial glossectomy. In a cross-sectional study conducted to assess tongue strength and oral outcomes with their relationship to performance status for speech, swallow, and QOL after partial glossectomy, researchers demonstrate the difference in tongue strength between patients who received a flap and those who had primary closure.[42] The cut-point for tongue strength after chemoradiation is identified as 30 kPa. Overall the data established that patients who had better tongue strength ($\geq$30 kPa) were eating a full, regular diet. Although patients with lower tongue strengths still take in a solid diet, it is less complex than their stronger tongue counterparts. Alternatively, a tongue pressure cutoff of $\geq$15 kPa can be used to detect dysphagia in patients who have had surgical resection for their HNC.[43] The dose and frequency of lingual strengthening programs have been reviewed extensively; however, the dysphagia literature does not currently recommend one particular protocol.[44–47]

MEASUREMENT OF APPEARANCE AND BODY IMAGE AMONG PATIENTS WITH HEAD AND NECK CANCER

Early strategies to measure appearance among patients with HNC used observer-rated scales of disfigurement such as the Dropkin Disfigurement scale[48] and the Observer Rated Disfigurement Scale (ORDS).[49] Over time, however, the field moved away from observer-rated measures of appearance (and disfigurement) toward PROMs of body image (and BID). This move to patient-reported measures of body image was driven by 3 emerging lines of evidence. First, a number of landmark clinical trials showed the benefit of harnessing the patient's voice through incorporation of PROMs into routine oncology clinical care.[50,51] As a result, there was a strong interest in harnessing the patient's voice to measure appearance and body image for patients with HNC. Second, researchers began to recognize that body image and appearance are conceptually different, and that BID is not due simply to treatment-related disfigurement.[52,53] According to these evolving conceptual frameworks, BID among patients with HNC is due to a combination of negative changes in appearance (disfigurement) and alterations in function (dysfunction) that collectively result in clinical impairment.[8,10,54,55] Third, researchers studying body image and appearance in HNC[56,57] and other cancer types (eg, breast cancer[58,59]) observed that observer-rated measures of disfigurement correlated poorly with PROMs of BID. As a result of these 3 converging lines of thinking, the field shifted to using PROMs to assess body image and BID among patients with HNC.[60]

Initially, the only PROMs available for measuring BID among patients with HNC were developed for, and validated in, non-HNC patient populations.[60,61] Although it was developed to measure body image among patients with breast cancer,[62] the Body Image Scale (BIS) became the most widely used PROM to assess BID among patients with HNC.[60,61] Studies utilizing the BIS made significant early contributions to our understanding of the epidemiology of BID among patients with HNC include its temporal trajectory and associated risk factors.[9,54,63,64] However, over time as researchers developed a more sophisticated understanding of BID among patients with HNC, they began to perceive a number of limitations to using the BIS in this population.[60] First, the BIS lacks content validity for HNC-related BID through its omission of key appearance (eg, drooling, facial asymmetry) and functional (eg, eating in public, speaking challenges) concerns. Second, the BIS includes items that lack relevance to patients with HNC (eg, "Did you find it difficult to look at yourself naked?"). Third, the BIS was limited for its longitudinal measurement of HNC-related BID from pre- to post-treatment through its inclusion of a question about dissatisfaction with a surgical scar.

To address these limitations of the BIS as a measure of HNC-related BID, a number of PROMs have recently been developed for, and validated among, patients with HNC. These measures include the Inventory to Measure and Assess image disturbance Head and Neck (IMAGE-HN), FACE-Q, and McGill Body Image Concerns Scale-Head and Neck Cancer (MBIS-HNC).[65-67] Of these new PROMs of HNC-related BID, the IMAGE-HN has been the most widely used in the research setting and is discussed in greater detail below.

The IMAGE-HN was developed in accordance with the Patient Reported Outcomes Measurement Information System (PROMIS) guidelines for the development and validation of PROMs.[68] Steps in the process include (1) comprehensive literature search to identify existing measures, (2) qualitative work to assess domain coverage, (3) cognitive interviewing of items for feedback on language and item clarity, (4) confirmation of domain factor structure and item analysis using Rasch analysis, and (5) validity testing of the final instrument. Following the systematic review,[60] qualitative work,[55] and cognitive interviewing, the IMAGE-HN underwent psychometric evaluation among 305 patients with HNC from 4 academic medical centers.[67]

The IMAGE-HN is a psychometrically acceptable 24-item PROM of HNC-related BID consisting of a global scale and 4 subscales measuring unique constructs and comprised independent items.[67] The IMAGE-HN subscales map to the conceptual domains of HNC-related BID identified in the researcher's qualitative work[55] and assess other-oriented appearance concerns, personal dissatisfaction with appearance, distress with functional impairments, and social avoidance and isolation. Global IMAGE-HN scores range from 0 to 84, with higher scores indicating more severe HNC-related BID.[67] The IMAGE-HN instrument and scoring manual are publicly available.[69]

Following psychometric validation of the IMAGE-HN, the researchers subsequently established clinically relevant cutoff scores.[12] In a separate multi-site cohort study of 250 HNC survivors from 6 academic centers, the researchers found that an IMAGE-HN score of ≥ 22 optimally distinguishes HNC survivors with and without clinically relevant BID.[12] The researchers also showed how the IMAGE-HN, with its content validity for BID among HNC survivors, improves accurate detection relative to PROMs of BID developed for other patient populations. Using the IMAGE-HN cutoff score of ≥ 22, the researchers identified 11% of the cohort as having HNC-related BID who would have been missed by measuring their BID using the BIS. As a result of its ability to successfully identify patients with HNC-related BID, the IMAGE-HN is now being used as an inclusion criterion in clinical trials evaluating BID among HNC survivors.[70]

The development of a psychometrically sound PROM of HNC-related BID has also furthered our understanding of the relationship between BID and disfigurement among patients with HNC. In a multi-site cross-sectional study, the researchers found no association between observer-rated disfigurement as measured by ORDS scores and

BID as measured by IMAGE-HN scores ($\beta = 1.6$; 95% CI, 0.9 to 2.4).[57] They also demonstrated that for a given level of observer-rated disfigurement, HNC survivors report a wide range of BID severity (**Fig. 1**).[57]

The authors suggested that their findings have 2 important considerations. First, the existing models of HNC-related BID, which have focused on clinical, demographic, and a limited number of psychosocial factors,[14] are inadequate to explain the variability in BID severity and lack of association with observer-rated disfigurement. These finding suggest that additional research is needed to refine existing conceptual models and identify the factors that moderate the relationship between disfigurement and BID among patients with HNC. Second, because of its poor correlation with HNC-related BID, observer-rated disfigurement (whether clinical assessment or using a validated scale) should not be used to identify HNC survivors with BID in clinical practice. These data suggest that if a clinician were to measure an HNC survivor's BID by assessing the severity of her/his disfigurement, the clinician could falsely miss patients who have minimal disfigurement but significant HNC-related BID and falsely identify patients with significant disfigurement but no clinically relevant HNC-related BID, Therefore, additional research is needed to develop formal screening protocols and instruments that can be implemented into clinical workflow to accurately identify HNC survivors with BID who may benefit from referral for supportive care interventions.

INTERVENTIONS TO IMPROVE BODY IMAGE DISTRESS AMONG HEAD AND NECK CANCER SURVIVORS

Management of BID among HNC survivors is a recommended part of survivorship care according to guidelines from the American Cancer Society[71] and American Head and Neck Society.[72] However, a recent national survey found that management of BID was the single most commonly omitted component of HNC survivorship care.[73] As discussed previously, BID is associated with a 6 fold increase in moderate–severe

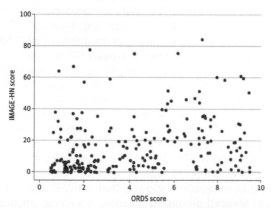

Fig. 1. Observer-Rated Disfigurement Scale (ORDS) versus Inventory to Measure and Assess image disturbance—Head and Neck (IMAGE-HN) Scores This scatterplot shows the association between observer-rated disfigurement (measured by ORDS scores) and body image–related distress (measured by IMAGE-HN scores) for 250 survivors of head and neck cancer. Each participant's ORDS value has been jittered horizontally by adding a random number between −0.5 and 0.5 to prevent overlap of data points along the x-axis. For a given level of observer-rated disfigurement (ORDS score), there is significant variability in the corresponding level of body image-related distress (IMAGE-HN score).

depressive symptoms, an 8 fold increase in moderate–severe anxiety symptoms, social isolation, stigmatization, and decreased QOL.[8–10,12–16] Furthermore, for the subset of patients who experience clinically significant HNC-related BID, the natural history suggests that it does not improve over time without treatment.[63]

The failure to address BID among HNC survivors is due in part to the limited evidence base supporting interventions in this population. Three published trials have evaluated different strategies to manage HNC-related BID. In a quasi-experimental study, Huang and colleagues[74] showed that a cosmetic rehabilitation intervention did not improve BID among HNC survivors relative to control. An Randomized Controlled Trial (RCT) by Chen and colleagues[75] evaluating a skin camouflage program among HNC survivors found no benefit relative to usual care. Finally, a single-arm pre-post study showed that MyChangedBody (MyCB), a web-based self-compassion expressive writing activity, failed to improve BID among HNC survivors.[76] The lack of efficacy of MyCB among HNC survivors with BID is important because MyCB improved BID among breast cancer survivors in a large RCT (N = 304) relative to the attention control arm.[77] Collectively, these trials confirm the need for novel strategies to improve BID among HNC survivors and suggest that a fundamentally different approach may be necessary.

An emerging line of research suggests that cognitive behavioral therapy (CBT) is a promising approach to manage HNC-related BID. Multiple meta-analyses have demonstrated that CBT produces durable reductions in BID in patients without visible disfigurement (eg, body dysmorphic disorder).[53,78–80] However, the evidence supporting CBT for BID in patients with visible disfigurement is weaker.[81–83] Whereas some studies have suggested that CBT may reduce BID among patients with disfigurement (eg, facial burns, craniofacial disorders, breast cancer),[84–87] 2 recent systematic reviews noted significant methodologic limitations in these studies including small sample size, nonrandomized allocation, and comparison to waitlist control.[88,89]

Based on the potential of CBT to manage BID among HNC survivors, researchers at the Medical University of South Carolina developed building a renewed image after head and neck cancer treatment (BRIGHT) as a brief telemedicine-based CBT intervention to manage HNC-related BID. The telemedicine design was chosen to address barriers to mental health care in this population (eg, travel burden, stigma, fatigue, treatment toxicity).[90,91] Based on stakeholder feedback from HNC survivors and clinicians, BRIGHT was developed as a brief (5 weekly 60-min sessions) CBT delivered one on one by a licensed clinical psychologist via video telemedicine platform to HNC survivors after completing treatment.[92] BRIGHT session topics include (1) psychoeducation about the cognitive model of body image; (2) self-monitoring about thoughts, feelings, and body image behaviors; (3) cognitive restructuring to identify and challenge unhelpful automatic HNC body image thoughts; (4) positive body image coping strategies; and (5) maintenance and relapse prevention.

Emerging evidence supports BRIGHT as having potential to be the first evidence-based treatment for HNC survivors with BID. In a single-arm pilot trial of n = 10 HNC survivors with BID, researchers showed that BRIGHT was feasible and acceptable.[92] BRIGHT also showed promising preliminary clinical efficacy BRIGHT with a 34.5% reduction in mean BIS scores at 1-month post-BRIGHT relative to baseline (mean decrease in BIS scores = 4.56; 95% CI 1.55 to 7.56)[92]; an effect that persisted at 3-month post-BRIGHT.[92]

BRIGHT was subsequently compared with a dose- and delivery-matched attention control (AC) condition in a pilot RCT of 44 HNC survivors with BID. At 1-month post-intervention, they found that BRIGHT improved HNC-related BID compared with AC (mean model-based difference in change in IMAGE-HN score = −7.9 [90% CI, −15.9

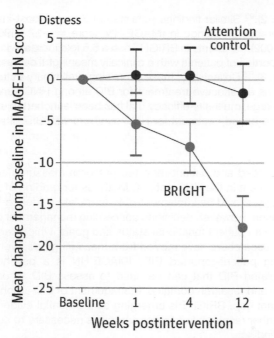

Fig. 2. Mean change from baseline of head and neck cancer (HNC)-related body image distress for patients in BRIGHT and attention control. Line graph demonstrating the mean change from baseline in IMAGE-HN scores over time by intervention allocation. Error bars represent 1 SE above and below the mean.

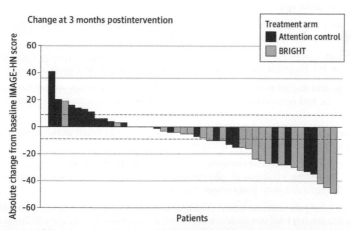

Fig. 3. Response of head and neck cancer (HNC)-related body image distress for patients in BRIGHT and attention control. Waterfall plot showing response to BRIGHT (Building a Renewed ImaGe after Head and neck cancer Treatment) and attention control, as measured by absolute change from baseline in IMAGE-HN scores at 3 months postintervention. The IMAGE-HN score ranges from 0 to 84, with higher scores indicating worse HNC-related body image distress (and negative bars thus indicating improvement in HNC-related body image distress). The dashed horizontal line at ±9 indicates a clinically meaningful change in IMAGE-HN score.

to 0.0] points; **Fig. 2**).[93] Similar findings persisted at 3 month post-intervention (mean model-based difference in change in IMAGE-HN score = −17.1 [90% CI, −25.6 to −8.6] points; P = .002).[94] Patients in BRIGHT had a 6.6 fold increase in the odds of clinical response (proportion of patients with a clinically meaningful decrease in IMAGE-HN scores of ≥ 9; **Fig. 3**).[93] Collectively, these promising preliminary data support the potential of BRIGHT as an effective treatment for BID among HNC survivors. Based on these pilot data, a large, multi-site efficacy trial has been launched to establish BRIGHT as the first evidence-based treatment for HNC survivors with BID.[70]

SUMMARY

Overall, clinician-graded and patient-reported outcome measures are necessary for dysphagia management in the HNC patient. Methods for grading of swallow severity and pathophysiology should be implemented to formulate evidence-based decisions regarding intervention. However, decisions concerning management of functional outcomes must align with patient functional status and goals, which can be captured by PROMs. Further, researchers have moved from measuring observer-rated disfigurement to assessing patient-reported BID. IMAGE-HN is a psychometrically valid PROM of HNC-related BID that can be used to assess BID among patients with HNC in the clinical and research domains. Management of BID among HNC survivors remains a significant gap. BRIGHT is emerging as a potential evidence-based treatment, although further research in a larger sample is necessary to confirm the promising preliminary findings.

CLINICS CARE POINTS

- Clinician-graded and patient-reported measures of communication and swallow function are critical aspects of a thorough clinical workup and contribute to evidence-based rehabilitation planning.

- The site, size, and nature of the defect and reconstruction impact the severity grade and physiologic drivers of postoperative dysphagia.

- Treatment of dysphagia should always match the underlying physiologic deficit that is identified in the objective swallowing evaluation or during clinical workup,

- Body image and appearance are conceptually different. Body image encompasses concepts of appearance and function and is more clinically relevant for patients with head and neck cancer.

- Functional outcomes among patients with HNC should be assessed using validated patient-reported outcome measures such as the MDADI and IMAGE-HN.

- Observer-rated disfigurement correlates poorly with body image disagrees among patients with HNC. Therefore, clinicians should not use their assessment of disfigurement to identify HNC survivors with body image distress.

- BRIGHT is a brief telemedicine-based cognitive behavioral therapy that has been effective at reducing BID among HNC survivors in small trials; a large multi-site RCT of BRIGHT is currently underway to determine whether BRIGHT should become the new standard of care for managing BID among HNC survivors.

DISCLOSURE

Dr E.M. Graboyes reports grants from National Cancer Institute related to this work, grants from the Triological Society, United States/American College of Surgeons,

National Cancer Institute, United States, and Castle Biosciences unrelated to this work, and personal fees from the National Cancer Institute and Castle Biosciences outside the submitted work. Dr C.E.A. Barbon receives salary and funding from the University of Texas MD Anderson Cancer Center, United States.

REFERECES

1. Hutcheson KA, Nurgalieva Z, Zhao H, et al. Two-year prevalence of dysphagia and related outcomes in head and neck cancer survivors: an updated SEER-Medicare analysis. Head Neck 2019;41(2):479–87.

2. García-Peris P, Parón L, Velasco C, et al. Long-term prevalence of oropharyngeal dysphagia in head and neck cancer patients: Impact on quality of life. Clinical Nutrition 2007;26(6):710–7.

3. Windon MJ, D'Souza G, Faraji F, et al. Priorities, concerns, and regret among patients with head and neck cancer. Cancer 2019;125(8):1281–9.

4. Huang ZS, Chen WL, Huang ZQ, et al. Dysphagia in tongue cancer patients before and after surgery. J Oral Maxillofac Surg 2016;74(10):2067–72.

5. Chang EI, Yu P, Skoracki RJ, et al. Comprehensive analysis of functional outcomes and survival after microvascular reconstruction of glossectomy defects. Ann Surg Oncol 2015;22(9):3061–9.

6. Dwivedi RC, Chisholm EJ, Khan AS, et al. An exploratory study of the influence of clinico-demographic variables on swallowing and swallowing-related quality of life in a cohort of oral and oropharyngeal cancer patients treated with primary surgery. Eur Arch Oto-Rhino-Laryngol 2012;269(4):1233–9.

7. Tassone P, Clookey S, Topf M, et al. Quality of life after segmental mandibulectomy and free flap for mandibular osteonecrosis: systematic review. Am J Otolaryngol 2022;43(5):103586.

8. Fingeret MC, Teo I, Goettsch K. Body image: a critical psychosocial issue for patients with head and neck cancer. Curr Oncol Rep 2015;17(1):422.

9. Fingeret MC, Yuan Y, Urbauer D, et al. The nature and extent of body image concerns among surgically treated patients with head and neck cancer. Psycho Oncol 2012;21(8):836–44.

10. Rhoten BA, Murphy B, Ridner SH. Body image in patients with head and neck cancer: a review of the literature. Oral Oncol 2013;49(8):753–60.

11. Fingeret MC, Nipomnick S, Guindani M, et al. Body image screening for cancer patients undergoing reconstructive surgery. Psycho Oncol 2014;23(8):898–905.

12. Macias D, Hand BN, Pipkorn P, et al. Association of Inventory to Measure and assess imaGe disturbance - head and neck scores with clinically Meaningful body image-related distress among head and neck cancer survivors. Front Psychol 2021;12:794038.

13. Melissant HC, Jansen F, Eerenstein SE, et al. Body image distress in head and neck cancer patients: what are we looking at? Support Care Cancer 2021; 29(4):2161–9.

14. Macias D, Hand BN, Maurer S, et al. Factors associated with risk of body image-related distress in patients with head and neck cancer. JAMA Otolaryngol Head Neck Surg 2021;147(12):1019–26.

15. Buckwalter AE, Karnell LH, Smith RB, et al. Patient-reported factors associated with discontinuing employment following head and neck cancer treatment. Arch Otolaryngol Head Neck Surg 2007;133(5):464–70.

16. Kissane DW, Patel SG, Baser RE, et al. Preliminary evaluation of the reliability and validity of the Shame and Stigma Scale in head and neck cancer. Head Neck 2013;35(2):172–83.

17. Hutcheson KA, Barrow MP, Barringer DA, et al. Dynamic Imaging Grade of swallowing Toxicity (DIGEST): scale development and validation. Cancer 2017;123(1): 62–70.

18. Hutcheson KA, Barbon CEA, Alvarez CP, et al. Refining measurement of swallowing safety in the dynamic Imaging Grade of swallowing Toxicity (DIGEST) criteria: validation of DIGEST version 2. Cancer 2022;128(7):1458–66.

19. Martin-Harris B, Brodsky MB, Michel Y, et al. MBS measurement tool for swallow impairment–MBSImp: establishing a standard. Dysphagia 2008;23(4):392–405.

20. Martin-Harris B, McFarland D, Hill EG, et al. Respiratory-swallow training in patients with head and neck cancer. Arch Phys Med Rehabil 2015;96(5):885–93.

21. Barbon CEA, Yao C, Alvarez CP, et al. Dysphagia profiles after primary transoral robotic surgery or radiation for oropharyngeal cancer: a registry analysis. Head Neck 2021;43(10):2883–95.

22. List MA, Ritter-Sterr C, Lansky SB. A performance status scale for head and neck cancer patients. Cancer 1996;66(3):564–9.

23. Eldridge RC, Pugh SL, Trotti A, et al. Changing functional status within 6 months posttreatment is prognostic of overall survival in patients with head and neck cancer: NRG Oncology Study. Head Neck 2019;41(11):3924–32.

24. Brady G, Leigh-Doyle L, Riva FMG, et al. Speech and swallowing outcomes following surgical resection with Immediate free Tissue Transfer reconstruction for Advanced Osteoradionecrosis of the Mandible following radiation treatment for head and neck cancer. Dysphagia 2022;37(5):1137–41.

25. Pauloski BR, Rademaker AW, Logemann JA, et al. Speech and swallowing in irradiated and nonirradiated postsurgical oral cancer patients. Otolaryngol Head Neck Surg 1998;118(5):616–24.

26. Yang ZH, Chen WL, Huang HZ, et al. Quality of life of patients with tongue cancer 1 year after surgery. J Oral Maxillofac Surg 2010;68(9):2164–8.

27. Lazarus CL, Husaini H, Jacobson AS, et al. Development of a new lingual range-of-motion assessment scale: normative data in surgically treated oral cancer patients. Dysphagia 2014;29(4):489–99.

28. Chepeha DB, Teknos TN, Shargorodsky J, et al. Rectangle tongue Template for reconstruction of the Hemiglossectomy Defect. Arch Otolaryngol Head Neck Surg 2008;134(9):993–8.

29. Taylor RJ, Chepeha JC, Teknos TN, et al. Development and validation of the neck dissection impairment Index: a quality of life Measure. Arch Otolaryngol Head Neck Surg 2002;128(1):44–9.

30. Hutcheson KA, Lewin JS, Barringer DA, et al. Late dysphagia after radiotherapy-based treatment of head and neck cancer. Cancer 2012;118(23):5793–9.

31. Aggarwal P, Goepfert RP, Garden AS, et al. Risk and clinical risk factors associated with late Lower Cranial Neuropathy in Long-term oropharyngeal squamous cell carcinoma survivors. JAMA Otolaryngol Head Neck Surg 2021;147(5): 469–78.

32. Aggarwal P, Zaveri JS, Goepfert RP, et al. Symptom Burden associated with late Lower Cranial Neuropathy in Long-term oropharyngeal cancer survivors. JAMA Otolaryngol Head Neck Surg 2018;144(11):1066–76.

33. Gibbons C, Porter I, Gonçalves-Bradley DC, et al. Routine provision of feedback from patient-reported outcome measurements to healthcare providers and patients in clinical practice. Cochrane Database Syst Rev 2021;10(10):Cd011589.

34. Chen AY, Frankowski R, Bishop-Leone J, et al. The development and validation of a dysphagia-specific quality-of-life Questionnaire for patients with head and neck cancer: the M. D. Anderson dysphagia Inventory. Arch Otolaryngol Head Neck Surg 2001;127(7):870–6.

35. Nichols AC, Theurer J, Prisman E, et al. Radiotherapy versus transoral robotic surgery and neck dissection for oropharyngeal squamous cell carcinoma (ORATOR): an open-label, phase 2, randomised trial. Lancet Oncol 2019; 20(10):1349–59.

36. Owadally W, Hurt C, Timmins H, et al. PATHOS: a phase II/III trial of risk-stratified, reduced intensity adjuvant treatment in patients undergoing transoral surgery for Human papillomavirus (HPV) positive oropharyngeal cancer. BMC Cancer 2015; 15(1):602.

37. Petkar I, Rooney K, Roe JWG, et al. DARS: a phase III randomised multicentre study of dysphagia- optimised intensity- modulated radiotherapy (Do-IMRT) versus standard intensity- modulated radiotherapy (S-IMRT) in head and neck cancer. BMC Cancer 2016;16(1):770.

38. Kazi R, Prasad V, Venkitaraman R, et al. Questionnaire analysis of swallowing-related outcomes following glossectomy. ORL (Oto-Rhino-Laryngol) (Basel) 2008;70(3):151–5.

39. Hutcheson KA, Barrow MP, Lisec A, et al. What is a clinically relevant difference in MDADI scores between groups of head and neck cancer patients? Laryngoscope 2016;126(5):1108–13.

40. Lam L, Samman N. Speech and swallowing following tongue cancer surgery and free flap reconstruction–a systematic review. Oral Oncol 2013;49(6):507–24.

41. Bschorer M, Schneider D, Hennig M, et al. Early intensive rehabilitation after oral cancer treatment. J Cranio-Maxillo-Fac Surg 2018;46(6):1019–26.

42. Lazarus CL, Husaini H, Anand SM, et al. Tongue strength as a predictor of functional outcomes and quality of life after tongue cancer surgery. Ann Otol Rhinol Laryngol 2013;122(6):386–97.

43. Hasegawa Y, Sugahara K, Fukuoka T, et al. Change in tongue pressure in patients with head and neck cancer after surgical resection. Odontology 2017;105(4): 494–503.

44. Krekeler BN, Rowe LM, Connor NP. Dose in exercise-based dysphagia Therapies: a Scoping review. Dysphagia 2021;36(1):1–32.

45. Robbins J, Gangnon RE, Theis SM, et al. The effects of lingual exercise on swallowing in older adults. J Am Geriatr Soc 2005;53(9):1483–9.

46. McKenna VS, Zhang B, Haines MB, et al. A systematic review of Isometric lingual strength-training Programs in adults with and without dysphagia. Am J Speech Lang Pathol 2017;26(2):524–39.

47. Smaoui S, Langridge A, Steele CM. The effect of lingual Resistance training interventions on adult swallow function: a systematic review. Dysphagia 2020;35(5): 745–61.

48. Dropkin MJ, Malgady RG, Scott DW, et al. Scaling of disfigurement and dysfunction in postoperative head and neck patients. Head Neck Surg 1983;6(1):559–70.

49. Katz M, Irish JC, Devins GM, et al. Reliability and validity of an observer-rated disfigurement scale for head and neck cancer patients. Head Neck 2000;22(2): 132–41.

50. Basch E, Deal AM, Kris MG, et al. Symptom Monitoring with patient-reported outcomes during Routine cancer treatment: a randomized controlled trial. J Clin Oncol 2016;34(6):557–65.

51. Basch E. Patient-Reported outcomes - Harnessing patients' Voices to improve clinical care. N Engl J Med 2017;376(2):105–8.

52. Rhoten BA. Body image disturbance in adults treated for cancer - a concept analysis. J Adv Nurs 2016;72(5):1001–11.

53. Fingeret MC, Teo I, Epner DE. Managing body image difficulties of adult cancer patients: lessons from available research. Cancer 2014;120(5):633–41.

54. Teo I, Fronczyk KM, Guindani M, et al. Salient body image concerns of patients with cancer undergoing head and neck reconstruction. Head Neck 2016;38(7):1035–42.

55. Ellis MA, Sterba KR, Day TA, et al. Body image disturbance in surgically treated head and neck cancer patients: a patient-Centered approach. Otolaryngol Head Neck Surg 2019;161(2):278–87.

56. Chen SC, Huang CY, Huang BS, et al. Factors associated with healthcare professional's rating of disfigurement and self-perceived body image in female patients with head and neck cancer. Eur J Cancer Care 2018;27(2):e12710.

57. Macias D, Hand BN, Zenga J, et al. Association between observer-rated disfigurement and body image-related distress among head and neck cancer survivors. JAMA Otolaryngol Head Neck Surg 2022;148(7):688–9.

58. Pezner RD, Lipsett JA, Vora NL, et al. Limited usefulness of observer-based cosmesis scales employed to evaluate patients treated conservatively for breast cancer. Int J Radiat Oncol Biol Phys 1985;11(6):1117–9.

59. Sneeuw KC, Aaronson NK, Yarnold JR, et al. Cosmetic and functional outcomes of breast conserving treatment for early stage breast cancer. 1. Comparison of patients' ratings, observers' ratings, and objective assessments. Radiother Oncol 1992;25(3):153–9.

60. Ellis MA, Sterba KR, Brennan EA, et al. A systematic review of patient-reported outcome measures assessing body image disturbance in patients with head and neck cancer. Otolaryngol Head Neck Surg 2019;160(6):941–54.

61. Shunmuga Sundaram C, Dhillon HM, Butow PN, et al. A systematic review of body image measures for people diagnosed with head and neck cancer (HNC). Support Care Cancer 2019;27(10):3657–66.

62. Hopwood P, Fletcher I, Lee A, et al. A body image scale for use with cancer patients. Eur J Cancer 2001;37(2):189–97.

63. Graboyes EM, Hill EG, Marsh CH, et al. Temporal Trajectory of body image disturbance in patients with surgically treated head and neck cancer. Otolaryngol Head Neck Surg 2020;162(3):304–12.

64. Fingeret MC, Hutcheson KA, Jensen K, et al. Associations among speech, eating, and body image concerns for surgical patients with head and neck cancer. Head Neck 2013;35(3):354–60.

65. Rodriguez AM, Frenkiel S, Desroches J, et al. Development and validation of the McGill body image concerns scale for use in head and neck oncology (MBIS-HNC): a mixed-methods approach. Psycho Oncol 2019;28(1):116–21.

66. Cracchiolo JR, Klassen AF, Young-Afat DA, et al. Leveraging patient-reported outcomes data to inform oncology clinical decision making: Introducing the FACE-Q Head and Neck Cancer Module. Cancer 2019;125(6):863–72.

67. Graboyes EM, Hand BN, Ellis MA, et al. Validation of a novel, Multidomain head and neck cancer Appearance- and Function-distress patient-reported outcome Measure. Otolaryngology-Head Neck Surg (Tokyo) 2020;163(5):979–85.

68. PROMIS. Instrument Development and Validation Scientific Standards Version 2.0. Periodical serial online. 2013.

69. Graboyes EM, Hand BN, Ellis MA, et al. Validation of a novel, Multidomain head and neck cancer Appearance- and Function-distress patient-reported outcome Measure. Otolaryngol Head Neck Surg 2020;163(5):979–85.

70. Graboyes EM. IMAGE-HN. Medical University of South Carolina College of Medicine. Available at: https://medicine.musc.edu/departments/otolaryngology/research/body-image/image-hn. Published 2021. Accessed August 30, 2021.

71. Building a Renewed ImaGe After Head & Neck Cancer Treatment (BRIGHT) Multi-Site RCT. U.S. National Library of Medicine ClinicalTrials.gov. Available at: https://clinicaltrials.gov/ct2/show/NCT05442957?term=graboyes&draw=2&rank=2. Accessed April 2, 2023.

72. Cohen EE, LaMonte SJ, Erb NL, et al. American cancer Society head and neck cancer survivorship care Guideline. CA Cancer J Clin 2016;66(3):203–39.

73. Goyal N, Day A, Epstein J, et al. Head and neck cancer survivorship consensus statement from the American Head and Neck Society. Laryngoscope Investig Otolaryngol 2022;7(1):70–92.

74. Cognetti DM, Villaflor VM, Fakhry C, et al. Survivorship support in head and neck cancer: American Head and Neck Society survey. Head Neck 2020;42(5): 939–44.

75. Huang S, Liu HE. Effectiveness of cosmetic rehabilitation on the body image of oral cancer patients in Taiwan. Support Care Cancer 2008;16(9):981–6.

76. Chen SC, Huang BS, Lin CY, et al. Psychosocial effects of a skin camouflage program in female survivors with head and neck cancer: a randomized controlled trial. Psycho Oncol 2017;26(9):1376–83.

77. Melissant HC, Jansen F, Eerenstein SEJ, et al. A structured expressive writing activity targeting body image-related distress among head and neck cancer survivors: who do we reach and what are the effects? Support Care Cancer 2021; 29(10):5763–76.

78. Sherman KA, Przezdziecki A, Alcorso J, et al. Reducing body image-related distress in women with breast cancer Using a structured Online writing exercise: Results from the My Changed body randomized controlled trial. J Clin Oncol 2018;36(19):1930–40.

79. Jarry JL, Ip K. The effectiveness of stand-alone cognitive-behavioural therapy for body image: a meta-analysis. Body Image 2005;2(4):317–31.

80. Jarry JL, Berardi K. Characteristics and effectiveness of stand-alone body image treatments: a review of the empirical literature. Body Image 2004;1(4):319–33.

81. Alleva JM, Sheeran P, Webb TL, et al. A meta-Analytic review of stand-alone interventions to improve body image. PLoS One 2015;10(9):e0139177.

82. Lewis-Smith H, Diedrichs PC, Halliwell E. Cognitive-behavioral roots of body image therapy and prevention. Body Image 2019;31:309–20.

83. Blashill AJ, Safren SA, Wilhelm S, et al. Cognitive behavioral therapy for body image and self-care (CBT-BISC) in sexual minority men living with HIV: a randomized controlled trial. Health Psychol 2017;36(10):937–46.

84. Newell RJ. Altered body image: a fear-avoidance model of psycho-social difficulties following disfigurement. J Adv Nurs 1999;30(5):1230–8.

85. Bessell A, Brough V, Clarke A, et al. Evaluation of the effectiveness of Face IT, a computer-based psychosocial intervention for disfigurement-related distress. Psychol Health Med 2012;17(5):565–77.

86. Faraji J, Mahdavi A, Samkhaniyan E, et al. A review of the effectiveness of cognitive-behavioral group therapy on the reduction of body image concern in patients with breast cancer. J Med Life 2015;8(Spec Iss 4):82–6.

87. Fadaei S, Janighorban M, Mehrabi T, et al. Effects of cognitive behavioral counseling on body Image following mastectomy. J Res Med Sci 2011;16(8):1047–54.

88. Hummel SB, van Lankveld J, Oldenburg HSA, et al. Efficacy of Internet-based cognitive behavioral therapy in improving sexual functioning of breast cancer survivors: Results of a randomized controlled trial. J Clin Oncol 2017;35(12): 1328–40.

89. Lewis-Smith H, Diedrichs PC, Rumsey N, et al. Efficacy of psychosocial and physical activity-based interventions to improve body image among women treated for breast cancer: a systematic review. Psycho Oncol 2018;27(12): 2687–99.

90. Bessell A, Moss TP. Evaluating the effectiveness of psychosocial interventions for individuals with visible differences: a systematic review of the empirical literature. Body Image 2007;4(3):227–38.

91. Massa ST, Rohde RL, McKinstry C, et al. An assessment of patient burdens from head and neck cancer survivorship care. Oral Oncol 2018;82:115–21.

92. Smith JD, Shuman AG, Riba MB. Psychosocial Issues in patients with head and neck cancer: an updated review with a Focus on clinical interventions. Curr Psychiatry Rep 2017;19(9):56.

93. Graboyes EM, Maurer S, Park Y, et al. Evaluation of a novel telemedicine-based intervention to manage body image disturbance in head and neck cancer survivors. Psycho Oncol 2020;29(12):1988–94.

94. Graboyes EM, Maurer S, Balliet W, et al. Efficacy of a brief tele-cognitive behavioral treatment vs attention control for head and neck cancer survivors with body image distress: a pilot randomized clinical trial. JAMA Otolaryngol Head Neck Surg 2023;149(1):54–62.

95. Rinkel RN, Verdonck-de Leeuw IM, Doornaert P, et al. Prevalence of swallowing and speech problems in daily life after chemoradiation for head and neck cancer based on cut-off scores of the patient-reported outcome measures SWAL-QOL and SHI. Eur Arch Otorhinolaryngol 2016;273(7):1849–55.

96. Rosenthal DI, Mendoza TR, Chambers MS, et al. Measuring head and neck cancer symptom burden: the development and validation of the M.D. Anderson symptom inventory, head and neck module. Head Neck 2007;29(10):923–31.

Improving Quality and Value in Head and Neck Reconstruction

Kiran Kakarala, MD[a,*], Matthew Mifsud, MD[b],
Peter Dziegielewski, MD, FRCSC[c]

KEYWORDS

- Quality • Value • Head and neck reconstruction • Free flap • Microvascular • ERAS
- Cost • Improvement

KEY POINTS

- Defining quality health care as Safe, Effective, Patient-centered, Timely, Efficient, and Equitable provides a framework for improving quality and value in head and neck reconstruction.
- Standardization of quality improvement efforts requires consensus around data collection and measurement of processes and outcomes.
- Significant opportunities exist to improve quality and value in head and neck reconstruction using this framework.

INTRODUCTION

Surgical and technological innovations have allowed reconstructive surgeons to address increasingly complex head and neck defects. Once a niche and relatively unreliable procedure, free tissue transfer has become widely available with ever-expanding indications and marked improvements in operative efficiency and outcomes. Technologies, such as implantable flap monitoring and virtual surgical planning, and care innovations, such as Enhanced Recovery After Surgery (ERAS), have been developed and implemented to improve outcomes. Comparatively little progress has been made in reaching a consensus on how to define and measure quality with respect to these reconstructions. Perhaps even less attention has been paid to accurately measuring costs associated with these procedures and understanding value

[a] Department of Otolaryngology-Head and Neck Surgery, University of Kansas Medical Center, 3901 Rainbow Boulevard, Kansas City, KS 66160, USA; [b] Department of Otolaryngology–Head and Neck Surgery, University of South Florida School of Medicine, 13330 USF Laurel Drive, Tampa, FL 33612, USA; [c] Department of Otolaryngology–Head and Neck Surgery, University of Florida School of Medicine, 1600 Southwest Archer Road, D1-121, Gainesville, FL 32608, USA
* Corresponding author.
E-mail address: kkakarala@kumc.edu

Otolaryngol Clin N Am 56 (2023) 853–858
https://doi.org/10.1016/j.otc.2023.04.019
0030-6665/23/© 2023 Elsevier Inc. All rights reserved.
oto.theclinics.com

(often defined as quality/cost). The Institute of Medicine has outlined 6 domains for health care quality: Safe, Effective, Patient-centered, Timely, Efficient, and Equitable (**Table 1**).[1] Using this framework, this brief review examines quality and value in head and neck reconstruction.

Safe

Safe care avoids harm to patients, a prerequisite to quality. Complex head and neck reconstruction is associated with varying rates and severity of complications. Attempts have been made to understand risk factors that might predict such complications.[2–5] Such efforts are important to allow for risk stratification and facilitate comparison of outcomes. The extent to which these complications are preventable or are the result of medical error (misdiagnosis, technical failure, medication error, and so forth) is unclear. Many health systems have attempted to foster a culture of safety that prioritizes learning from and thereby preventing medical errors using scientific, transparent, and nonpunitive methods. Standardization of perioperative care in the form of ERAS protocols has been an important advance in providing safer, more consistent care to reconstructive patients.[6] Intraoperative interventions, such as standardizing communication (eg, surgical time outs and sign outs) and creating and supporting high-performing teams for head and neck reconstruction, including surgeons, nurses, and surgical technologists, may also play a role in facilitating safety.[7–9]

Effective

In the early days of free tissue transfer, flap survival was a primary measure of success. With improvements in experience and techniques, most high-volume centers have now achieved flap survival rates of greater than 95%.[10] Thus, although measuring flap survival is still necessary, it is important to develop and implement new measures of effectiveness.[11] As outlined in the articles of this issue, other rungs of the reconstructive ladder also play a critical role in head and neck reconstruction, underlining the importance of developing measures to compare the effectiveness of different reconstructive modalities for similar defects. Objective outcome measures might include operative time, length of stay, reoperations, readmissions, flap survival, tracheostomy and gastrostomy tube dependence, and complications, among others.[12] Patient-reported outcome measures are at least equally important to judging the effectiveness of a reconstruction. Numerous head and neck–specific quality-of-life instruments have been developed, with some focusing on specific domains, such as swallowing and cosmesis.[13,14] Many high-volume centers have developed prospective registries to track outcomes for free tissue transfer patients. However, there is little standardization in the methodology behind these efforts, making comparison of outcomes between surgeons and institutions difficult.[15]

Patient-Centered

Patient-centered care is defined as "care that is respectful of and responsive to individual patient preferences, needs, and values and ensuring that patient values guide all clinical decisions. "[1] Optimizing shared decision making and informed consent can be challenging in complex head and neck surgery with reconstruction. Barriers may include time constraints, limited patient health literacy, and complexity of the planned procedure.[16] However, optimizing patient education and partnering with patients in surgical decision making is critically important to optimizing patient experience and outcomes. Failures in this regard may increase patient distress and the likelihood of decision regret following reconstructions.[17] A successful outcome from the surgeon's perspective may differ in important ways from the patient's perspective.

Table 1
Institute of Medicine's 6 domains of quality[1] defined with possible head and neck reconstruction quality measures

Domain	Definition	Possible Head and Neck Reconstruction Quality Measures
Safe	Avoiding harm to patients from the care that is intended to help them	*Structure:* Training of high-performing teams, availability of technologies (flap monitoring), patient safety and quality improvement culture, training, and infrastructure *Process:* Adherence to structured surgical time out, structured sign-out, ERAS perioperative measures *Outcome:* Risk-adjusted incidence of medical and surgical complications, rates of reoperations and readmissions
Effective	Providing services based on scientific knowledge to all who could benefit and refraining from providing services to those not likely to benefit (avoiding underuse and misuse, respectively)	*Outcome:* Flap survival, tracheostomy and feeding tube dependence, bony union, occlusion and mouth opening, speech, diet, patient-reported outcomes (quality of life, swallowing, appearance)
Patient-centered	Providing care that is respectful of and responsive to individual patient preferences, needs, and values and ensuring that patient values guide all clinical decisions	*Structure:* Creation of patient advisory boards *Process:* Structured patient education and shared decision making *Outcome:* Patient satisfaction, patient-reported outcomes (decision certainty, decision regret, perioperative anxiety)
Timely	Reducing waits and sometimes harmful delays for both those who receive and those who give care	*Process:* Timely reconstructive consultation and surgery, initiation of adjuvant radiation within 6 wk of surgery when indicated
Efficient	Avoiding waste, including waste of equipment, supplies, ideas, and energy	*Structure:* Staff training in quality improvement methods, such as Lean *Outcome:* Operative time, length of stay, cost, supply, and technology utilization
Equitable	Providing care that does not vary in quality because of personal characteristics, such as gender, ethnicity, geographic location, and socioeconomic status	*Structure:* Staff training in health equity and cultural competency *Process:* Availability of interpreter services, screening for social risk factors and health literacy, measuring and addressing disparities in process by gender, ethnicity, and so forth *Outcome:* Measuring and addressing disparities in risk-adjusted outcomes by gender, ethnicity, and so forth

As mentioned above, patient-reported outcomes are therefore deservedly receiving increasing attention with respect to head and neck reconstruction. Ensuring patient input and involvement in quality improvement efforts across the spectrum of care (eg, Patient Advisory Councils) will be critical to achieving patient-centered care.

Timely

Delays in accessing head and neck reconstructive procedures can be devastating for patients who suffer from conditions affecting both function and cosmesis. As advanced reconstructive procedures such as free tissue transfer have become more widely available, patients have benefited from better access to care. Timely access to reconstruction is even more critical in cancer cases. The ability to immediately reconstruct defects from advanced cancer resections has improved both survival and quality of life for these patients. Recent studies have highlighted the vital importance of both timely access to cancer surgery (with concurrent reconstruction) and timely initiation of adjuvant treatment; patients who experience delays in cancer care have worse survival.[17,18] The Commission on Cancer has recently established initiation of adjuvant radiation within 6 weeks of surgery as a quality measure for head and neck cancer treatment.[19,20] Thus, quality measures in head and neck reconstruction will increasingly include metrics of timeliness of surgery and adjuvant treatment, and avoidance of complications that might cause delays.

Efficient

Efficient care avoids waste. Head and neck reconstruction, especially procedures involving free tissue transfer, may utilize many resources, including people and materials. There is the potential for a great deal of waste if attention is not paid to maximizing efficiency. Time is an important target for cutting waste in surgery. Studies have demonstrated the importance of reducing operative time, especially in potentially long surgeries involving free flaps; longer procedures result in more postoperative complications.[21,22] Operating room time is also a highly valuable and limited hospital resource. Efforts to make reconstructions more time efficient will thus provide value to both patients and health systems and may be a logical choice for future quality measures. Lean methodology has become increasingly prevalent in health care and provides a useful framework for cutting waste from complex procedures like head and neck reconstruction.[8,23]

With respect to materials, technologies such as implantable flap monitors and virtual surgical planning have become increasingly commonplace in head and neck reconstruction. Although some effort has been made to investigate cost-effectiveness of these technologies, judgments regarding their value (defined as quality/cost) have been largely left to individual surgeons and hospitals.[24,25] As outlined earlier, there are no widely accepted metrics for judging effectiveness in head and neck reconstruction, which further confounds measurement of value. Future measures of quality and value in head and neck reconstruction will undoubtedly have to confront the cost of these and other emerging technologies and their relative value in optimizing outcomes.

Equitable

Although disparities in the delivery of health care and health outcomes have long been recognized, the past few years have seen renewed interest and energy into taking concrete steps to address this problem. There is a growing literature highlighting disparities in head and neck cancer care and outcomes with respect to ethnicity, geographic location, and socioeconomic status. Less attention has been paid to disparities in head and neck reconstruction availability, delivery, and outcomes. Future quality measures for reconstruction should incorporate equity considerations, but it is not immediately obvious how to do so. The National Quality Forum has developed a road map for eliminating health care disparities and endorsed quality measures specific to health equity (eg, measurement of health literacy, provision of interpreter services, cultural competency) that may provide a useful starting point.[26]

SUMMARY

Despite rapid advances in surgical techniques and technology, significant opportunities for improving quality and value in head and neck reconstruction remain. These efforts should start with building consensus and standardization around the development and collection of outcomes data. Standardized outcomes data would allow for fair comparisons between surgeons, hospitals, and health systems; reliable comparative data could in turn drive quality improvement projects. Many head and neck reconstruction centers of excellence have begun this process, using measures such as those outlined in **Table 1**, but efforts remain largely siloed. The ongoing shift in health care financing away from fee-for-service toward value-based purchasing will provide resources and motivation for coordination of these efforts. The domains described above offer a useful framework for quality improvement in head and neck reconstruction.

DISCLOSURE

K. Kakarala, M. Mifsud, and P. Dziegielewski have no relevant disclosures.

REFERENCES

1. Institute of Medicine (IOM). Crossing the quality chasm: a new health system for the 21st Century. Washington, D.C: National Academy Press; 2001.
2. Suh JD, Sercarz JA, Abemayor E, et al. Analysis of outcome and complications in 400 cases of microvascular head and neck reconstruction. Arch Otolaryngol Head Neck Surg 2004;130:962–6.
3. Osborn HA, Rathi VK, Tjoa T, et al. Risk factors for thirty-day readmission following flap reconstruction of oncologic defects of the head and neck. Laryngoscope 2018;128(2):343–9.
4. Tam S, Dong W, Adelman DM, et al. Risk-adjustment models in patients undergoing head and neck surgery with reconstruction. Oral Oncol 2020;111:104917.
5. Dooley BJ, Karassawa Zanoni D, Mcgill MR, et al. Intraoperative and postanesthesia care unit fluid administration as risk factors for postoperative complications in patients with head and neck cancer undergoing free tissue transfer. Head Neck 2020;42(1):14–24.
6. Dort JC, Farwell DG, Findlay M, et al. Optimal Perioperative Care in Major Head and Neck Cancer Surgery With Free Flap Reconstruction: A Consensus Review and Recommendations From the Enhanced Recovery After Surgery Society. JAMA Otolaryngol Head Neck Surg 2017;143(3):292–303.
7. Doherty C, Nakoneshny SC, Harrop AR, et al. A standardized operative team for major head and neck cancer ablation and reconstruction. Plast Reconstr Surg 2012;130(1):82–8.
8. Ibrahim A, Ndeti K, Bur A, et al. Association of a Lean Surgical Plan of the Day With Reduced Operating Room Time for Head and Neck Free Flap Reconstruction. JAMA Otolaryngol Head Neck Surg 2019;145(10):926–30.

9. Sawaf T, Renslo B, Virgen C, et al. Team Consistency in Reducing Operative Time in Head and Neck Surgery with Microvascular Free Flap Reconstruction. Laryngoscope 2023. https://doi.org/10.1002/lary.30542.

10. Shen AY, Lonie S, Lim K, et al. Free Flap Monitoring, Salvage, and Failure Timing: A Systematic Review. J Reconstr Microsurg 2021;37(3):300–8.

11. Shaw RJ. Defining success and failure in head and neck reconstruction: is flap survival the ultimate measure? Front Oral Maxillofac Med 2021;3:32.

12. Vila PM, Rich JT, Desai SC. Defining Quality in Head and Neck Reconstruction. Otolaryngol Head Neck Surg 2017;157(4):545–7.

13. Hutcheson KA, Barrow MP, Lisec A, et al. What is a clinically relevant difference in MDADI scores between groups of head and neck cancer patients? Laryngoscope 2016;126(5):1108–13.

14. Graboyes EM, Hand BN, Ellis MA, et al. Validation of a Novel, Multidomain Head and Neck Cancer Appearance- and Function-Distress Patient-Reported Outcome Measure. Otolaryngol Head Neck Surg 2020;163(5):979–85.

15. Mady LJ, Poonia SK, Baddour K, et al. Consensus of free flap complications: Using a nomenclature paradigm in microvascular head and neck reconstruction. Head Neck 2021;43(10):3032–41.

16. Turkdogan S, Roy CF, Chartier G, et al. Effect of Perioperative Patient Education via Animated Videos in Patients Undergoing Head and Neck Surgery: A Randomized Clinical Trial. JAMA Otolaryngol Head Neck Surg 2022;148(2):173–9.

17. Nallani R, Smith JB, Penn JP, et al. Decision regret 3 and 6 months after treatment for head and neck cancer: Observational study of associations with clinicodemographics, anxiety, and quality of life. Head Neck 2022;44(1):59–70.

18. Goel AN, Frangos MI, Raghavan G, et al. The impact of treatment package time on survival in surgically managed head and neck cancer in the United States. Oral Oncol 2019;88:39–48.

19. Chen MM, Harris JP, Orosco RK, et al. Association of Time between Surgery and Adjuvant Therapy with Survival in Oral Cavity Cancer. Otolaryngol Head Neck Surg 2018;158(6):1051–6.

20. Graboyes EM, Divi V, Moore BA. Head and Neck Oncology Is on the National Quality Sidelines No Longer-Put Me in, Coach. JAMA Otolaryngol Head Neck Surg 2022;148(8):715–6.

21. Brady Jacob S, Desai Stuti V, Crippen MM, et al. Association of Anesthesia Duration With Complications After Microvascular Reconstruction of the Head and Neck. JAMA Facial Plastic Surgery 2018;188–95.

22. White LJ, Zhang H, Strickland KF, et al. Factors Associated With Hospital Length of Stay Following Fibular Free-Tissue Reconstruction of Head and Neck Defects: Assessment Using the American College of Surgeons National Surgical Quality Improvement Program (ACS NSQIP) Criteria. JAMA Otolaryngol Head Neck Surg 2015;141(12):1052–8.

23. Bahethi RR, Gold BS, Seckler SG, et al. Efficiency of microvascular free flap reconstructive surgery: An observational study. Am J Otolaryngol 2020;41(6):102692.

24. Fatima A, Hackman TG, Wood JS. Cost-Effectiveness Analysis of Virtual Surgical Planning in Mandibular Reconstruction. Plast Reconstr Surg 2019;143(4):1185–94.

25. Poder TG, Fortier PH. Implantable Doppler in monitoring free flaps: a cost-effectiveness analysis based on a systematic review of the literature. Eur Ann Otorhinolaryngol Head Neck Dis 2013;130(2):79–85.

26. Anderson AC, O'Rourke E, Chin MH, et al. Promoting Health Equity And Eliminating Disparities Through Performance Measurement And Payment. Health Aff 2018;37(3):371–7.

Moving?

Make sure your subscription moves with you!

To notify us of your new address, find your **Clinics Account Number** (located on your mailing label above your name), and contact customer service at:

Email: journalscustomerservice-usa@elsevier.com

800-654-2452 (subscribers in the U.S. & Canada)
314-447-8871 (subscribers outside of the U.S. & Canada)

Fax number: 314-447-8029

Elsevier Health Sciences Division
Subscription Customer Service
3251 Riverport Lane
Maryland Heights, MO 63043

*To ensure uninterrupted delivery of your subscription, please notify us at least 4 weeks in advance of move.

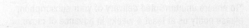

Printed and bound by CPI Group (UK) Ltd, Croydon, CR0 4YY

03/10/2024

01040470-0009